ACTA PÆDIATRICA

Vol. XXIX

MCMXLI

Almqvist & Wiksells Boktryckeri-Aktiebolag

UPPSALA 1942

INDEX ACTORUM

VOL. XXIX.

Pag.

S. van Creveld: Sporadic Hemophilia and Pseudo-Hemophilia 37
— —: and A. Grunbaum: Renal rickets and cystinuria . 183
Torfinn Denstad: Some Remarks on the X-Ray Appearance and Prognosis of Infant Tuberculosis 303
Erik Frisell: Missbildungen der Harnwege mit familiärem Auftreten von Doppelureter bei Kindern 418
V. Gaustad: Vide H. F. Lange and V. Gaustad.
A. Grunbaum: Vide S. van Creveld and A. Grunbaum.
Curt Gyllenswärd: Physiologische Temperaturerhöhung bei Neugeborenen 107
Bertil Hamne: Über die tuberkulotoxische Meningitis beim Kinde 285
C. W. Herlitz: Über Dosierung und Nebenwirkungen bei der Behandlung von Kindern mit Sulfathiazol 1
Gillis Herlitz: Zur Kenntnis der anämischen und polyzytämischen Zustände bei Neugeborenen sowie des Icterus gravis neonatorum 211
— —: Vide Supplementum I.
G. J. Huët: Diphteria, Anatoxine and Tuberculosis . . . 75
H. F. Lange and V. Gaustad: Epidemiology of scarlet fever illustrated through typing of hemolytic streptococci in a primary case and its return cases 254
Nils Malmberg: Erfahrungen bei der Rachitisprophylaxe frühgeborener Kinder. II: Die Schutzdosis von Vitamin D_3 für Kinder mit einem Geburtsgewicht bis 2 000 g. 367
Chr. R. Roesgaard: Pneumococcal peritonitis typed by precipitation of the urine 387
Paul E. Sjöquist: Experimental (osteo-dentino-)amelo-dystrophia in rats 59
Bertil Sourander: Über Scharlach und Diphterie in Finnland und Schweden wärend der letzten Dezennien . . 96

Folke Thuresson: Zweiterkrankung an Scharlach 266
Chr. Uldall: Comparative Studies on Feces of Healthy Breast-, Bottle- and Spoon-fed Infants 339
Arvid Wallgren: The Neonatal Mortality in Sweden, from a Pediatric Point of View 372
Olof S. Wåhlin: Vide Supplementum II.
Y. Åkerrén: Physiological Enlargement of the Spleen in the Newborn Child 395

SUPPLEMENTA.

I. Gillis Herlitz: Studien über die sog. initialen Fieberkrämpfe bei Kindern . . . . 1—142
II. Olof S. Wåhlin: Über die Methodik bei der Ausführung der Tuberkulinreaktionen sowie über die Verbreitung der Tuberkulinallergie bei Schulkindern im nördlicben Schweden (Västerbotten). Eine statistische Analyse I—VIII . . . . 1—165

AUS DER KINDERKLINIK DES KAROLINISCHEN INSTITUTS IM KRANKENHAUS NORRTULL, STOCKHOLM. CHEF: DOZENT C. W. HERLITZ.

Über Dosierung und Nebenwirkungen bei der Behandlung von Kindern mit Sulfathiazol.

Von

C. W. HERLITZ.

Während der kurzen Zeit, welche verstrichen ist, seitdem das 2-Sulfanilylaminothiazol (Sulfathiazol) von FOSBINDER und WALTER sowie LAUDON und SJÖGREN in die Therapie eingeführt wurde, sind verschiedene Autoren zu der Ansicht gelangt, dass dieses Präparat gewisse Vorzüge dem Sulfapyridin gegenüber besitzt. Was die klinische Erprobung betrifft, so hat man noch nicht genügend Material für eine erschöpfendere Beurteilung sammeln können. Es ist indessen schon jetzt von klinischer Seite die Aufmerksamkeit auf den Umstand gelenkt worden, dass die toxischen Nebenwirkungen beim Gebrauch von Sulfathiazol auffallend leicht zu sein scheinen, leichter als nach Anwendung von Sulfapyridin, während das therapeutische Resultat den Eindruck erweckte, den bei Verwendung des letzteren Mittels erzielten Ergebnissen gleichwertig zu sein. Zu diesen Resultaten gelangen u. a. SCOTT und JONES bei der Behandlung der Pneumonie bei Kindern.

In einer vorausgehenden Arbeit (Acta Pædiatrica 1941, S. 173) hatten wir Gelegenheit, zu zeigen, dass, wenn auch bei Anwendung von Sulfanilamid und Sulfapyridin im Kindesalter die hierbei auftretenden toxischen Nebenwirkungen im allgemeinen als leicht und rasch vorübergehend zu bezeichnen sind, doch in einem nicht allzu kleinen Prozentsatz der Fälle beachtenswerte Störungen in der Myelopoese auftreten, und zwar schon bei einer verhältnismässig zurückhaltenden Dosierung und nach sehr kurzer Behandlungsdauer (48—144 Stdn.). Im Hinblick auf die soeben geschilderte Lage der Dinge ist es offenbar, dass eine eingehende Prüfung der Nebenwirkungen und der Dosierung des Sulfathiazols sehr wichtig ist. Insbesondere ist der Einfluss des Mittels auf die Leukopoese bei Kindern höchst unvollständig bekannt, was u. a. natürlich darauf beruht, dass diejenigen Infektionen, bei welchen das Mittel im allgemeinen Verwendung findet, an und für sich das Knochenmark und das Blutbild beeinflussen.

I. **Material.**

Das vorliegende Material besteht aus 125 hauptsächlich an Infektionen der Luftwege (Bronchitiden, kapillare Bronchitiden, Bronchopneumonien, Pneumonien vom kroupösen Typ und Mittelohrentzündungen) leidenden Kindern (siehe *Tab. 1*). Von den Kindern befanden sich 48 im Alter von 0—1 Jahr und 77 im Alter von 1—13 Jahren.

Ausserdem sind zwei Kinder im Alter von 2 Monaten mit schwerem, nichtluetischem Hydrocephalus internus ohne nennenswerte Anzeichen einer akuten Infektion mit Sulfathiazol behandelt worden. Die Patienten waren sämtlich in den Jahren 1940/41 in der Kinderklinik des Karolinischen Instituts im Krankenhaus Norrtull stationär behandelt worden.

Den Herren Dozenten H. Nordenson, E. Segerdahl und J. Waldenström danke ich für ihre wertvolle Hilfe bei der Untersuchung von Knochenmarkpräparaten. Das verwendete Präparat war Sulfathiazol in Tablettenform zum Gebrauch per os, welches uns von der A.-G. Astra in Södertälje wohlwollend zur Verfügung gestellt wurde.

II. **Dosierung.**

Es ist selbstverständlich mit grossen Schwierigkeiten verbunden, zu beurteilen, welche Dosierung am geeignetsten ist, da es ja im frühen Kindesalter meistens Fälle von Infektionen der Luftwege sein dürften, die zur Erprobung des Sulfathiazols

Tab. 1.

Sulfathiazoldosierung im vorliegenden Material und Übersicht der Nebenwirkungen.

Fall Nr.	Alter	Diagnose	Körpergew. in kg	Durchschn. Tagesdosis in g	Durchschn. Tagesdosis pro kg Körpergew. in g	Anzahl d. Beh.-Tage	Ges.-Dos. in g	Nebenwirkungen
1	20 *T.*	Pemphigus	3,10	0,40	0,13	2	0,80	Unerhebl. Erbrechen (Ursache?)
2	15 »	Bronchitis	3,12	0,30	0,09	5	1,50	—
3	30 »	Sepsis	3,90	0,22	0,06	8	1,75	—
4	30 »	Bronchit. capill.	3,75	0,53	0,14	6	3,20	—
5	17 »	D:o + Vit. org. cord. + Pemphigus + Deb. cong.	2,06	0,43	0,21	8	3,40	Unerhebl. Erbrechen (Ursache?)
6	19 »	Bronchit. cap + Deb. congen.	1,72	0,25	0,15	7	1,75	—
7	21 »	Br. capill.	2,58	0,58	0,22	8	4,60	Erbrechen
8	27 »	Br. capill.	4,14	0,30	0,07	7	2,10	—
9	4 »	Pharyngitis	3,12	0,43	0,11	4	1,70	Hämaturie
10	23 »	Br. capill.	2,80	0,50	0,18	5	2,50	—
11	5 *M.*	Bronchitis	6,20	0,60	0,09	3	1,80	— *Sternalpunktion* unmittelbar vor u. nach d. Beh.: normale Verh.
12	5 »	Pertussis	7,10	0,60	0,08	6	3,60	—
13	2 »	Pylorosp. + Pertussis	3,50	0,28	0,08	8	2,20	Neutropenie. Weiss. Blk. gingen von 25 000 auf 15 800 zurück, die neutrophilen polynukl. von 26 % auf 10 %, davon 2 % stabkernige
14	5 »	Meningitis cerebr. ep. + Bronchit. + Otit. med.	6,60	1,13	0,17	15	17,00	— (gesund)
15	3 »	Pertussis + Bronchit. + Rachitis + Dystrophia	4,35	0,40	0,09	5	2,00	—
16	4 »	Pertussis + Br. pneum.	3,90	0,56	0,14	7	3,90	—
17	4 »	Br. asthmat.	5,88	0,52	0,09	10	5,20	—
18	2 »	Pertussis + Br. capill.	3,30	0,36	0,11	8	2,90	—
19	2 »	Br. capill.	3,60	0,46	0,13	10	4,60	—

Tab. 1. (Forts. 1.)

Fall Nr.	Alter	Diagnose	Körpergew. in kg	Durchschn. Tagesdosis in g	Durchschn. Tagesdosis pro kg Körpergew. in g	Anzahl d. Beh.-Tage	Ges.-Dos. in g	Nebenwirkungen
20	2 *M.*	Br. capill.	3,70	0,45	0,12	13	5,80	— 14 Tage n. Abschl. d. Beh. *Sternalpunktion*: normaler Befund
21	4 »	Br. capill. + Dystrophia	3,90	0,54	0,14	12	6,50	*Exanthem* am 3. Tage
22	3 »	Bronchit.	5,80	0,65	0,11	6	3,90	Unerhebl. Erbrechen.
23	5 »	Br.-pneum.	6,20	0,60	0,10	7	4,20	—
24	8 »	Pseudocr.	9,50	0,75	0,08	3	2,25	*Erbrechen.* Sternalp. am letzten Tage zeigt Infektionsmark
25	10 »	Bronchit.	9,40	0,60	0,06	3	1,80	—
26	9 »	Br. capill. + Vit. org. cord.	5,90	0,66	0,11	7	4,65	—
27	11 »	Pemphigus + Otit. m.	8,20	1,25	0,15	6	7,50	—
28	10 »	Br.-pneum.	7,10	0,80	0,11	2	1,60	—
29	9 »	Pseudocr.	8,70	1,20	0,14	3	3,60	—
30	7 »	Otit. med.	7,50	1,20	0,16	5	6,00	—
31	8 »	Pertussis + Bronchit.	9,70	0,66	0,07	5	3,30	—
32	8 »	Otit. med.	8,10	0,52	0,06	5	2,60	—
33	8 »	Pneum. cr.	7,85	0,57	0,07	3	1,70	—
34	10 »	Otit. m. + Vit. org. c.	8,00	0,39	0,05	5	1,95	—
35	11 »	Br. asthm.	8,65	0,60	0,07	2	1,20	—
36	7 »	Br. capill.	7,00	0,35	0,05	4	1,40	Erbrechen. Zyanose
37	8 »	Br.-pneum.	7,20	0,40	0,06	6	2,40	—
38	9 »	» »	8,40	0,49	0,06	14	6,80	—
39	6 »	Pneum. cr.	7,50	0,55	0,07	4	2,20	Erbrechen
40	7 »	Pyelitis	7,42	0,36	0,05	7	2,50	Schweres Erbrechen
41	10 »	Br.-Pneum.	9,45	0,65	0,07	4	2,60	Neutropenie. Weiss. Blk. gingen von 32 000 auf 7 600 zurück. Wert f. neutr. polynukl.: vor d. Beh.: 23 % stabk. 45 % segm. am letzt. Tag: 3 % » 7 % » am Tage nach Schluss d. Beh.: 1 % stabk. 5 % segm. Nach 1 Monat zus. 12 % neutrophile. Nach weiteren 3 Wochen 35 %.
42	11 »	Bronchit.	8,40	0,73	0,09	8	5,80	—

Tab. 1. (Forts. 2.)

Fall Nr.	Alter	Diagnose	Körpergew. in kg	Durchschn. Tagesdosis in g	Durchschn. Tagesdosis pro kg Körpergew. in g	Anzahl d. Beh.-Tage	Ges.-Dos. in g	Nebenwirkungen
43	11 *M.*	Bronchit.	10,00	0,56	0,06	8	4,50	—
44	8 »	»	7,76	0,57	0,07	6	3,40	— Sternalpunktion nachher neg.
45	8 »	Br. capill. + Otit. med.	7,96	0,52	0,07	21	11,00	—
46	7 »	Bronchitis	6,50	0,52	0,08	9	4,70	—
47	9 »	Otit. med.	10,10	0,70	0,07	5	3,50	—
48	9 »	Bronchit.	7,42	0,42	0,06	4	1,80	—
49	1—2 J.	Vit. org. cord. + Otit.	8,30	1,50	0,18	4	6,00	—
50	»	V. o. c. + Bronchit.	8,50	0,75	0,09	14	10,45	—
51	»	Pneum. cent. + Otit. med. + Mastoid. + Myocard.	10,00	1,10	0,11	3	3,30	— *Sternalpunktion* unmittelbar vor u. nach der Beh.: normale Verhältnisse.
52	»	Otit. med. + Bronchit.	10,00	0,50	0,05	3	1,50	—
53	»	Pharyngit + Dyspepsi	9,70	0,48	0,05	5	2,40	—
54	»	Br.-pneum.	12,60	0,64	0,05	5	3,20	Unerhebl. Zyanose u. Erbrechen
55	»	Otit. med.	11,50	0,95	0,08	3	2,85	—
56	»	» »	10,00	0,56	0,06	4	2,25	—
57	»	Tbc. hili + Bronchit. + Otit. med.	9,00	0,48	0,05	4	1,90	Neutropenie. Weiss. Blk. vor u. nach d. Beh.: 10 400 bzw. 5 600; Hämogramm: siehe *Anm. 1.*
58	»	Lymphadenit. colli sept.	8,60	0,75	0,09	4	3,00	—
59	»	Pneum. cr. + Otit. med.	12,60	1,50	0,12	3	4,50	—
60	»	Pneum. cr.	10,00	1,04	0,10	5	5,20	—
61	»	Bronchitis	12,00	1,30	0,11	3	3,90	—
62	»	»	10,80	0,90	0,08	2	1,80	—
63	»	Otit. med.	10,70	0,72	0,07	5	3,60	Neutropenie: siehe *Anm. 2.*
64	»	Pneum. cr. + Pertussis	9,20	1,00	0,11	6	6,00	Schweres Erbrechen.

Tab. 1. (Forts. 3.)

Fall Nr.	Alter	Diagnose	Körpergew. in kg	Durchschn. Tagesdosis in g	Durchschn. Tagesdosis pro kg Körpergew. in g	Anzahl d. Beh.-Tage	Ges.-Dos. in g	Nebenwirkungen
65	1—2 J.	Deb. cong. + v. o. c. + Br.-pneum.	7,00	0,90	0,13	5	4,50	Unerhebl. Erbrechen,
66	»	Pseudocr.	10,40	0,71	0,07	4	2,85	—
67	»	Pneum. cr.	10,80	0,60	0,06	2	1,20	—
68	»	Br.-pneum.	9,80	0,70	0,07	6	4,20	—
69	»	» »	12,50	0,34	0,03	4	1,35	—
70	»	Pneum. cr. + Otit. med.	9,00	0,54	0,06	5	2,70	—
71	»	Bronchitis	8,40	0,48	0,06	10	4,75	Erbrechen.
72	»	Br.-pneum.	8,10	0,53	0,07	8	4,20	Erbrechen.
73	»	» »	10,40	0,83	0,08	7	5,80	Neutropenie. Weiss. Blk. gingen von 9 200 auf 4 900 zurück. Die neutroph. polynukl. von 35 % auf 7 %. Nach einer weiteren Woche, vom letzten Beh.-Tag. ab gerechnet, 44 %.
74	»	» »	11,00	0,47	0,04	10	4,70	—
75	»	» »	8,70	1,03	0,12	6	6,20	Erbrechen.
76	»	» »	12,40	0,84	0,06	5	4,20	—
77	»	» » + Emp. pleur.	9,70	1,00	0,10	12	12,00	—
78	»	Pneumokokken-meningit.	9,70	1,32	0,14	13	17,10	—
79	2—3 J.	Lymphadenit. coll. sept.	12,00	0,54	0,05	5	2,70	—
80	»	Diab. mell. + Pharyng.	12,80	0,67	0,05	3	2,00	—
81	»	Tbc. lgl. br. + Angina foll.	13,00	0,80	0,06	4	3,20	—
82	»	Pneum. cr.	14,00	1,20	0,09	4	4,80	—
83	»	Pharyngit.	13,80	0,37	0,03	6	2,20	—
84	»	Bronchit. + Otit. med.	15,00	0,56	0,04	4	2,25	—
85	»	Br.-pneum.	11,50	0,73	0,06	6	4,40	Starke Unruhe.
86	»	Pneum. cr.	11,80	0,65	0,06	3	1,95	—
87	»	Br.-pneum. + V. o. c.	10,50	0,71	0,07	8	5,70	—

Tab. 1. (Forts. 4.)

Fall Nr.	Alter	Diagnose	Körpergew. in kg	Durchschn. Tagesdosis in g	Durchschn. Tagesdosis pro kg Körpergew. in g	Anzahl d. Beh.-Tage	Ges.-Dos. in g	Nebenwirkungen
88	2—3 J.	Pneum. cr.	11,50	1,54	0,13	6	9,25	Leukopenie. Siehe *Anm. 3.*
89	3—4 J.	Angina retronas.	15,00	1,08	0,07	12	12,90	— *Sternalpunktion* unmittelbar nach Schluss der Beh. ergab normale Verhältnisse.
90	»	Angina tons. + Otit. med.	15,60	1,80	0,12	2	3,60	—
91	»	Angina tons. + Myocardit.	12,00	1,36	0,11	5	6,80	—
92	»	Bronchitis	16,20	0,80	0,05	6	4,80	—
93	»	Br.-pneum.	13,50	0,52	0,04	5	2,60	—
94	»	» » + Pertussis	15,00	0,60	0,04	6	3,60	Erbrechen. Unruhe.
95	»	Br.-pneum.	13,20	0,96	0,07	6	5,70	Leukopenie. Siehe *Anm. 4.*
96	»	» »	14,00	0,88	0,06	10	8,80	—
97	»	» »	13,60	1,37	0,10	10	13,70	Recht erhebliches Erbrechen. Sternalpunktion 8 Tage nach Abschluss d. Beh.: Geringe Linksverschiebung in d. Myelopoese, sonst o. B.
98	»	Bronchit. + Otit. med.	19,70	0,80	0,04	6	4,30	—
99	4—5 J.	Pneum. cr.	15,00	2,00	0,13	4	8,00	—
100	»	Angina t.	20,00	1,53	0,08	3	4,60	—
101	»	Pharyngit.	16,00	0,70	0,04	2	1,40	—
102	»	Bronchit. + Pertussis	17,60	1,00	0,06	3	3,00	—
103	»	Br. pneum. + Pertussis	12,50	1,11	0,09	13	14,40	—
104	5—6 J.	Pneum. cr.	20,50	1,53	0,07	6	9,20	—
105	»	Angina retronas.	20,50	1,30	0,06	3	3,90	—
106	»	Otit. med.	17,00	0,92	0,05	5	4,60	—
107	»	Bronchit. + Endocard.	17,00	1,06	0,06	4	4,25	—
108	»	Br.-pneum. + Otit. med.	18,50	1,29	0,07	15	19,40	—
109	»	Br.-pneum.	20,00	2,58	0,13	6	15,50	—

Tab. 1. (Forts. 5.)

Fall Nr.	Alter	Diagnose	Körpergew. in kg	Durchschn. Tagesdosis in g	Durchschn. Tagesdosis pro kg Körpergew. in g	Anzahl d. Beh.-Tage	Ges.-Dos. in g	Nebenwirkungen
110	6—7 J.	Diab. mell. + Pertussis + Bronchitis	29,00	1,20	0,04	7	8,40	Unerhebl. Zyanose (Blutzucker unbeeinflusst).
111	»	Otit. med.	20,00	1,00	0,05	4	4,00	—
112	7—8 J.	Bronchitis + Otit. m.	18,60	1,80	0,09	5	9,00	—
113	»	Pneum. cr.	28,50	1,24	0,04	5	6,20	Mikroskopisch nachweisbare Hämaturie.
114	»	Angina foll.	26,00	1,70	0,07	6	10,20	—
115	8—9 J.	Morb. Feer + Lymphadenit. colli sept.	25,00	1,50	0,06	3	4,50	—
116	»	Br.-pneum.	28,50	2,67	0,09	6	16,00	—
117	»	» »	20,50	2,42	0,12	12	29,00	— (Anzahl d. weiss. Blk. vor der Beh. 20 700 und während der ganzen Beh. 19 000—212 000).
118	9—10 J.	Pneum. cr.	22,50	1,62	0,07	9	14,60	—
119	10-11 J.	» »	28,00	2,08	0,07	6	12,50	—
120	»	Br.-pneum.	24,50	2,75	0,11	4	11,00	—
121	11-12 J.	Polyarthrit. ac.	28,00	0,86	0,03	9	7,75	—
122	12-13 J.	Pneum. cr.	33,00	2,64	0,08	7	18,50	—
123	»	Br.-pneum.	28,50	1,88	0,07	4	7,50	—
124	»	Pneum. cr.	32,00	4,67	0,15	3	14,00	—
125	»	» »	45,00	2,50	0,06	10	25,00	—

Gelegenheit geben, also eine Krankheitsgruppe, wo der klinische Verlauf bei den einzelnen Fällen ganz verschiedenartig ist, und wo demzufolge die Beurteilung des chemotherapeutischen Effekts schwierig sein muss. Nach von verschiedenen Seiten stammenden Untersuchungen dürfte man davon ausgehen können, dass Sulfathiazol rascher als Sulfapyridin resorbiert und ausgeschieden wird. Daraus folgt, dass, wenn Sulfathiazol in derselben Dosierung wie Sulfapyridin bei kontinuierlicher Medikation gegeben wird, die Blutkonzentration des ersteren Präparats niedriger wird als die des letzteren (FRISK, LONG). Der Gedanke hieran hat dazu geführt, dass man beim Sulfathiazol etwas grössere und dichter aufeinanderfolgende Dosen als beim Sulfapyridin empfohlen hat. Diese theoretisch begründeten Überlegungen zur Erzielung einer hohen und gleichmässigen Blutkonzentration des Thiazols müssen selbstverständlich klinisch nachgeprüft werden. Entscheidend bei der Stellungnahme in der Dosierungsfrage sind diejenigen Erfahrungen, welche man am Krankenbett machen kann. Einerseits wünscht man natürlich einen guten therapeutischen Effekt, und andererseits muss man versuchen, das Zustandekommen toxischer Nebenwirkungen nach Möglichkeit zu vermeiden. Wir gingen bei der Planung der Sulfathiazolbehandlung von derjenigen Dosierung des Sulfapyridins aus, welche wir in 199 Fällen von Infektionen der Luftwege bei Kindern angewendet hatten (siehe Acta Pædiatrica 1941, S. 193). Wir empfahlen da:

bei	Kindern	im	Alter	von	1—3 M.	ca.	0,6—0,8 g	als	Tagesdosis	(24 Stdn.)
»	»	»	»	»	6 »	»	0,5—1,0 »	»	»	» »
»	»	»	»	»	2 J.	»	1,0—2,0 »	»	»	» »
»	»	»	»	»	6 »	»	2,0—2,5 »	»	»	» »

Die Gesamtdosis der ganzen Behandlung war:

bei	Kindern	im	Alter	von	1—3 M.	ca.	1,5—3,5 g
»	»	»	»	»	6 »	»	2,0—4,0 »
»	»	»	»	»	1 J.	»	3,0—5,0 »
»	»	»	»	»	4 »	»	3,0—6,0 »

Zur Beurteilung der Grösse und des Effekts der therapeutischen Dosis wurden zunächst die im Material enthaltenen Fälle von Pneumonie des lobären (kroupösen) Typs ausgewählt, einer Krankheit, bei welcher ja der im allgemeinen ziemlich gleichartige Verlauf verhältnismässig gute Möglichkeiten zur Beurteilung des therapeutischen Effekts bietet (*Tab. 2*).

In sämtlichen Fällen ist die Diagnose röntgenologisch verifiziert. Das Material enthält 19 Fälle von kroupöser Pneu-

Tab. 2.

Sulfathiazoldosierung, Nebenwirkungen und Behandlungsresultate bei 19 Pneumoniefällen vom kroupösen Typ.

Fall Nr.	Alter in Jahren und Monaten	Körpergew. in kg	durchschn. Tagesdosis in g	durchschn. Tagesdosis pro kg Körpergew.	Anzahl der Beh.-Tage	Ges.-Dosis in g	Behandlungsresultat. Nebenwirkungen
51	1,3	10,00	1,10	0,11	3	3,30	Kritischer Temp.-fall in 48 Stdn. am 4.–5. Fiebertage. Keine Nebenwirkungen
99	4,2	15,00	2,00	0,13	4	8,00	Kritischer Temp.-fall in 24 Stdn. am 3.–4. Fiebertage. Keine Nebenwirkungen
122	12,5	33,00	2,64	0,08	7	18,50	Kritischer Temp.-fall in 24 Stdn. am 3. Fiebertage. Keine Nebenwirkungen
104	5,6	20,50	1,53	0,07	6	9,20	Kritischer Temp.-fall in 24 Stdn. am 2.–3. Fiebertage. Keine Nebenwirkungen
82	2,2	14,00	1,20	0,09	4	4,80	Kritischer Temp.-fall in 24 Stdn. am 6. Fiebertage. Keine Nebenwirkungen
118	9,1	22,50	1,62	0,07	9	14,60	Kritischer Temp.-fall in 48 Stdn. am 4.–5. Fiebertage. Keine Nebenwirkungen
59	1,1	12,60	1,50	0,12	3	4,50	Kritischer Temp.-fall in 48 Stdn. am 3.–4. Fiebertage. Keine Nebenwirkungen
60	1,7	10,00	1,04	0,10	5	5,20	Kritischer Temp.-fall in 24 Stdn. am 7. Fiebertage. Keine Nebenwirkungen
33	0,8	7,85	0,57	0,07	3	1,70	Kritischer Temp.-fall in 24 Stdn. am 2. Fiebertage. Keine Nebenwirkungen
113	7,0	28,50	1,24	0,04	5	6,20	Kritischer Temp.-fall in 24 Stdn. am 3.–4. Fiebertage. Mikroskopisch nachweisbare *Hämaturie* während einiger Tage
64	1,3	9,20	1,00	0,11	6	6,00	Kritischer Temp.-fall in 48 Stdn. am 4.–5. Fiebertage. *Erbrechen*
124	13,0	32,00	4,67	0,15	3	14,00	Kritischer Temp.-fall in 24 Stdn. am 4. Fiebertage. Keine Nebenwirkungen
67	1,9	10,80	0,60	0,06	2	1,20	Kritischer Temp.-fall in 24 Stdn. am 3.–4. Fiebertage. Keine Nebenwirkungen
86	2,11	11,80	0,65	0,06	3	1,95	Kritischer Temp.-fall in 24 Stdn. am 2.–3. Fiebertage. Keine Nebenwirkungen
39	0,6	7,50	0,55	0,07	4	2,20	Kritischer Temp.-fall in 24 Stdn. am 3. Fiebertage. *Erbrechen*
70	1,4	9,00	0,54	0,06	5	2,70	Kritischer Temp.-fall in 24 Stdn. am 2.–3. Fiebertage. Keine Nebenwirkungen

Tab. 2. (Forts.).

Fall Nr.	Alter in Jahren und Monaten	Körpergew. in kg	durchschn. Tagesdosis in g	durchschn. Tagesdosis pro kg Körpergew.	Anzahl der Beh.-Tage	Ges.-Dosis in g	Behandlungsresultat. Nebenwirkungen
119	10,0	28,00	2,08	0,07	6	12,50	Kritischer Temp.-fall in 24 Stdn. am 2.–3. Fiebertage. Keine Nebenwirkungen
125	13,0	45,00	2,50	0,05	10	25,00	Die Behandlung wurde am 9. Fiebertage begonnen, worauf im Laufe von 5 Tagen Fieberfreiheit eintrat. Die Krankheit hatte mit einer Angina tonsillaris eingesetzt
88	2,5	11,50	1,54	0,13	6	9,25	Die Behandlung wurde am 4. Fiebertage begonnen, worauf im Laufe von 4 Tagen Fieberfreiheit eintrat. *Leukopenie*

monie. Aus *Tab. 2* und anderen Umständen geht hervor, dass man bei wenigstens 16 Fällen die therapeutische Wirkung als gut bezeichnen muss. Bei den drei übrigen Fällen (Nr. 60, 88 u. 125) ist es nicht so sicher, ob und in welchem Grade das Medikament bei dem auch hier günstigen klinischen Verlauf eine Rolle gespielt hat. Eine nähere Betrachtung der Dosierung bei diesen 19 Pneumoniefällen ergibt, dass alle Kinder im Alter von 6 M.—13 J. durchschnittlich ungefähr dieselbe Dosis pro kg Körpergewicht pro Tag (24 Stdn.) erhalten hatten (*Tab. 3*).

Die Tagesdosis pro kg Körpergewicht variierte zwischen 0,04 und 0,15, die Gesamtdosis pro Behandlung zwischen 0,11 und 0,80 g. Hieraus ziehen wir den Schluss, dass man mit Vorteil etwa 0,10 g Sulfathiazol pro kg Körpergewicht pro Tag (24 Stdn.) bei Kindern im Alter von 6 M.—13 J. geben kann. Das Medikament wurde in diesen Fällen im allgemeinen 5mal in 24 Stunden verabreicht, und die erste Dosis war nicht grösser als die übrigen. In der Regel wurde das Mittel während einer Zeit von 3—6 Tagen gegeben. Da gewöhnlich binnen 24—48 Stdn. ein kritischer Temperaturfall erzielt wurde, so bedeutet dies, dass Sulfathiazol am besten 48—96 Stdn. weiterverabfolgt wird, nachdem der Patient fieberfrei geworden ist.

Tab. 3.

Sulfathiazoldosierung bei Fällen von kroupöser Pneumonie. Material in Altersgruppen eingeteilt.

Alter in Jahren	Anzahl der Fälle	Tagesdosis pro kg Körpergewicht in g	Gesamtdosis pro kg Körpergewicht in g
6/12—1	2	0,07	0,22—0,29
1—2	6	0,06—0,12	0,11—0,66
2—4	3	0,06—0,13	0,17—0,80
4—6	2	0,07—0,13	0,45—0,53
6—9	1	0,04	0,22
9—13	5	0,05—0,15	0,44—0,65

Sa. 19 Fälle.

Die Erfahrung lehrt, dass manchmal eine neuerliche Temperatursteigerung eintritt, wenn man die medikamentöse Behandlung am Zeitpunkt des kritischen Temperaturfalls abschliesst. Über die Nebenwirkungen sei an dieser Stelle nur bemerkt, dass sie während der Behandlung dieser Fälle von kroupöser Pneumonie unerheblich waren.

Wenn man also 0,10 g Sulfathiazol pro kg Körpergewicht pro Tag (24 Stdn.) gibt, so ist die Gesamtdosis Sulfathiazol pro Tag bei normalentwickelten Kindern ungefähr wie folgt:

Kinder im Alter von	6 M.	Tagesdosis	ca.	0,7	g	=	0,15 × 5 (ungef.)
» » » »	1 J.	»	»	1,0	»	=	0,20 × 5
» » » »	2 »	»	»	1,25	»	=	0,25 × 5
» » » »	3 »	»	»	1,50	»	=	0,30 × 5
» » » »	5 »	»	»	2,00	»	=	0,40 × 5
» » » »	8 »	»	»	2,50	»	=	0,50 × 5
» » » »	10 »	»	»	3,00	»	=	0,60 × 5
» » » »	13 »	»	»	4,00	»	=	0,80 × 5

Aus *Tab. 4* wird ersichtlich, dass bei dem Gesamtmaterial (also nicht nur bei kroupösen Pneumonien) etwa dieselbe Tagesdosis (24 Stdn.) pro kg Körpergewicht gewählt worden ist wie bei den Pneumoniefällen. Die Grösse der Dosis wechselte zwischen 0,03 und 0,22 g.

Das Gesamtmaterial gibt zum Unterschied von dem Pneumoniematerial auch Aufschluss über die Dosierung in den Altersgruppen 0—1 M. und 1—6 M. Bei den insgesamt 23 Fällen in diesen Altersstufen betrug die Dosis pro kg Körpergewicht pro Tag 0,06—0,22 g oder im Durchschnitt ebenso viel wie die entsprechende Dosis in den übrigen Altersgruppen. Auch in diesen niedrigsten Altersstufen (0—6 M.) kann man

Tab. 4.

Sulfathiazoldosierung bei dem vorliegenden Material, in Altersgruppen eingeteilt. Nebenwirkungen.

Alter in Jahren	Anzahl der Fälle	Tagesdosis in g	Tagesdosis pro kg Körpergew. in g	Anzahl d. Beh.-Tage	Gesamtdosis in g	Nebenwirkungen
0—1/12	10	0,22—0,58	0,06—0,22	2—8	0,80— 4,60	1 Fall Erbrechen 1 » Hämaturie
1/12—6/12	13	0,28—1,13	0,09—0,17	3—15	1,80—17,0	1 » Erbrechen 1 » Exanthem 1 » Neutropenie
6/12—1	25	0,52—1,25	0,05—0,16	2—21	1,20—11,00	3 » Erbrechen 1 » Zyanose u. Erbr. 1 » Neutropenie
1—2	30	0,34—1,50	0,03—0,18	2—14	1,20—17,1	5 » Erbrechen 1 » Zyanose u. Erbr. 3 » Neutropenie
2—4	20	0,52—1,80	0,03—0,13	3—12	1,95—13,7	1 » Erbrechen 1 » Unruhe 2 » Leukopenie 1 » Unruhe u. Erbr.
4—6	11	0,70—2,58	0,04—0,13	2—15	1,40—15,0	Keine
6—9	8	1,00—2,67	0,04—0,12	3—12	4,00—29,0	1 Fall Zyanose 1 » Hämaturie
9—13	8	0,86—4,67	0,03—0,15	3—10	7,50—25,0	Keine

Sa. 26 Fälle.

mit Vorteil etwa 0,10 g Sulfathiazol pro kg Körpergewicht pro Tag (24 Stdn.) geben.

Was speziell die Fälle in der Altersgruppe 0—1 M. betrifft (Fall 1—10 in *Tab. 1*), so betrug die Tagesdosis pro kg Körpergewicht im Durchschnitt 0,13 g, und die Anzahl der Behandlungstage durchschnittlich 6. Bei einer solchen Dosierung ist die Gesamtdosis Sulfathiazol pro Tag bei normalentwickelten Kindern ungefähr folgende:

Kinder im Alter von	1	M.	Tagesdosis	ca.	0,40 g	$=0,08 \times 5$
» » » »	3	»	»	»	0,50 »	$=0,10 \times 5$

III. **Nebenwirkungen.**

In insgesamt 26 von den 125 behandelten Fällen (= 20,8 v. H.) traten Nebenwirkungen auf. Nach den Symptomen lassen sich dieselben folgendermassen einteilen:

11	Fälle von	Erbrechen
2	» »	Erbrechen und Zyanose
1	» »	Erbrechen und Unruhe
2	» »	mikroskopisch nachweisbarer Hämaturie
1	» »	Exanthem
1	» »	Unruhe
1	» »	Zyanose
5	» »	Neutropenie
2	» »	Leukopenie

Summa: 26 Fälle. Siehe *Tab. 5*.

Da man sich denken könnte, dass die Gesamtdosis Sulfathiazol pro kg Körpergewicht pro Behandlung bei denjenigen Fällen, wo Nebenwirkungen auftraten, höher lag als bei den übrigen, wurde ein diesbezüglicher statistischer Vergleich angestellt (siehe *Tab. 6*, *7*, *u. 8*).

Die Differenz zwischen den Fällen mit Nebenwirkungen und den ohne solche beträgt, wie aus *Tab. 8* ersichtlich wird, $0,03 \pm 0,09$ und ist also kleiner als ihr mittlerer Fehler.

Tab. 5.

Sulfathiazoldosierung bei den 26 Fällen, wo Nebenwirkungen auftraten (Material: 125 Fälle).

Fall Nr.	Alter	Diagnose	Körpergew. in kg	Tagesdosis pro kg Körp.-gew. in g	Anzahl der Beh.-Tage	Ges.-Dosis pro kg Körp.-gew.	Ges.-Dosis in g	Nebenwirkungen
7	21 T.	Br. cap.	2,58	0,22	8	1,78	4,60	Erbrechen
9	4 »	Pharyngit.	3,12	0,11	4	0,55	1,70	Hämaturie
13	2 M.	Pertussis Pylorosp.	3,50	0,08	8	0,63	2,20	Neutropenie
21	4 »	Br. cap. Dystrophie	3,90	0,14	12	1,67	6,50	Exanthem
22	3 »	Bronchit.	5,80	0,11	6	0,67	3,90	Erbrechen
24	8 »	Pseudocr.	9,50	0,08	3	0,24	2,25	Erbrechen
36	7 »	Br. capill.	7,00	0,05	4	0,20	1,40	Erbrechen u. Zyanose
39	6 »	Pneum cr.	7,50	0,07	4	0,29	2,20	Erbrechen
40	7 »	Pyelitis	7,42	0,05	7	0,35	2,50	Erbrechen
41	10 »	Br.-pneum.	9,45	0,07	4	0,28	2,60	Neutropenie
54	1–2 J.	Br.-pneum.	12,60	0,05	5	0,25	3,20	Erbrechen u. Zyanose
57	»	Tbc. hili Bronchitis Otit. med.	9,00	0,05	4	0,21	1,90	Neutropenie
63	»	Otit. med.	10,70	0,07	5	0,35	3,60	Neutropenie
64	»	Pneum. cr. Pertussis	9,20	0,11	6	0,66	6,00	Erbrechen
65	»	Br.-pneum. Vit. org. c. Debil. cong.	7,00	0,13	5	0,64	4,50	Erbrechen
71	»	Bronchit.	8,40	0,06	10	0,57	4,75	Erbrechen
72	»	Br.-pneum.	8,10	0,07	8	0,52	4,20	Erbrechen
73	»	Br.-pneum.	10,40	0,08	7	0,56	5,80	Neutropenie
75	»	Br.-pneum.	8,70	0,12	6	0,71	6,20	Erbrechen
85	2–3 J.	Br.-pneum.	11,50	0,06	6	0,38	4,40	Unruhe
88	»	Pneum. cr.	11,50	0,13	6	0,80	9,25	Leukopenie
94	3–4 J.	Br.-pneum. Pertussis	15,00	0,04	6	0,24	3,60	Erbrechen und Unruhe

Tab. 5. (Forts.).

Fall Nr.	Alter	Diagnose	Körpergew. in kg	Tagesdosis pro kg Körp.-gew. in g	Anzahl der Beh.-Tage	Ges.-Dosis pro kg Körp.-gew.	Ges.-Dosis in g	Nebenwirkungen
95	3–4 J.	Br.-pneum.	13,20	0,07	6	0,43	5,70	Leukopenie
97	»	Br.-pneum.	13,60	0,10	10	1,01	13,70	Erbrechen
110	6–7 J.	Diab. mell. Bronchitis Pertussis	29,00	0,04	7	0,29	8,40	Zyanose
113	7–8 J.	Pneum. cr.	28,50	0,04	5	0,22	6,20	Hämaturie

Sa. 26 Fälle.

Dies bedeutet, dass das Material der Annahme keine Stütze bietet, Dosen innerhalb der erprobten Grenzen seien von Bedeutung für die Entstehung der untersuchten Nebenwirkungen.

Von den 14 Fällen mit *Erbrechen* können nur 3 als schwere Fälle klassifiziert werden (Nr. 40, 64 und 97, d. h. 3 von 125 untersuchten Fällen). Beim Aussetzen des Medikaments verschwand das Erbrechen rasch. Die *Unruhe* war bei den beiden Fällen mit diesem Symptom als schwer zu bezeichnen, liess aber bald nach, als das Mittel weggelassen wurde. Den Erscheinungen *Hämaturie*, *Zyanose* und *Exanthem* konnte man bei den insgesamt 4 Fällen, wo sie vorkamen, keine nennenswerte klinische Bedeutung beimessen.

Nun noch einige Worte über die 5 Fälle (Nr. 13, 41, 57, 63 und 73 in *Tab. 1*) mit *Neutropenie*. Bei diesen Fällen erreichte die Anzahl der neutrophilen polynukleären Blutkörperchen ihre niedrigsten Werte wie folgt:

Fall 13: 10 %; am letzten der 8 Behandlungstage.
» 41: 6 %; 24 Stdn. nach Abschluss der 4tätigen Behandlung.
» 57: 6 %; 72 » » » » » » .
» 63: 2 %; am letzten der 5 Behandlungstage.
» 73: 7 %; » » » 7 »

Tab. 6.

Gesamtdosis des Sulfathiazols pro kg Körpergewicht bei Fällen mit und ohne Nebenwirkungen.

Fälle ohne Nebenwirkungen						Fälle mit Nebenwirk.	
Fall Nr.	Dosis	Fall Nr.	Dosis	Fall Nr.	Dosis	Fall Nr.	Dosis
1	0,26	44	0,45	87	0,54	7	1,78
2	0,48	45	1,38	89	0,86	9	0,55
3	0,45	46	0,72	90	0,23	13	0,63
4	0,85	47	0,35	91	0,57	21	1,67
5	1,65	48	0,24	92	0,29	22	0,67
6	1,02	49	0,72	93	0,19	24	0,24
8	0,51	50	1,23	96	0,63	36	0,20
10	0,89	51	0,33	98	0,24	39	0,29
11	0,29	52	0,15	99	0,53	40	0,35
12	0,51	53	0,25	100	0,23	41	0,28
14	2,58	55	0,25	101	0,09	54	0,25
15	0,46	56	0,23	102	0,17	57	0,21
16	1,00	58	0,35	103	1,15	63	0,35
17	0,88	59	0,36	104	0,45	64	0,66
18	0,88	60	0,52	105	0,19	65	0,64
19	1,28	61	0,33	106	0,27	71	0,57
20	1,57	62	0,17	107	0,25	72	0,52
23	0,68	66	0,27	108	1,05	73	0,56
25	0,19	67	0,11	109	0,78	75	0,71
26	0,78	68	0,43	111	0,20	85	0,38
27	0,91	69	0,11	112	0,48	88	0,80
28	0,23	70	0,30	114	0,40	94	0,24
29	0,41	74	0,43	115	0,18	95	0,43
30	0,80	76	0,34	116	0,56	97	1,01
31	0,34	77	1,24	117	1,42	110	0,29
32	0,32	78	1,76	118	0,65	113	0,22
33	0,22	79	0,23	119	0,45		
34	0,24	80	0,16	120	0,45		
35	0,14	81	0,25	121	0,28		
37	0,33	82	0,34	122	0,56		
38	0,81	83	0,16	123	0,26		
42	0,57	84	0,15	124	0,44		
43	0,45	86	0,17	125	0,56		

Tab. 7.

Dosis	Anzahl der Fälle	
	Ohne Nebenwirkung.	Mit Nebenwirkung.
—0,20	16	1
0,21—0,40	32	11
0,41—0,60	23	5
0,61—0,80	8	6
0,81—1,00	8	—
1,01—1,20	3	1
1,21—1,40	4	—
1,41—1,60	2	—
1,61—1,80	2	2
1,81—2,00	—	—
2,01—2,20	—	—
2,21—2,40	—	—
2,41—2,60	1	—
Summa	99	26

Tab. 8.

	n	$M \pm \varepsilon(M)$	σ
Fälle ohne Nebenwirk. .	99	0,53 ± 0,04	0,42
» mit » .	26	0,56 ± 0,08	0,00

Differenz 0,03 ± 0,09

Hierbei ist besonders zu beachten, dass bei zwei Fällen der niedrigste Wert erst 24—72 Stdn. nach Abschluss der Behandlungsperiode auftrat, woraus die Notwendigkeit einer Kontrolle der Blutwerte während der ersten Woche nach dem Aussetzen des Medikaments deutlich hervorgeht. Die Einzelheiten der Hämogramme sind bezüglich der Fälle 13, 41 und 73 aus *Tab. 1* und hinsichtlich der Fälle 57 und 63 aus *Tab. 1 b* zu ersehen.

Anmerkungen zu Tab. 1.

Anm. 1. (Fall 57).

Zeitpunkt	weisse Blk.	stabk. %	segmk. %	eos. %	basoph. %	Mono. %	Lympho. %
Vor d. Behandlung	10 400	15	20	0	0	3	62
letzter (4.) Beh.-Tag	5 600	6	2	0	0	3	89
3. Tag n. Schluss d. Beh. . . .	5 900	3	3	0	0	1	93
4. Tag n. Schluss d. Beh. . . .	8 600	2	6	1	1	1	89
5. Tag n. Schluss d. Beh. . . .	8 000	5	9	0	0	3	83

Anm. 2. (Fall 63).

Zeitpunkt	weisse Blk.	stabk. %	segmk. %	eos. %	basoph. %	Mono. %	Lympho. %
Vor d. Behandlung	19 000	29	44	0	0	2	25
letzter (5.) Beh.-Tag	4 800	0	2	0	0	2	96
24 Stdn. n. Schluss d. Beh.	4 900	1	5	0	0	2	92
48 Stdn. n. Schluss d. Beh.	7 800	0	6	0	0	4	90
72 Stdn. n. Schluss d. Beh.	5 600	5	16	0	0	1	78
96 Stdn. n. Schluss d. Beh.	6 300	9	31	1	0	2	57
6. Tag n. Schluss d. Beh. . . .	10 600	1	23	0	0	1	75
8. Tag n. Schluss d. Beh. . . .	12 900	6	35	0	0	2	57

Anmerkungen zu Tab. 1.

Sternalpunktion 24 Stdn. nach Abschluss der Behandlung:

»Zellreiches Präparat. Auffallend starke Linksverschiebung in der Myelopoese, aber keine direkte Sperre im Reifungsprozess, wenn auch segmentkernige Zellen recht selten sind. Sonst nichts merkbar Pathologisches». (Nordenson).

Sternalpunktion 8 Tage nach Abschluss der Behandlung:

»Zellreiches Präparat. In der Myelopoese etwas Linksverschiebung. Erythropoese o. B. Retikel im grossen ganzen o. B.» (Nordenson).

Das Kind wurde gesund.

Anm. 3. (Fall 88).

Zeitpunkt	weisse Blk.	stabk. %	segmk. %	eos. %	basoph. %	Mono. %	Lympho. %
2. Beh.-Tag . .	8 000	11	28	0	0	1	60
3. Beh.-Tag . .	4 300	12	35	0	0	0	53
4. Beh.-Tag . .	4 700	3	28	0	0	3	56
5. Beh.-Tag . .	4 600	8	21	0	0	0	71
24 Stdn. n. Schluss d. Beh.	3 300	2	10	0	0	2	86
48 Stdn. n. Schluss d. Beh.	5 000	3	9	0	0	1	87
4. Tag n. Schluss d. Beh. . . .	5 500	1	13	2	0	1	83
6. Tag n. Schluss d. Beh. . . .	7 400	9	40	0	0	1	50

Sternalpunktion am 4. Tage nach Schluss der Behandlung:

»Relativ zellreiches Präparat. Recht starke Linksverschiebung in der Myelopoese ohne merkbare Sperre. Sonst keine Veränderungen.» (Nordenson).

Anm. 4. (Fall 95).

Vor Beginn der Behandlung betrug die Anzahl der weissen Blutkörperchen 10 900, am Schluss derselben (am 6. Behandlungstage) 3 400. 48 Stdn. nach Abschluss der Behandlung war die Anzahl 4 700 und nach weiteren 72 Stdn. 6 200. Hierbei wurde keine Neutropenie beobachtet; als die Anzahl der weissen Blutkörperchen 3 400 betrug, machten die stabkernigen neutrophilen 5 %, die segmentkernigen 26 % und die Lymphozyten 67 % aus.

Bei keinem der fünf Fälle mit Neutropenie lag eine Leukopenie vor. Bei 4 von den 5 Fällen war die Neutropenie ohne besondere Massregeln innerhalb einer Woche verschwunden, während bei dem fünften Fall noch 1 Monat später eine Neutropenie bestand (Fall 41). Die Sternalpunktionen, welche vor und nach der Behandlung bei einem der Fälle (Fall 63, *Tab. 1 b*) ausgeführt wurden, ergaben keinen mit Sicherheit pathologishen Befund von Bedeutung.

Schliesslich ein Bericht über die beiden Fälle mit *Leukopenie* (Fall 88 und 95 in *Tab. 1* und *Tab 1 b*).

Bei dem ersten Fall (Nr. 88) handelte es sich um einen 2 $^1/_2$-jährigen Knaben mit kroupöser Pneumonie. Er erhielt täglich (in 24 Stdn.) 0,13 g Sulfathiazol pro kg Körpergewicht während insgesamt 6 Tagen oder eine Gesamtmenge von 9,25 g. Hämogramm siehe *Tab. 1 b*. Die Anzahl der weissen Blutkörperchen sank am tiefsten, auf 3 300, ungefähr 24 Stunden nach Abschluss der Behandlung. Bereits am folgenden Tage war der Wert auf 5 500 gestiegen. Während der Zeitperiode 24—96 Stdn. nach Abschluss der Behandlung lag Neutropenie vor. Die erst am 4. Tage nach Abschluss der Behandlung vorgenommene Sternalpunktion ergab eine starke Linksverschiebung in der Myelopoese, aber keine wahrnehmbare Sperre (NORDENSON). Die Rekonvaleszenz verlief normal. Andere toxische Symptome, welche auf die Medikation zurückzuführen wären, traten nicht auf.

Es handelte sich also um eine Neutropenie und eine Leukopenie nach einer niedrigen therapeutischen Dosis von Sulfathiazol.

Der andere Fall (Nr. 95, *Tab. 1* und *1 b*) betraf ein 3jähriges Mädchen mit Bronchopneumonie. Sie erhielt nur 0,07 g Sulfathiazol pro kg Körpergewicht pro Tag während insgesamt 6 Tagen oder eine Gesamtdosis von nur 5,70 g. Vor Beginn der Behandlung hatte die Anzahl der weissen Blutkörperchen 10 900 betragen, und am 6. Behandlungstage (dem letzten) erreichte der diesbezügliche Wert sein Minimum oder 3 400. Schon 120 Stdn. nach Abschluss der Behandlung war die Anzahl ohne besondere Massnahmen auf 6 200 gestiegen. Während des Verlaufs trat keine Neutropenie auf.

Als die Anzahl der weissen Blutkörperchen 3 400 betrug, war der Prozentsatz der neutrophilen polynukleären 31. Dieser Befund ist von prinzipieller Bedeutung.

Die bei diesen beiden Fällen auftretende Leukopenie kam also vor, ohne dass eine besonders niedrige Anzahl weisser Blutkörperchen vor dem Einsetzen der Behandlung vorlag, und zwar nach einer sehr mässigen Sulfathiazoldosis. Die Leukopenie verschwand in beiden Fällen nach einigen Tagen, ohne dass sich irgendein schädlicher Einfluss auf den Allgemeinzustand des Patienten entdecken liess. Ebensowenig wurden andere toxische Erscheinungen beobachtet.

Als abschliessendes Urteil über die bei den vorliegenden 125 sulfathiazolbehandelten Fällen beobachteten Nebenwirkungen mag angeführt werden, dass sie zwar in 20,8 v. H. oder bei 26 Fällen auftraten, dass sie aber leicht waren und rasch ohne merkbare Folgen für die Patienten zurückgingen. Die geschilderten Fälle von Neutropenie und Leukopenie dürften auf das Medikament als Ursache zurückzuführen sein, wenn sich auch der Einfluss der Infektion beim Zustandekommen der Blutveränderungen nicht gänzlich ausschliessen lässt. (Siehe ferner bezüglich dieser Frage Verf.s Arbeit über andere Sulfanilamidpräparate und deren Wirkungen, Acta Pæd. 1941, S. 173).

Wie oben gesagt wurde, hat man verschiedentlich das Sulfathiazol dem Sulfapyridin vorziehen wollen, da es den Eindruck erweckte, als ob jenes Präparat leichtere Nebenwirkungen habe als dieses. Die soeben zitierte Arbeit enthält eine Zusammenstellung von bei Sulfanilamid- und Sulfapyridinmedika-

Tab. 9.

Präparat	Anzahl der beh. Fälle	Anzahl der Fälle mit					
		Erbrechen	Zyanose	Exanthem	Hämaturie	Störg. der Leukopoese	Unruhe
Sulfapyridin (»Septipulmon»)	102	—	—	0	0	3	4
M & B 693 . . .	97	—	—	1	2	1	6
Sulfanilamid . .	70	—	—	0	0	0	3
Sulfathiazol . .	125	14	2	1	2	7	3

tion gefundenen Nebenwirkungen. Die Dosen der besagten Chemotherapeutika, welche da angewendet worden sind, waren ungefähr dieselben, wie die Sulfathiazoldosen, die in dem hier vorliegenden Material Verwendung gefunden haben. *Tab. 9* gibt einen Vergleich der Frequenz von Nebenwirkungen bei Anwendung der verschiedenen Präparate.

Bei diesem Vergleich ergibt sich, dass das Sulfathiazol Nebenwirkungen hat, von welchen man nicht sagen kann, dass sie seltener vorkommen oder leichter sind als die beim Gebrauch von Sulfapyridin auftretenden, wenn sie auch in dem vorliegenden Material nicht an und für sich schwer waren. Doch kamen bei Anwendung von Sulfathiazol in 7 von 125 Fällen Störungen innerhalb der Leukopoese vor, welche freilich rasch vorübergingen.

IV. **Untersuchung der Nebenwirkungen bei Sulfathiazolbehandlung zweier Fälle ohne Anzeichen einer akuten Infektion.**

Da Sulfanilamidpräparate im Kindesalter nach Massgabe üblicher klinischer Indikationen verabfolgt werden, d. h. meistens bei akuten Infektionen der Luftwege, bleibt man oft im ungewissen über die Ursache des Krankheitsausgangs, aber auch über die Ursache für das Auftreten derartiger Nebenwirkungen, welche mit von der Krankheit als solcher verursachten Symptomen verwechselt werden können. Es muss also äusserst erwünscht sein, den Effekt der Präparate bei Fällen erproben zu können, wo keine Infektion der ebenerwähnten oder anderer Art vorliegt. Wir hatten bei zwei Fällen Gelegenheit, eine solche Untersuchung auszuführen. Hierzu wurden zwei Kinder gewählt, beide ca. 2 Monate alt, welche beide an sehr hochgradigem, nichtleutischem Hydrocephalus internus mit begleitender schwerer Demenz litten. Speziell wurde der Einfluss des Sulfathiazols auf die Leukopoese untersucht.

Erster Fall. (*Tab. 10* u. *Tab. 11*).

(Krankenhaus Norrtull, Jr.-Nr. 617/1940).

Bevor Sulfathiazol eingesetzt wurde, untersuchten wir das weisse Blutbild (*Tab. 10*, Hämogramm vom 19.11), welches ebenso wie

Tab. 10.

Fall L. W., Krankenhaus Norrtull, Jr.-Nr. 617/1940.
(Hydrocephalus int.)
Alter beim Beginn der Untersuchung 2 Monate. Körpergewicht 4 170 g.

Zeitperioden der Sulfathiazolbeh. Dosis	Datum	Weisses Blutbild						
		Anzahl d. weiss. Blk.	stabk. neutr. %	segmk. neutr. %	eosinoph. polynukl. %	basoph. polynukl. %	Lympho. %	Mono. %
	19.11.	6 400	5	26	1	0	64	4
20.–26.11. 7 gr.	22.11.	5 800	5	10	4	0	78	3
	25.11.	4 700	3	13	4	1	72	7
	27.11.	6 000	4	31	4	0	55	5
	29.11.	6 500	1	22	2	1	69	4
	2.12.	4 500	2	20	0	0	74	4
	4.12.	4 900	6	24	2	0	64	4
	6.12.	4 900	4	18	4	0	70	4
	9.12.	4 600	6	32	2	0	60	0
11.–26.12. 15,6 gr.	11.12.	3 900	3	22	2	0	71	2
	12.12.	5 800	2	17	0	0	78	1
	27.12.	4 000	4	12	0	0	80	4
4.–11.1. (septipulmon) 11,5 gr.	4.1.	7 000	1	20	10	0	67	2
	7.1.	8 200	1	15	3	0	78	3
	11.1.	5 400	1	14	0	0	82	3
	17.1.	6 000	1	20	1	0	77	1
	31.1.	8 000	1	27	0	0	69	3
	10.2.	9 000	5	32	0	0	58	5
11.–14.2. 3,4 gr.	12.2.	5 700	7	22	2	0	65	4
	14.2.	5 000	6	6	0	0	83	5
10.–18.3. 9,4 gr.	10.3.	7 700	7	20	0	0	72	1
	12.3.	6 400	4	20	1	0	75	0
	14.3.	3 200	4	12	0	0	81	3
	17.3.	2 900	2	9	0	0	86	3
	19.3.	3 300	3	7	0	0	88	2

Tab. 10. (Forts.).

Zeitperioden der Sulfathiazolbeh. Dosis	Datum	Weisses Blutbild						
		Anzahl d. weiss. Blk.	stabk. neutr. %	segmk. neutr. %	eosinoph. polynukl. %	basoph. polynukl. %	Lympho. %	Mono. %
	21.3.	7 400	2	8	1	0	88	1
	28.3.	7 100	1	18	3	0	78	0
	31.3.	4 300	5	15	1	0	76	0
	2.4.	6 100	2	11	1	0	85	1
	7.4.	4 600	2	11	1	0	83	3
	12.4.	10 100	4	66	0	0	34	2
	15.4.	12 400	4	32	2	0	60	1
	21.4.	7 500	2	33	3	0	59	3
	30.4.	7 600	2	43	1	0	53	1
	7.5.	8 100	3	31	6	0	57	3
	14.5.	7 700	1	28	0	0	70	1
	16.5.	8 000	2	14	3	0	78	3
17.–27.5. 12,2 gr.	19.5.	7 300	0	24	0	0	75	1
	21.5.	8 000	0	29	1	0	68	2
	23.5.	9 200	4	24	0	0	71	1
	26.5.	12 000	2	30	3	0	73	2
	28.5.	12 000	1	43	4	0	50	2
	30.5.	12 000	0	28	4	0	66	2
	3.6.	7 900	1	25	6	0	67	1
	5.6.	10 200	7	62	0	0	29	2
	7.6.	19 000	2	71	0	0	25	2
	9.6.	14 000	0	39	3	0	56	2
	11.6.	15 100	6	27	5	0	60	2
	20.6.	6 400	—	—	—	—	—	—
	27.6.	8 000	6	28	5	0	60	1
	4.7.	16 500	7	40	0	0	53	0

das rote normal befunden wurde. An demselben Tage wurde eine Sternalpunktion vorgenommen. Das Punktat wurde von E. SEGERDAHL untersucht, welcher hierüber folgendes Gutachten abgab: »Zellreiches Präparat. Völlig normale Verhältnisse in bezug auf Erythro- und Leukopoese und die diesbezüglichen Relationen. Das einzig Bemerkenswerte im Präparat ist ein an gewissen Stellen wahrnehmbares reichliches Vorkommen von Leukozyten, wie es von Lichtenstein und Nordenson bei Frügeborenen beschrieben worden ist. Dasselbe beruht hier wahrscheinlich auf zufälliger Aspiration eines Nodulus lymphaticus im Knochenmark. Die Erythrozyten im Präparat weisen eine leichte Anisozytose und eine leichte Polychromasie auf.»

Dann wurde während insgesamt 7 Tagen (20.—26.11. 1940) eine Gesamtmenge Sulfathiazol von 7 g = 0,24 g pro kg Körpergewicht pro Tag (24 Stdn.) gegeben. Die Dosis war also doppelt so gross wie die oben als durchschnittliche therapeutische Dosis empfohlene, aber nicht grösser als diejenigen, welche oft verabreicht zu werden pflegen und auch in meinem Material einige Male zu therapeutischen Zwecken gegeben worden sind. Die nach der Behandlungsperiode vorgenommene Sternalpunktion misslang leider technisch. Wie aus *Tab. 10* hervorgeht, wurde das Blutbild von der Behandlung nicht beeinflusst. Auch sonst kamen keine Nebenwirkungen vor. Während ca. 2 Wochen nach Abschluss der Behandlung wurde das Blutbild regelmässig untersucht, wobei sich normale Verhältnisse konstatieren liessen (bis zum 9.12.).

Am Ende dieser Periode ohne Chemotherapeutika (am 6. 12.) wurde eine Sternalpunktion ausgeführt, welche folgendes Resultat hatte: ». . . Sowohl Leuko- wie Erythropoese normal. Das Präparat enthält jetzt eine verhältnismässig grosse Menge von retikuloendothelialen Elementen, was man indessen ab und zu in normalem Knochenmark sieht.» (E. SEGERDAHL).

In einer zweiten Periode wurde Sulfathiazol 15 Tage lang (11.—26.12.) in einer Gesamtmenge von 15,6 g = 0,24 g pro kg Körpergewicht pro Tag im Durchschnitt gegeben. Die Dosis war also dieselbe wie während der vorhergehenden Behandlungsperiode. Auch jetzt traten keine Nebenwirkungen auf. Das weisse Blutbild blieb normal. Am letzten Behandlungstage wurde eine Sternalpunktion mit folgendem Ergebnis vorgenommen: »Das Präparat weist nichts pathologisches auf. Das Knochenmark ist sehr lymphozytenreich, aber dies dürfte durch das Alter des Patienten erklärt werden.» (JAN WALDENSTRÖM).

Neun Tage nach Abschluss der Behandlung wurde eine neuerliche Untersuchung des weissen Blutbildes ausgeführt, welches normal befunden wurde, mit 7 000 weissen Blutkörperchen und 21 % neutrophilen polynukleären. Die gleichzeitig (am 4.1.) vorgenommene Sternalpunktion hatte ein unerwartetes und sehr merkwürdiges Resultat: »Relativ zellreiches Präparat. Stark geschädigte Myelopoese mit ausgesprochenen degenerativen Veränderungen. Ausserdem etwas Linksverschiebung und eine hypoplastische Myelopoese. Erythropoese o. B. Lymphozyten spärlich. Retikel recht stark hyperplastisch.» (NORDENSON).

Das Bemerkenswerte ist selbstverständlich, dass die schwere Schädigung der Myelopoese erst 9 Tage nach Abschluss der Behandlung auftrat, oder, genauer ausgedrückt: dieselbe war unmittelbar nach Schluss der Behandlung nicht vorhanden. Daneben ist es von grosser prinzipieller Bedeutung, dass das weisse Blutbild keinerlei Veränderungen aufwies, während gleichzeitig ein pathologisches Knochenmarksbild vorlag.

Da das soeben erwähnte Resultat der letzten Knochenmarkpunktion nicht vorauszusehen war, und da wir die Absicht hatten, zu prüfen, ob sich bei diesem Patient irgendein Unterschied des Resultates nach Behandlung mit Sulfathiazol und Sulfapyridin (Septipulmon) beobachten lassen würde, wurde leider schon am 4.1. das letztere Medikament eingesetzt, welches der Patient dann während insgesamt 8 Tagen (4.—11.1.) in einer Gesamtdosis von 11,5 g oder einer durchschnittlichen Tagesdosis (in 24 Stdn.) von 0,28 g pro kg Körpergewicht erhielt (Pat. war jetzt 4 Monate alt und wog 5 170 g). Hierbei verhielt sich das weisse Blutbild normal. Die neutrophilen Leukozyten betrugen jedoch am Ende der Behandlungsperiode nur 15 %. Fünf Tage nach Abschluss der Septipulmonbehandlung (am 17.1.) wurde von neuem eine Sternalpunktion mit folgendem Resultat ausgeführt: »Zellreiches Präparat. Nach wie vor recht ausgesprochene degenerative Veränderungen bei der Myelopoese, doch etwas geringer als voriges Mal. Starke Linksverschiebung und gewisse Sperre mit Herabsetzung der Anzahl von segmentierten. Erythropoese o. B. Retikel leicht hyperplastisch. Megakaryozyten o. B.» (NORDENSON).

Nun wurde während einer Zeit von 4 Wochen (12.1—10.2. 41) kein Medikament gegeben. Am 30.1. oder ca. 3 Wochen nach Schluss der Septipulmonbehandlung wurde eine neuerliche Sternalpunktion mit folgendem Ergebnis vorgenommen: »Zellreiches Präparat. Im grossen ganzen normale Verhältnisse. Bemerkenswerte Zunahme des Retikels.» (NORDENSON). Das Verhalten des Hämogramms wird aus *Tab. 10* ersichtlich. Sonstige toxische Symptome wurden nicht beobachtet.

Während des Zeitabschnitts 11.—14.2. wurde aufs neue während insgesamt 4 Tagen Sulfathiazol in einer Gesamtdosis von 3,4 g = 0,13 g pro kg Körpergewicht pro Tag (24 Stdn.) verabreicht. Während dieser Zeit war die Anzahl der weissen Blutkörperchen normal, während die der neutrophilen polynukleären von 29 auf 12 % zurückging. Sonst keine Nebenwirkungen. Am letzten Behandlungstage (14.2.) Sternalpunktion: »Zellreiches Präparat. Bei der Myelopoese machen sich unerhebliche toxische Einflüsse geltend. Erythropoese o. B. Ungewöhnlich zahlreiche Lymphozyten. Retikel leicht hyperplastisch. Diagnose: im grossen ganzen normales Mark.» (NORDENSON).

Vom 15.2. bis zum 9.3. wurde kein Medikament gegeben, und während dieser ganzen Zeit war das Kind bezüglich der Sulfathiazolwirkung erscheinungsfrei; das weisse Blutbild war normal.

Am 10.3. wurde eine erneute Sternalpunktion mit folgendem Resultat vorgenommen: »Zellreiches Präparat. In der Myelopoese Linksverschiebung und gewisse Sperre nach den Metamyelozyten. Erythropoese o. B. Retikel stark hyperplastisch.» (NORDENSON). Hier lagen demnach von neuem, trotz der vorausgehenden 3wöchigen Ruhepause, gewisse toxische Einflüsse bei der Myelopoese vor.

Während der Periode 10.—18.3. 41 wurde aufs neue Sulfathiazol in einer Gesamtmenge von 9,4 g = 0,16 g pro kg Körpergewicht pro Tag verabfolgt. In dieser Periode hatte das Kind während einiger Tage subfebrile Temperatur und Husten. Am Schluss der Behandlungsperiode (14.—17.3.) trat eine Leukopenie (2 900 weisse Blutkörperchen) sowie eine Neutropenie (11 %) auf, welche 2—3 Tage nach dem Aussetzen der Behandlung verschwanden. (Während der Behandlung stellte sich Erbrechen ein, von welchem man aber wohl annehmen könnte, dass es auf der leichten Infektion als solcher beruhte.). Am letzten Tage der Behandlung (18.3.) Sternalpunktion: »Zellreiches Präparat. Im grossen and ganzen dasselbe Bild, keine merkbare Verschlimmerung. Diagnose: Mark vom Granulozytopenietyp.» (NORDENSON).

Während des Zeitabschnitts 19.3.—16.5. wurde kein Sulfathiazol gegeben. In dieser ganzen Periode wurden keine Erscheinungen beobachtet, welche man mit der Sulfathiazolmedikation in Zusammenhang bringen könnte. Am 9.4., also 3 Wochen nach Schluss der letzten Behandlungsperiode, wurde eine neuerliche Sternalpunktion vorgenommen, welche folgendes ergab: »Zellreiches Präparat. Myelopoese toxisch und mit leichter Linksverschiebung. Keine Anzeichen einer gröberen Störung im Reifungsprozess. Erythropoese o. B. Retikel im grossem ganzen o. B.» (NORDENSON). Am 13.5. wiederum Sternalpunktion: »Zellreiches Präparat. Keine merkbaren morphologischen Veränderungen.» (NORDENSON).

Vom 17. bis zum 27.5. wurde von neuem Sulfathiazol in einer Gesamtmenge von 12,2 g = 0,14 g pro kg Körpergewicht pro Tag (24 Stdn.) gegeben. Hierbei traten klinisch keine Nebenwirkungen auf; das weisse Blutbild war normal. Am letzten Behandlungstage wurde eine Sternalpunktion ausgeführt: »Zellarmes Präparat. In der Hauptsache toxische Veränderungen. Keine Reifungsstörung.» (NORDENSON). Am 3.6. wurde noch eine Sternalpunktion vorgenommen: »Relativ zellarmes Präparat. Verringerung reiferer myeloischer Zellen. Keine direkte Sperre, aber deutliche Linksverschiebung. Retikel leicht hyperplastisch.» (NORDENSON). Während weiterer 5 Wochen wurde das Blutbild kontrolliert, welches normale Verhältnisse aufwies. Allgemeinzustand des Patienten (bis auf die schweren Symptome von Hydrozephalus) o. B.

Tab. 11.

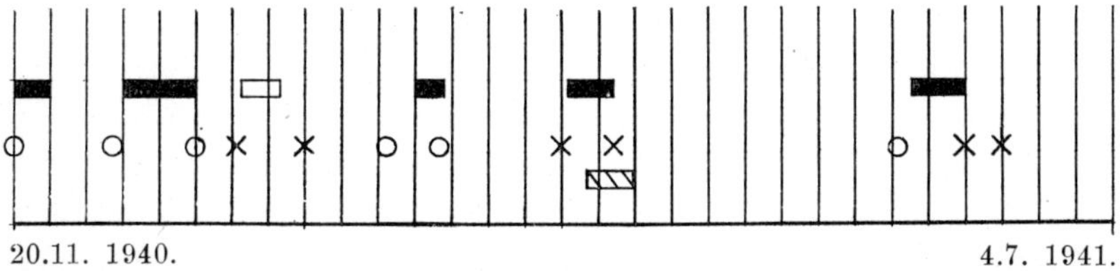

Die Abstände der senkrechten Linien stellen je eine Woche dar.
Diejenigen Perioden, während welcher Sulfathiazol gegeben wurde, sind mit ▬ bezeichnet;
diejenige Periode, während welcher Septipulmon verabreicht wurde, ist mit ▭ markiert;
Normaler Knochenmarkbefund: O
Pathologischer » : X
Periode der Leukopenie: ▨

Zusammenfassung: Es handelt sich also um ein Kind, welches im Alter von 2—8 Monaten, während einer Zeit von insgesamt 6 Monaten in 5 Perioden von 7 bzw. 15, 4, 9 und 11 Tagen oder zusammen 46 Tagen 47,6 g Sulfathiazol erhalten hatte. Die 24Stundendosis war 0,13—0,24 g pro kg Körpergewicht. Ausserdem bekam der Patient während 8 Tagen insgesamt 11,5 g Sulfapyridin (Septipulmon). (Siehe *Tab. 11*).

Der Allgemeinzustand war während der ganzen Zeit gut. Andere als die Leukopoese betreffende Nebenwirkungen traten nicht auf.

Es wurde Knochenmark von charakteristischem Granulozytopenietyp beobachtet, nachdem der Patient zuerst 7 Tage lang insgesamt 7 g Sulfathiazol erhalten hatte, dann 2 Wochen ohne Medikament gewesen war und später wieder während insgesamt 15 Tagen 15,6 g dieses Mittels bekommen hatte. Es war bemerkenswert, dass das Mark unmittelbar nach Abschluss dieser Behandlung ein normales morphologisches Bild aufwies, während 9 Tage später eine stark geschädigte Myelopoese beobachtet wurde. Sulfathiazol wurde während der beiden besagten Perioden in einer Menge von 0,24 g pro kg Körpergewicht pro Tag (24 Stdn.) gegeben.

Es war noch ein weiteres Mal während des Verlaufs zu konstatieren, dass eine Schädigung der Myelopoese erst diagnostizierbar wurde, nachdem eine gewisser Zeitraum (ca. 3 Wochen) nach dem Abschluss der Sulfathiazolbehandlung verstrichen war (siehe *Tab. 11*).

Bei einer Gelegenheit trat während einer Zeit von zusammen ca. 4 Tagen beim Abschluss einer 9 Tage langen Sulfathiazolperiode Leukopenie auf, wobei auch eine Neutropenie bestand (*Tab. 10*).

Sonst kam bei den Gelegenheiten, wo eine geschädigte Myelopoese beobachtet wurde, keine Schädigung des weissen Blutbildes vor.

Der wichtigste Punkt bei diesen Versuchen ist der, dass man *hier keine Veranlassung hat, den Einfluss einer behandelten Infektion auf die Entstehung von Granulozytopeniemark bei der Sulfathiazoltherapie in Betracht zu ziehen.* Die ausgeführte Untersuchung wirft kein Licht auf die Frage, ob die Sulfanilamidtherapie bei Fällen von Infektion oder bei gewissen Fällen von Infektion ebenso leicht, leichter oder weniger leicht zu Schädigungen im Bereich der Myelopoese führt, als wenn das Medikament Individuen ohne Infektion verabreicht wird.

Zweiter Fall. (*Tab. 12*).

(Krankenhaus Norrtull, Jr.-Nr. 363/1941).

Sulfathiazol wurde während 8 Tagen in einer Gesamtmenge von 8,4 g = 0,20 g pro kg Körpergewicht pro Tag (24 Stdn.) gegeben. Bei der Ausführung des Versuchs hatte das Kind einen leichten Husten, war aber fieberfrei. Aus *Tab. 11* geht hervor,

Tab. 12.

Fall G. A., Krankenhaus Norrtull, Jr.-Nr. 363/1941.
(Hydrocephalus int.)
Alter beim Beginn der Untersuchung 2 Monate. Körpergewicht 5,310 g.

Zeitperiode der Sulfathiazolbeh. Dosis	Datum	Weisses Blutbild						
		Anzahl d. weiss. Blk.	stabk. neutr. %	segmk. neutr. %	eosinoph. polynukl. %	basoph. polynukl. %	Lympho. %	Mono. %
	13.5.	14 500	4	46	2	0	40	8
17.–24.5. 8,4 gr.	17.5.	7 600	—	—	—	—	—	—
	19.5.	8 200	11	27	0	0	60	2
	21.5.	10 300	4	22	1	0	70	3
	23.5.	10 000	0	18	1	0	80	1
	26.5.	11 600	4	24	3	0	67	2
	28.5.	17 200	4	32	0	0	62	2
	31.5.	22 700	0	12	1	0	87	0
	3.6.	10 100	2	28	1	0	69	0
	5.6.	8 800	1	30	0	0	66	3
	7.6.	12 000	10	56	0	0	31	3
	9.6.	9 600	0	18	0	0	80	2
	4.7.	5 800	2	14	2	0	80	2

dass das Blutbild vor dem Versuch normal war und die Sternalpunktion bei derselben Gelegenheit folgendes ergab: »Zellreiches Präparat mit im grossen ganzen normalem Knochenmark.» (NORDENSON).

Am 7. Tage der Behandlung wurde eine mikroskopisch nachweisbare Hämaturie festgestellt (30—40 rote Blutkörperchen pro Gesichtsfeld), nachdem der Patient eine Sulfathiazolmenge von insgesamt 7,1 g erhalten hatte. Die Hämaturie verschwand binnen 7 Tagen vollständig. Drei Tage nach Abschluss der Behandlung wurde eine Sternalpunktion ausgeführt: »Zellreiches Präparat. Linksverschiebung und toxische Veränderungen.» (NORDENSON).

Wie bei dem obenbeschriebenen Fall liessen sich auch hier toxische Einflüsse auf das Knochenmark nachweisen, nachdem

Sulfathiazol in einer therapeutischen, üblichen Dosis während nur 8 Tagen gegeben worden war, wobei auch eine Hämaturie entstand. Wie aus *Tab. 12* ersichtlich wird, blieb trotz Vorkommens eines toxisch veränderten Knochenmarks das weisse Blutbild unverändert normal.

V. Zusammenfassung und Schlussfolgerungen.

Patientenmaterial:

125 Kinder mit in der Hauptsache akuten Infektionen der Luftwege. 48 waren im Alter von 0—1 Jahr und 77 im Alter von 1—13 Jahren. (Die Untersuchung schliesst sich an eine andere von uns über u. a. Dosierung und Nebenwirkungen von Sulfapyridin ausgeführte an. Dieses Material enthielt 199 Kinder, von welchen 128 im Alter von 0—1 Jahr und 71 im Alter von über 1 Jahr waren. Siehe Acta Pædiatrica 1941, S. 173). Sämtliche Fälle waren im Krankenhaus Norrtull, Stockholm, stationär behandelt worden.

Ausserdem wurde der Sulfathiazoleffekt bei zwei Kindern im Alter von 2 Monaten untersucht, welche an schwerem, nichtluetischem Hydrocephalus internus litten, aber keine nennenswerten Symptome einer akuten Infektion aufwiesen.

Dosierung:

Dieselbe Dosierung fand bei Kindern in allen Altersgruppen, auch bei den jüngsten im Alter von 0—1 Monat (10 Kinder in diesem Alter befanden sich in dem Gesamtmaterial), Anwendung.

Diejenige Dosierung, welche verwendet wurde und die jetzt empfohlen wird, ist: 0,10 g pro kg Körpergewicht pro Tag (24 Stdn.). In gewissen Fällen wurde mit gutem Resultat ungefähr die Hälfte dieser Dosis und in einigen Fällen, ebenfalls mit gutem Resultat, die doppelte Dosis gegeben. Es wurde statistisch nachgewiesen, dass innerhalb der angegebenen Grenzen die Grösse der Dosis offenbar ohne Einfluss auf die Entstehung toxischer Nebenwirkungen ist. Dies schliesst selbstverständlich nicht aus, dass man bei grösseren als den hier verwendeten Dosen wohl stärkere Nebenwirkungen als in dem vorliegenden Material erwarten kann.

Das Sulfathiazol wurde im allgemeinen 5mal im Laufe der 24 Stundenperiode verabfolgt, jedesmal dieselbe Menge. Es wurde im Durchschnitt während 3—6 Tagen und bei kritischem Temperaturfall im Anschluss an Pneumonien vom lobären Typ ca. 2—4 Tage nach dem Temperaturfall gegeben.

Bei der angegebenen Durchschnittsdosis pro kg Körpergewicht pro Tag (0,10 g) gestaltet sich das Dosierungsschema folgendermassen:

Kinder im Alter von	1 M.:	24Stundendosis	0,40 g = 0,08 × 5
» » » »	3 »	»	0,50 » = 0,10 × 5
» » » »	6 »	»	0,70 » = 0,15 × 5 (ungef.)
» » » »	1 J.	»	1,00 » = 0,20 × 5
» » » »	2 »	»	1,25 » = 0,25 × 5
» » » »	3 »	»	1,50 » = 0,30 × 5
» » » »	5 »	»	2,00 » = 0,40 × 5
» » » »	8 »	»	2,50 » = 0,50 × 5
» » » »	10 »	»	3,00 » = 0,60 × 5
» » » »	13 »	»	4,00 » = 0,80 × 5

Nebenwirkungen: (siehe *Tab. 9*).

Bei der angewendeten Dosierung traten in 26 von 125 untersuchten Fällen (20,8 v. H.) toxische Nebenwirkungen auf (siehe die tabellarische Zusammenstellung hierüber auf S. 14). Von diesen Nebenwirkungen mögen hier nur die 14 Fälle von *Erbrechen*, darunter 3 schwerere, sowie 5 Fälle von Neutropenie und 2 Fälle von Leukopenie (von welchen einer gleichzeitig Neutropenie aufwies) erwähnt werden. Die grösste Beachtung verdienen die Fälle mit geschädigter Leukopoese.

Die 5 *Neutropeniefälle*: Die Neutropenie trat bei kurzdauernder Behandlung mit Sulfathiazol in üblicher therapeutischer Dosis auf. Bei keinem der Fälle war die Gesamtanzahl der weissen Blutkörperchen vor Beginn der Behandlung besonders niedrig, was wohl zu beachten ist. In keinem Fall trat Leukopenie auf. Es wurde konstatiert, dass die Zahl der neutrophilen polynukleären in einigen Fällen ihren niedrigsten Wert nicht eher als mehrere Tage nach dem Aussetzen der Behandlung erreichte, woraus die Wichtigkeit einer Kontrolle des weissen Blutbildes während der auf die Sulfathiazolzufuhr folgenden Zeitperiode klar ersichtlich wird. Die Neutropenie verschwand bei 4 von den 5 Fällen binnen einiger Tage; bei dem fünften bestand die Neutropenie noch nach einem Monat weiter. In einem der Fälle war der Knochenmarkbefund vor und nach der Behandlung normal. Bei den übrigen 4 Fällen wurde das Knochenmark nicht untersucht.

Die 2 *Leukopeniefälle*: Die in diesen Fällen verwendete Dosis war niedrig, sie betrug nur 0,13 bzw. 0,07 g pro kg Körpergewicht pro 24 Stdn. während bei beiden Fällen nur 6 Tagen (9,25 bzw. 5,70 g Sulfathiazol bei einem 2 1/2- bzw. 3jährigen Kinde). Die Feststellung, dass bei keinem dieser beiden Fälle die Gesamtanzahl der weissen Blutkörperchen vor Beginn der Behandlung besonders niedrig war, ist von grosser Bedeutung. Einer der Fälle wies während einiger Tage auch Neutropenie auf, aber bei dem anderen war dies nicht der Fall, was Beachtung verdient. Einige Tage nach dem Aussetzen der Medikation war die Leukopenie verschwunden. Etwaige andere toxische Symptome wurden nicht beobachtet.

Untersuchung über den Sulfathiazoleffekt bei 2 Säuglingen ohne nennenswerte Anzeichen einer akuten Infektion:

Bei beiden Fällen entstand nach Behandlung mit Sulfathiazol in der gewöhnlich angewendeten therapeutischen Dosis das Bild eines toxischen Knochenmarks vom Granulozytopenietyp. Bei dem einen Falle stellte sich daneben eine vorübergehende Leukopenie mit Neutropenie ein. Bei dem anderen war gelegentlich des pathologischen Knochenmarkbefundes das weisse Blutbild normal. In einem der Fälle trat eine Hämaturie flüchtigen Charakters auf. Aus den erhobenen Befunden wurden einige besondere Schlussfolgerungen gezogen:

1. Bei Granulozytopeniemark (nach Sulfathiazolbehandlung) kann das weisse Blutbild völlig normal sein.
2. Neutropenie braucht bei von Sulfathiazol hervorgerufener Leukopenie nicht vorzuliegen.
3. Pathologisch verändertes Knochenmark kann nach einem wochenlangen Interwall nach dem Aussetzen der Sulfathiazolbehandlung auftreten. Diese Befunde besitzen klinische Bedeutung.

Vergleich zwischen dem Effekt des Sulfathiazols und des Sulfapyridins:

Nebenwirkungen sind bei klinischem Gebrauch von Sulfathiazol und Sulfapyridin nach den oben angegebenen Richtlinien im Kindesalter ungefähr ebenso häufig und unterscheiden sich nicht hinsichtlich ihres Schweregrades. In dem untersuchten Material waren sie als leicht zu klassifizieren. Beide Präparate führen indessen nicht selten zu Schädigungen der Leukopoese. Es erscheint uns ziemlich sicher, dass man viel häufiger toxische, von den besagten Präparaten verursachte Schädigungen der Myelopoese finden würde, wenn Knochenmarkuntersuchungen nach Sulfapyridin- und Sulfathiazolbehandlung öfter vorgenommen werden würden, als es heutzutage bei der klinischen Arbeit aus begreiflichen Gründen der Fall sein kann. Dies mahnt zweifelsohne zu grösster Vorsicht bei der Anwendung, und zwar nicht nur dort, wo niedrige Leukozytenwerte vor der Behandlung vorliegen und während derselben Leukopenie auftritt, sondern überhaupt bei allen behandelten Fällen. Therapeutisch scheint die Wirkung beider Präparate in bezug auf Infektionen der Luftwege bei Kindern ungefähr gleich gut zu sein. Besonders gut ist der Effekt bei Pneumonien vom lobären Typ.

Da Sulfathiazol ein erheblich billigeres Präparat ist als Sulfapyridin muss das erstere Mittel vor dem Sulfapyridin empfohlen werden, wenn es sich um Infektionen der Luftwege im Kindesalter handelt.

VI. Literaturverzeichnis.

FOSBINDER, R. J. und WALTER, L. A., J. Am. Chem. Soc. 61, 2032, 1939. — FRISK, R. A., Nordisk Medicin 7, 1483, 1940. — HERLITZ, C. W., Acta Pædiatrica XXVIII, 173, 1941 (siehe auch Literaturverzeichnis dort). — LAUDON, J. und SJÖGREN, B., Svensk kemisk Tidskrift 52, 64, 1940. — SCOTT, JOHN P. und JONES, A. M., J. of Pediatr. 17, 423, 1940. — LONG, P. H. et al., J. A. M. A. 115, 364, 1940.

Sporadic Hemophilia and Pseudo-Hemophilia.

By

S. VAN CREVELD, M. D., Amsterdam.

Our knowledge of the causes of the prolonged coagulation-time of blood in hemophilia has of late greatly extended. According to researches performed especially in Holland (1) and in the United States (2) there can be derived from normal blood, from citrated plasma and from fresh normal serum a substance, which in vitro and in vivo exerts a strong coagulation-promoting influence on hemophilic plasma and on hemophilic blood. The same substance can also be obtained from plasma which is freed of the bloodplatelets, from plasma of patients with thrombopenic purpura, and also from plasma free from fibrinogen and prothrombin (3). This substance is for the greater part absent from hemophilic blood. The well known favourable effect of a blood transfusion and that of injection of plasma or of fresh serum on the prolonged coagulation-time in hemophilia must be ascribed in the first place to the fact that by these actions the shortage of this coagulation-promoting substance is completed. Thus hemophilia can to a certain degree be regarded as being a deficiency disease.

The coagulation-promoting substance in plasma and in fresh serum is attached to the coarse-disperse protein fractions. We learned this a. o. from ultrafiltration experiments, in which membranes were used with an increased permeability. The ultrafiltrate of normal plasma, obtained by means of such membranes, appeared to have no coagulation-promoting influence on hemophilic blood, when the membranes only allowed the passing of albumen and pseudo-globulin. As soon as the ultrafiltrate contained euglobulin it exerted a coagulation-promoting influence.

The coagulation-promoting substance present in normal plasma and in normal fresh serum was further investigated by us in adsorption- and in precipitation experiments. The last mentioned researches have learned amongst others that the coagulation-promoting activity is attached to a protein fraction which can be precipitated from plasma and from fresh serum after a tenfold dilution with destilled water, followed by acidification with weak acetic acid till P_H is about 5.6. We called this fraction when obtained from fresh serum *coagulation-globulin*. Dissolved in the same quantity of NaCl 0.9 % as equaled the quantity of serum from which was started, a solution was obtained with a protein content of 4—5 %. This solution when added to hemophilic blood and plasma had a coagulation-promoting effect equal to that of the original serum. — From hemophilic plasma and serum in an analogous way could be precipitated a fraction of about the same protein content; however, after redissolving in the same amount of NaCl 0.9 %, this fraction was not able to produce a coagulation-promoting activity. From these findings which have been confirmed by the american authors and which also have been applied in vivo, we concluded that the protein itself is only the carrier of the coagulation-promoting factor in plasma and in fresh serum. In examining the parents of hemophilic patients it appeared that here the coagulation-promoting factor was present in the blood in a normal way (see table I and II).

From the more recent studies on this clotting-promoting substance in normal blood we mention here only two points. The first one regards the behaviour of this and other clotting-promoting factors present in blood and plasma during preservation of both. The prothrombin content of blood decreases fairly rapidly after keeping the blood for some days (4). — From this fact results that stored blood and plasma are al-

Table I.

Coagulation time of plasma of a hemophiliac after addition of different quantities of serum, plasma and solutions of coagulation-globulin (prepared from this serum and plasma), all originating from blood of the *father of this hemophiliac.*

			coagulation-time:
hemophilic plasma			lasts hours
»	»	+ 1/5 *plasma* of the father	5—25[1] minutes
»	»	+ 1/10 » » » »	20— »
»	»	+ 1/25 » » » »	20— »
»	»	+ 1/50 » » » »	lasts hours
»	»	+ 1/10 coag.-glob., prepared from plasma (c.-g. dissolved in 1/3 of the original volume)	12—20 minutes
»	»	+ 1/25 coag.-glob.	12—20 »
»	»	+ 1/50 » »	15— »
»	»	+ 1/125 » »	25— »
»	»	+ 1/5 *serum* of the father	5—25 »
»	»	+ 1/10 » » » »	10—25 »
»	»	+ 1/25 » » » »	25— »
»	»	+ 1/50 » » » »	30— »
»	»	+ 1/125 » » » »	lasts hours
»	»	+ 1/10 coag.-glob., prepared from serum (c.-g. dissolved in 1/9 of the original volume)	2— 5 minutes
»	»	+ 1/25 coag.-glob.	3— 5 »
»	»	+ 1/50 » »	5—15 »
»	»	+ 1/125 » »	7—15 »
»	»	+ 1/250 » »	12— »
»	»	+ 1/500 » »	1 hour—

[1] »5—25 minutes» means the beginning and the end of the coagulation. We considered the coagulation complete, when the surface, after the test-tube was cautiously turned, did not break.

Table II.

Coagulation-time of plasma of a hemophiliac after addition of different quantities of serum, plasma and solutions of coagulation-globulin (prepared from this serum), all originating from blood of the *mother of this hemophiliac.*

	coagulation-time:
hemophilic plasma + 1/5 *serum* of the mother	3—10 minutes
» » + 1/10 » » » »	5—11 »
» » + 1/25 » » » »	7—12 »
» » + 1/50 » » » »	8—14 »
» » + 1/125 » » » »	15—40 »
» » + 1/5 *plasma* of the mother	7—15 »
» » + 1/10 » » » »	8—15 »
» » + 1/25 » » » »	10—20 »
» » + 1/50 » » » »	15—40 »
» » + 1/125 » » » »	15—40 »
» »	15—40 »
hemophilic plasma	60 »
» » + 1/5 coag.-glob. prepared from serum (c.-g. dissolved in NaCl 0.9 %, in 3/4 of the original volume)	3—10 »
» » + 1/10 coag.-glob.	5—15 »
» » + 1/25 » »	10—25 »
» » + 1/50 » »	10—40 »
» » + 1/125 » »	30— »

ready after some days unsuitable to control hemorrhages which are caused by a shortage of prothrombin. So this blood and plasma cannot be used to control hemorrhages in patients with an obstructive jaundice, nor in many new-borns showing symptoms of a hemorrhagic diathesis (provided no vitamin K was given). However, the clotting-promoting activity of preserved blood and plasma on hemophilic blood is maintained for a much longer time (5). —

Secondly, in recent studies the dialysis method was also used for the isolation of the protein fractions to which the coagulation-promoting product present in plasma and in fresh serum is attached. In dialyzing citrated plasma in cellophane tubes PATEK, LOZNER and TAYLOR (6) obtained precipitates which after treatment exerted in vitro and in vivo a strong coagulation-promoting activity on hemophilic blood. Together with G. G. A. MASTENBROEK (7) we have repeated and confirmed these results in vitro with a modified technic.

In the old question on the cause of the prolonged coagulation-time in hemophilia these researches have thus availed new arguments in favour of the plasma-theory as far as this theory assumed that in hemophilia a plasma-factor should be lacking which is indispensable for the coagulation. The theory of the increased resistence of the bloodplatelets in hemophilia — according to which elements necessary for the coming about of the coagulation are liberated from the bloodplatelets in a retarded tempo — has lost a good deal of its value.

Recent studies which could point into the opposite direction are especially those of BRINKHOUS (8) and of DAM and VENNDT (9).

BRINKHOUS studied the prothrombin-conversion-time in five patients with hemophilia. He concluded from his experiments that in hemophilia prothrombin is converted slowly into thrombin. This slow thrombin formation should allow the thrombin to be destroyed by antithrombin almost as rapidly as it is formed. The bloodplatelets in hemophilia should play an important role in this process as the thromboplastin should be liberated from them more slowly than in normal blood. — Two facts just mentioned, namely the presence of a clotting-promoting factor in plasma of patients with thrombopenic purpura, and the presence of this factor in normal plasma freed from bloodplatelets, are more in favour of the plasma theory.

DAM and VENNDT concluded, that the abnormal clotting of hemophilic plasma is based on the decreased power of the plasma to coagulate in the presence of small quantities of tissue extract. If instead of tissue extract suspensions of bloodplatelets were used, the difference in coagulation-power between normal and hemophilic plasma was still more distinct. — In our opinion also these experiments are not in defiance of the plasma theory to which we adhere. According to FEISSLY (10) hemophilic plasma exerts a particular protecting influence on the bloodplatelets. The principal cause of the retarded coagulation in hemophilia is, also according to FEISSLY, dependant of a quantitative shortage of a plasma-factor, namely plasma-thrombokinase.

In agreement with our conception that in hemophilia a plasma-factor is lacking, it is obvious to accept that there also should exist a form of hemorrhagic diathesis, greatly resembling hemophilia, where the cause of the important prolongation of the coagulation-time lies in a disturbance in the function of the bloodplatelets; potent activators for clotting have been obtained from the platelets (a. o. in 1936 from horse blood-platelets by CHARGAFF (11) c. s.). WEISFELT (12) recently gave a description of such a patient, a women 26 years old. Her disease showed resemblance to hemophilia (greatly prolonged coagulation-time) and next to this also to the thrombasthenia of GLANZMANN (retraction of the bloodclot was disturbed in a high degree). The bleeding-time was normal as also the number of platelets. Morphologically these platelets showed only slight changes. The determination of the prothrombin-time after QUICK or after SMITH, ZIFFREN, OWEN and HOFFMAN gave a highly prolonged »prothrombin-time» when a surplus of (tissue) thromboplastin was used. When, however, instead of this tissue-thromboplastin, 0.1 cc of a normal suspension of bloodplatelets was added, the coagulation occurred within some minutes. As in this case the existence of a shortage of vitamin K could be excluded, this result thus pointed to a difference between the tissue-thromboplastin and the thromboplastin of the bloodplatelets.

Deficiency of one or more of the normal clotting-factors may theoretically spoken cause a disturbance in the coagulation of the blood. Without further examination into different directions patients with a prolonged clotting-time of the blood may be mistaken for (hereditary) hemophilia.

Until yet the following causes of a prolonged coagulation-time must be considered (compare QUICK (23):

I deficiency of thromboplastic substances
  a) derived from bloodplatelets (thrombopenia; case of WEISFELT);
  b) derived from plasma (hemophilia);
II deficiency of prothrombin, caused by
  a) insufficient production of vitamin K (hypoprothrombinemia neonatorum), or
  b) insufficient resorption of this vitamin (obstructive jaundice and several intestinal disorders), or
  c) a greatly disturbed liver function, giving rise to faulty formation of prothrombin;
III hemophilia calcipriva[1] (HESS (15));
IV afibrinogenemia, fibrinopenia and fibrinasthenia (FANCONI (16));
V rare cases of disturbed clotting procedure caused by the presence of an excess of inhibitory factors like heparin. — To these rare cases belongs that described by LOZNER, JOLLIFFE and TAYLOR (17). The inhibitory factor in this case was not heparin, because it was not neutralized by salmine.

What we have told thus far was given as introductory remarks to the clinical descriptions which follow now.

One of the questions which we bore in mind from the very beginning of our researches was, in how far the above-mentioned findings could be of help in analyzing diseases whose relations to hereditary hemophilia is doubted. As such we want to discuss here some cases, partly belonging to the so-called sporadic hemophilia, partly cases for which the name pseudo-hemophilia often is used. By the name »pseudo-hemophilia» various conditions are indicated which have all in common with hemophilia a more or less prolonged coagulation-time of the blood, but where next to this agreement also exist distinct differences with hemophilia. The name is given to two rare condi-

[1] It must be doubted, however, whether such a decrease of the calcium content of the serum or of the calcium ion concentration of the blood occurs which in itself may be responsible for a prolonged coagulation-time of the blood.

tions: congenital fibrinopenia and afibrinogenemia. (The use of the term pseudo-hemophilia for these conditions is confusing, as in hemophilia the fibrinogen content of the plasma is normal.) Further it is given to the rare cases of hemophilia in the females and thirdly to some hereditary forms of hemorrhagic diathesis to which attention has been drawn by several publications, a. o. by the articles of v. WILLEBRAND (13) and of FARBER (14). The heredity in these conditions is different from that in hemophilia; the clotting-time is either normal or only slightly prolonged (36), the bleeding-time is usually distinctly prolonged, the number of bloodplatelets is normal as also the retraction of the bloodclot. Joint hemorrhages do not occur in these latter diseases and the clotting-promoting effect of plasma and fresh serum of these patients on hemophilic blood is normal. The exact mechanism of the cause of the prolonged bleeding in these conditions is not yet understood, though it is possible that there is question of an abnormal agglutinability of the platelets (v. WILLEBRAND and JÜRGENS (37)).

By sporadic hemophilia are meant isolated cases of hemophilia without a known heredity. A very extensive family-history is always necessary in such cases, owing to the fact that the disease may skip several generations. When such a case of hemophilia with absence of hereditary anamnesis occurs, there have been assumed two different explanations:

a) either the case must be a mutation from the normal condition into that existing in hemophilia, or
b) there was existing a latent inclination to hemophilia which has been inherited throughout different generations without manifest clinical symptoms, until now this inclination becomes clinically manifest in an individual who showed a special predisposition.

The geneticists do not agree which explanation should be regarded as being the right one (see a. o. FONIO (18), BIRCH (19), HALDANE (20), SIRKS (21)). In order to judge the problem we have also to consider clinical and experimental data. As to the clinical findings the literature also here shows a disagreement. Some authors say that in sporadic hemophilia the condition generally is more serious than in hereditary hemophilia, but others declare positively (a. o. Fonio) that clinically there does not exist any difference, and this is also our opinion.

Our three observed cases of sporadic hemophilia are the following.

I. A. G., a boy, now eight years old, is the third child of healthy parents and has two normal sisters. He was born full term and was breast fed. Nothing particular happened during the first months of life. Teeth came in due time without hemorrhages. At the normal age the child could go. When five months old thick blue spots appeared on the skin apparently occurring spontaneously and disappearing slowly. Later on these hemorrhages mostly occurred after a fall or a push. When we saw the boy for the first time (then he was one year old), his skin at different places showed more or less extensive intracutaneous hemorrhages, partly resembling the so-called purpura urticans. As the anamnesis of the family revealed no particularities the diagnosis hemophilia seemed to be highly improbable. The Pirquet- and Wassermann-tests were negative. The mucous membranes of mouth and throat were normal as well as the internal organs. A thorough examination of the blood learned that the coagulation-time of the blood was greatly prolonged[1] and that the cause of this prolongation had to be the same as in hereditary hemophilia. An extensive blood examination, especially of the coagulation-factors in the parents of the patient, in two brothers of the mother and in the two sisters of the patient also availed no particularities. The patient's bloodgroup was the same as his mother's one (group B). So this fact is in agreement with the observation of Kubányi (22) (1926), that in families with hemophilia the bloodgroup of the affected male members always is the same as that of the mother. In other patients suffering from hemophilia we could, however, not always confirm this conception (see also a. o. Fonio and Birch).

The »rétractilité du caillot» of the boy's blood and the aspect of his bloodplatelets always were normal. Also the calcium content of the serum and the fibrinogen content of the plasma

[1] We always determine the coagulation-time (in triplicate) of our patients at 37° C with blood, obtained by venous puncture.

(method of CULLEN and VAN SLYKE) gave normal values. The bleeding-time always remained within normal limits. Just as in hereditary hemophilia also our patient never kept on bleeding after a venous puncture, nor was there any formation of hematoma under such condition. We further found that plasma (citrated) and fresh serum of this patient did not exert any coagulation-promoting influence on the blood of a patient with hereditary hemophilia. The prothrombin-time of the blood of our boy determined after the method of QUICK (23) and of ZIFFREN, OWEN, HOFFMAN and SMITH (24), gave normal values just as in hereditary hemophilia (25).

The clinical symptoms of our patient since the first observation have been the same as in hereditary hemophilia. So f. i. after careful sounding of the left lacrimal duct, necessary with a view to an existing chronic dacryocystitis, the child got a large hematoma in the left cheek which disappeared only after ten days. Till yet he has had nearly no hemorrhages of nose and gums, but already repeatedly hemorrhages of the joints (knees), much dreaded in hemophilia. The most serious hemorrhage he got some years ago after a rather slight trauma was a very severe intrathoracal hemorrhage; then the child living outside of Amsterdam in a small house, was in a deplorable condition and a blood transfusion performed at home in a small garretroom, saved his life. Since then we only once have seen an analogous large intrathoracal hemorrhage in a case of hereditary hemophilia.

II. A boy, now 4 years old, showed his first apparently spontaneous hematoma of the skin of different sizes at the age of eight months; later on they occurred more frequently and especially after slight traumata. About a year ago he got the first joint hemorrhage (right knee) and also now and then hemorrhages of the mucous membranes (a. o. of the frenulum). The anamnesis of the family up till four generations back, shows no cases of hemorrhagic diathesis. No consanguinity between the parents; only the grandparents of the paternal side were second cousins. A younger brother of the patient, now nearly two years old, has till yet been quite normal. Also in this patient the coagulation-time of the blood was greatly prolonged. The »rétractilité du caillot» of his blood and the number and aspect of the bloodplatelets were normal; also the fibrinogen content of the plasma and the prothrombin-time of the blood (QUICK) were normal. In this case the bloodgroup corresponded to that of the father (A), whereas the mother's bloodgroup was O. Also here the citrated plasma of the patient did not exert a coagulation-promoting influence on the blood of a patient with hereditary hemophilia.

III. The third patient with sporadic hemophilia, now seven years old, has from the prime childhood been suffering from hemorrhages after slight traumata, and cutting wounds remained bleeding for a very long time. Two years ago a wound of the lip kept on bleeding in such a way that a blood transfusion was necessary. Of late he also had hemorrhages of the joints. No bleeders in the family for three generations. A sister of the patient, five years old, is normal. Also in this case the clotting-time of the venous blood was greatly prolonged, the prothrombin-time (QUICK) was normal, the number and aspect of the bloodplatelets was normal, the fibrinogen content of the plasma and the calcium content of the serum was also normal. The citrated plasma did not exert a coagulation-promoting influence on the blood of a patient with hereditary hemophilia.

All three above mentioned patients thus showed a strikingly prolonged coagulation-time, a normal prothrombin-time, absence of a coagulation-promoting activity of their plasma when added in different dilutions to blood of a patient with hereditary hemophilia, normal fibrinogen and calcium content resp. of plasma and of serum, normal number and aspect of the thrombocytes.

In the first patient we more especially studied the effect of addition of the solution of coagulation-globulin obtained from the serum and plasma of the patient (after tenfold dilution with distilled water followed by acidification till p_H of about 5.6, and dissolving the precipitate in the same quantity of NaCl 0.9 % as equaled the quantity of plasma or serum from which was started) to hemophilic blood, and to hemophilic citrated plasma obtained from a patient with hereditary hemophilia. This solution of coagulation-globulin practically did not exert any coagulation-promoting activity on the blood or plasma of the patient with hereditary hemophilia.

As to the clinical particularities of the three patients we already mentioned the severe intrathoracal hemorrhage observed in the first case. Symptoms of hemorrhages in spinal marrow or brain were not noted. That localisation of hemorrhages in thorax and in the central nervous system is relatively rare in hemophilia can also be seen from the statistics of BIRCH (1937): in 98 patients with hemophilia he saw 83 hemorrhages in joints, whereas he noted 6 in brains and spinal marrow and 5 in lungs and pleurae. Also FONIO, in observing 59 patients with hemophilia, noted only four times a hemorrhage in the central nervous system (twice followed by epilepsia), and only once a pleural-abdominal hemorrhage. —

In other diseases with hemorrhagic diathesis hemorrhages in the central nervous system are more frequent; f. i. in the acute form of morbus Werlhofii. Splenectomy generally causes a diminution of the hemorrhages. Till yet we only once observed that some time after the splenectomy symptoms of a hemorrhage of the spinal marrow occurred. This took place in a girl of seven years old in which splenectomy had been performed on account of m. Werlhofii. After the operation the number of blood-platelets showed a temporary rise up to more than 400.000, but soon afterwards it decreased rather quickly to a very low number. Four months after the splenectomy the girl came back to the hospital with new spontaneous hemorrhages and other symptoms of Werlhoff's disease. — Moreover, the normal reflexes of the legs had disappeared and Babinski's reflex was present, first unilateral, later on bilateral. These symptoms were explained as being the consequences of a hemorrhage of the spinal marrow. After some months the normal reflexes reappeared.

In the following case the diagnosis (sporadic?) hemophilia is until yet uncertain.

IV. B. Z., a boy now eight years old, is the youngest of three children. The eldest is a girl of fifteen years, suffering from asthma bronchiale, the second a healthy boy of twelve years old. The mother is 48 years old and formerly has stayed twice in a sanatorium on account of tuberculosis of the lungs. She always kept bleeding for a long time after traumata such as extraction of teeth, and also her father had long lasting traumatic hemorrhages. The patient's father died at the age of 47 years of carcinoma hepatis. In the anamnesis of the family we find epilepsia and insanity but no other cases of hemorrhagic diathesis.

The boy was born spontaneously, in due time; he was breast fed till the age of 6 months. He was rather late in going, speaking and cutting of teeth. He has had rubeola, measles and varicella. From the age of 6 years on he now and then had epileptiform attacks. The first symptoms of hemorrhagic diathesis became manifest at the circumcision at the age of 3 weeks; the wound kept on bleeding and had to be sewed up. After that now and then occurred long lasting bleedings of the nose and of wounds, and after a fall there always were many blue spots. Till yet joint hemorrhages did not occur. At the age of 7 years when he came for the first time into the clinic blood examination demonstrated a slightly prolonged coagulation time, a normal number of thrombocytes, a normal bleeding- and prothrombin-time, and a normal retraction of the bloodclot. The Pirquet-test was negative. At the end of July 1940 he came for the second time into the clinic; four weeks before his gums had been bleeding for three days at a stretch. One week later the gums began to bleed again after a trauma. The bleeding was stopped each time to be followed by a renewed hemorrhage. Five days before the entrance into the hospital a blood examination learned that he had no anemia, a normal number of thrombocytes, a scarcely prolonged coagulation-time (13 minutes) and a normal prothrombin-time (micromethod of KATO (26)). In the night after this investigation the bleeding of the gums started again and kept on for two days. When taken into the hospital the boy was very anemic (Sahli 33 %); after a blood transfusion (200 cc) the hemorrhage stopped and the anemia soon disappeared. The patient's bloodgroup was AB, that of his mother B. The dentist was of opinion that the repeated hemorrhages of the gums were supported by the bad condition of the teeth. During his stay in the clinic at three different times some carious elements were extracted; each time the extraction wounds were treated by means of renewed tampons soaked with coagulation-globulin. (This local treatment of hemorrhages by coagulation-globulin, especially those arising after tooth-extraction, has given good results in hemophilic patients (35). The coagulation-globulin used in these cases was mostly prepared from cow's plasma in the way as indicated in the introduction of this article and used in powdered form.) Twice the extraction wound with this treatment healed in due time without any hemorrhage; the third time the alveolus was shallow so that tampon could not properly be fixated and the wound kept on bleeding past the tampon. For that reason a blood transfusion (150 cc) was given with prompt success.

During a period when any influence of a blood transfusion could be excluded we found in this boy:

a) for the coagulation-time of the venous blood at 37° C the following values: 13, 8, 11, 11, 10 1/2, 8 1/2 and 14 minutes. The value of 8 minutes can be laid aside as it was obtained after a severe hemorrhage.
b) for the prothrombin-time a normal value;
c) for the fibrinogen content of the plasma (CULLEN and VAN SLYKE) a normal value (4.4 ‰);
d) for the calcium content of the serum a value of 10.6 mgr %;
e) a normal number of thrombocytes;
f) the citrated plasma of the patient exerted in different dilutions a practically normal coagulation-promoting activity on fresh hemophilic blood.

In this case it is not easy to make an exact diagnosis. The possibility that we have to deal with a case of (sporadic) hemophilia cannot be excluded though we found, at periods when no hemorrhages were present, values for the coagulation-time which could be called normal or only slightly prolonged. We have observed some patients with hereditary hemophilia in which at different times normal or scarcely prolonged values for the coagulation-time of the venous blood were found, whereas clinically these patients do not differ from hemophiliacs with a prolonged coagulation-time. To this category our patient might belong, and with regard to prophylaxis and therapy of his hemorrhages he is treated as a hemophilic and with success. It is remarkable, however, that our boy, now ten years old, till yet never has had joint hemorrhages, though in the milder cases joint hemorrhages are often initiated during puberty (Birch). Moreover it is very peculiar that the mother and the maternal grandfather (no longer alive) have a history of habitual bleeding following slight injuries; and further that the coagulation-time of the mother's blood is prolonged. At two different periods her coagulation-time was 15 and 16 1/2 minutes respectively, the normal maximum value being 12 minutes; a nearer study of the clotting-factors of her blood did not reveal the cause of this prolongation of the clotting-time. — The possibility thus remains that we have to do here with a definite form of hereditary pseudo-hemophilia.

A case such as that of this boy once more points to the necessity of a repeated determination of the coagulation-time, if there is a history of habitual bleeding following slight traumata in a patient where an operation is to be performed. Only in this way as small prolongation of the clotting-time can be ascertained.

In the literature we find several cases mentioned in which deviations of one or more clotting-factors established shortly after birth and giving rise to a tendency to bleeding, had partly or totally disappeared at a later age. Here we exclude of course the physiological changes in the clotting-factors taking place during the first days of life. As examples of the above mentioned changes according to age, we can give some cases of thrombopenia (hereditary or not) in the new born (see a. o. Davidson (27), Moncrieff and Whitby (28), and Greenwald (29)), and thrombopenia often combined with afibrinogenemia and fibrinopenia. In the case of afibrinogenemia described by Macfarlane (30), thrombocytopenia and afibrinogenemia were present for several years. At the age of 8 years the number of platelets had risen to a normal value, but fibrinogen still remained absent from the blood. — An analogous increase of the platelets, but occurring in a much shorter time, was further observed in one of the cases of Glanzmann c. s. (31).

Many writers are of opinion that in hemophilia great improvement also takes place at or after adolescence and that the patient may even appear normal during middle life. Critical discussion of this question by other authors has not given support to this opinion (compare Birch) and also our experience is not in agreement with this conception. Neither in hereditary nor in sporadic hemophilia however, it has been observed that the prolonged coagulation-time became normal at a very early age. The following case may in this regard be of some interest in so far as there was a history of a severe hemorrhage after a minor operation at an early age and a distinct prolongation of the coagulation-time was established at the age of 4 months. Later on, when the child was 8 resp. 20 months old, a normal coagulation-time was found and no further hemorrhage occurred in this child.

V. S. A., a boy, was born in April 1939. He was a full term child, weighing 4150 gram. At the age of 8 days circumcision was performed. In the night of this day bleeding from the wound occurred which continued slightly during next day. Two days later renewed severe hemorrhage occurred. Since then there were no clinical symptoms of a hemorrhagic diathesis. The family history gave no particularities. At the age of 4 months the baby was taken into a surgical clinic for the removal of a large angioma on an upper arm. With a view to the history of a long lasting bleeding, the clotting-time of the blood was determined and found to be slightly but distinctly prolonged (16 minutes). For a nearer study the baby was transported to the Pediatric Department. Clinically no particularities were found with the exception of the large angioma. The following investigations were made in the blood:

haemoglobin 90 %
red cells 4.550.000 (per c.mm)
colour index 0.99
white cells 8.800 (per c.mm)
rod formed leucocytes 6 %
segmented formed leucocytes 9 %
lymphocytes 84 %
monocytes 1 %
platelets count 305.000 (Fonio)
coagulation-time, at 37° C, *20* minutes (normal maximum 12 min.)
bleeding-time normal
fibrinogen content of plasma 3.5 ‰
calcium content of the serum 11.9 mgr %
clotting-promoting activity of citrated plasma on fresh hemophilic blood: slight.
Prothrombin-time normal.
Retraction of the bloodclot: normal.
Galactose test: within normal limits.

In the blood of the mother and in that of a sister and of a maternal uncle clotting-time and prothrombin-time were normal.

With regard to these results, the diagnosis sporadic hemophilia seemed to be justified and radium-therapy of the angioma was recommanded.

Clinically this boy, now two years old, has nevermore shown any tendency to bleeding. The clotting-time of his blood determined again at the age of 8 months and 1 $^1/_2$ years were found to be normal. It is difficult to give an exact explanation of this case, but it illustrates the difficulties of diagnosis.

To the conditions from which hemophilia must be differentiated belong those in which there is a strong diminution or absence of fibrinogen from the bloodplasma. Afibrinogenemia is a constitutional congenital anomaly of which only a restricted number of cases has been published. Fibrinopenia occurs as a secondary phenomenon in certain conditions, especially in extensive liver diseases, and as a rare constitutional deviation. A survey of the literature on these rare morbid pictures together with a detailed description of one case of afibrinogenemia and of one case of acquired fibrinopenia was recently given by GLANZMANN, STEINER and KELLER (31). We may refer to these excellent articles for full particularities.

In hemorrhagic diseases of the new born temporary fluctuations of the fibrinogen content of the plasma not rarely do occur. However, only sporadically this content is decreased in such a way that this factor alone or in combination with other abnormal clotting factors (hypoprothrombinemia) causes a disturbed clot formation. The name »hemophilia neonatorum temporaria» given to such conditions, and of which we could observe one case (32), is badly chosen, as in hemophilia the fibrinogen content of the plasma is not decreased.

The following case may probably be reckoned to the cases of congenital afibrinogenemia, and was observed with Dr. N. E. HEYBROIK.

VI. The patient, a boy, was born in March 1935. He was a prematurely born infant, youngest of a twin; birthweight 1210 gram. The mother was healthy. The condition of the baby at birth was good. One day after birth cyanotic attacks with convulsions occurred. Tube feeding was started beginning with fatpoor mother's milk. On the third day of life 5 cc of pregnant-serum was given subcutaneously, this was repeated orally on the following nine days. The cyanotic attacks and convulsions stopped after one day. During the following weeks nothing particular happened. When six weeks old the baby looked pale and showed a tendency to the occurrence of bleeding. Liver and spleen not enlarged. The coagulation-time of the blood appeared to be indefinitely long. (The modern methods for the determination of the prothrombin time then were still unknown.) Hemoglobin 50 %; red cells 2.390.000 per c.mm.; leucocytes 10.800. Number of *thrombocytes normal.* There was further anisocytosis and slight poikilocytosis; the differential count gave nothing particular, with 4 normoblasts on 100 leucocytes. Wassermann test negative. Sedimentation rate low. In urine trace of urobilin, no bile substances. No sulf- or methemoglobin in plasma or in urine; plasma not icteric. With the exact method of Cullen and van Slyke *no fibrinogen* could be demonstrated in two determinations in the bloodplasma. — The baby remained bleeding from small prick wounds. A blood transfusion (20 cc) and blood injections only had a temporary effect (vitamin K was still unknown). The anemia was progressive. Two days before death at the age of 7 weeks the fontanel was bulging and lumbar puncture gave a sanguinolent spinal fluid; culture negative. The day before death the Sahli had decreased till 30. A second lumbar puncture also gave sanguinolent spinal fluid. Injections of hémostyl and of calcium gluconate were also given, but had no success. The early death of the infant made a more thorough examination of the blood impossible, such as had been performed in analogous cases, especially by MACFARLANE, and by GLANZMANN and co-workers. — In the twin-child (birthweight 2.000 gm) the blood was examined shortly after the death of the other child. The coagulation-time of this blood was normal, as also the fibrinogen content of the plasma. — In the family of the mother no cases of hemorrhagic tendency occurred. The father was unknown.

At the necropsy performed in the Pathologic Institute of the University of Amsterdam (director prof. dr. H. T. DEELMAN) the following was found:

The body was emaciated and the skin had a pale-yellow tint. Hypostatis was slight. At the left lower leg and on the head the skin was bluish, caused by subcutaneous haematomata. All internal organs and muscles were very pale. The lower margin of the liver reached 1 cm. below the right costal margin and below the xiphoid process. The peritoneal cavity contained some blood and bloody fluid. The pleura covering each lung was free from adhesions. The heart weight 17 Gm.; its form and size were normal. Valvules and ostia normal; D. Botalli obliterated. Heart muscle pale. Lungs pale-grey, elastic. Under the pleura was one large and numerous stippled hemorrhages. Cut surface:

pale-grey, at pressure clear foam appears. Lymph, nodes, vessels and bronchi nothing particular.

Thymus: size and form normal; pale-yellow, nothing particular.

Spleen: weight 9 Gm., form normal. There is an accessory spleen of the size of a pea. The spleen was purplish red and rather firm, elastic. Cut surface: follicles visible, purple red pulp, which could not be scraped off. — Adrenals: normal form and size. Urinary tract no particularities. — *Liver: normal form*, weight 65 Gm., pale-brownish, rather firm, elastic, cut surface was green-brown. Vessels and bile-ducts nothing particular. Bile-bladder normal. — Kidneys normal. — Bone marrow (vertebral column) pale red. Brain section was not allowed.

Microscopic studies were made of liver, spleen and bone marrow. *Liver:* much bile-substance in bile capillaries and in liver cells. Numerous myeloid spots, diffusely spread. *Further no particularities.*

Spleen: the red pulp contains little blood, but numerous large cells with great irregular nucleolus and ungranulated protoplasma.

Bone-marrow of a vertebra: myeloblasts, myelocytes, normoblasts, etc. Nothing particular.

The essential findings at necropsy thus were: very severe anemia, uncoagulated blood in the peritoneal cavity, subcutaneous and subpleural hemorrhages. Brain section could not be performed so that the presence of hemorrhages at different places of the central nervous system, which could be expected according to the findings at the spinal puncture and to those in the case of Schönholzer (33), could not be controlled. The numerous myeloid spots found in the liver at the microscopic examination in this young prematurely born infant may be regarded as reaction to the severe anemia. It is a well-known fact that extra-medullary haemopoetic activity in the liver of a prematurely born infant may be retained for a long time and may be intensified by severe bleeding or increased haemolysis (34). — The significance of the numerous large cells in the pulp of the spleen for the arise of the afibrinogenemia is uncertain. The *marrow picture* was *normal*.

We could compare the results of this necropsy with those obtained at the necropsy of the twin-brother (binovular twins) which took place 5 weeks later. The birth weight of this child was 2.000 Gm. At birth the condition of this infant was excellent and during the first two months nothing abnormal occurred in this infant. When it was two months old, a slight anemia existed, but the fibrinogen content of the plasma and the clotting time of the blood were normal. Shortly afterwards the child got an acute dyspepsia which took a serious course and caused the death of the baby. Two days before death the fontanel was bulging, but the spinal fluid was clear. — At the necropsy there were no hemorrhages, no distinct anemias of the organs. The principal changes were found in the colon, where the mucosa had practically disappeared and there was slight cell-infiltration of all layers. Further the liver showed a fairly strong perifer fatty infiltration. The large number of myeloid spots in the liver and the peculiar large cells in the spleen of the first case failed here.

The observation of this case of afibrinogenemia gives rise to the following remarks: the two symptoms characteristic for afibrinogenemia were present here, namely absence of any trace of bloodclotting, and prolonged bleeding-time. In contrast to other cases bleeding did not start here directly after birth. Thrombopenia, which in other cases of afibrinogenemia constantly or intermittently accompanied the afibrinogenemia, failed here. As far as could be ascertained there was no question of a hereditary affection. Liver and spleen were not enlarged.

Summary:

A short survey is given of the results of some recent studies on the causes of the prolonged coagulation-time of blood in hemophilia. Different factors which may cause a prolonged coagulation-time of blood are mentioned. Three cases of sporadic hemophilia are described in detail. A fourth case is added in which the diagnosis sporadic hemophilia is still uncertain. Attention is drawn to those rare cases in which deviations of one or more clotting factors existed for a fairly long time after birth and partly or totally disappeared at a later age; an example is given. Finally a case of (congenital) afibrinogenemia is communicated.

References.

1. See a. o. BENDIEN, W. M. and CREVELD, S. VAN, Acta Brevia Neerland. V, 135, 1935, Am. J. Dis. Children *54,* 713, 1937 and Acta Med. Scand. *99,* 12, 1939. — 2. See a. o. PATEK, A. J. and STETSON, R. P., J. Clin. Investig. *15,* 531, 1936; POHLE, F. J. and TAYLOR, F. H. L., J. Clin. Investig. *16,* 741, 1937; HOWELL, W. H., Bull. New York Acad. Medicine *15,* 3, 1939. — 3. LOZNER, E. L., KARK, R. and TAYLOR, F. H. L., J. Clin. Investig. *18,* 603, 1939. — 4. RHOADS, J. E. and PANZER, L. M., J. A. M. A. *112,* 309, 1939. ZIEGLER, E. R., OSTERBERG, A. E. and HOVIG, M., J. A. M. A. *114*, 1341, 1940; QUICK, A. J., J. A. M. A. *114,* 1342, 1940. — 5. CREVELD, S. VAN, Acta Brevia Neerland. X, 191, 1940. — 6. See a. o. LOZNER, E. L. and TAYLOR, F. H. L., J. Clin. Investig. *18,* 821, 1939. — 7. To be published elsewhere. — 8. BRINKHOUS, K. M., Am. J. Med. Sciences *198,* 509, 1939. — 9. DAM, H. and VENNDT, H., The Lancet 1940 I, p. 70. — 10. FEISSLY, R., Helvetica Medica Acta *7,* 583, 1940/41. — 11. CHARGAFF, E., BANCROFT, I. W. and STANLEY-BROWN, M., J. Biol. Chem. *116,* 237, 1936. — 12. WEISFELT, L. R., Nederl. Tydschr. v. Geneesk. *85,* 2423, 1941. — 13. WILLEBRAND, E. A. v., Acta Med. Scand. *76,* 521, 1931. — 14. FARBER, J. E., Am. J. Med. Sciences *188,* 815, 1934. — 15. HESS, A. F., Arch. Int. Med. *17,* 203, 1916. — 16. FANCONI, G., Schweiz. med. Wchschr. *71,* 55, 1941. — 17. LOZNER, E. L., JOLLIFFE, L. S. and TAYLOR, F. H. L., Am. J. Med. Sciences *199,* 318, 1940. — 18. FONIO, A., a. o. Ergebn. inn. Med. u. Kinderh. *51,* 443, 1936, and Arch. Julius Klaus-Stiftung f. Vererbungsforsch. etc. *12,* 495, 1937. — 19. BIRCH, C. LA FLEUR, Illinois Med. and Dental Monographs vol. 1, no. 4, 1937. — 20. HALDANE, J. B. S., Journ. of Genetics *31,* 317, 1935. — 21. SIRKS, M. J., Genetica *19,* 417, 1937. — 22. KUBÁNYI, A., Klin. Wchschr. *5,* 321, 1926. — 23. QUICK, A. J., Am. J. Physiol. *118,* 260, 1937; and Am. J. Med. Sciences *199,* 118, 1940. — 24. ZIFFREN, S. E., OWEN, C. A., HOFFMAN, G. R. and SMITH, H. P., Proc. Soc. Exp. Biol. Med. *40,* 595, 1939. — 25. See a. o. DAM, H., SCHÖNHEYDER, F. and TAGE-HANSEN, E., Biochem. J. *30,* 1075, 1936; SNELL, A. M., J. A. M. A. *112,* 1457, 1939; and personal experience. — 26. See KATO, K. and PONCHER, H. G., J. A. M. A. *114,* 749, 1940. — 27. DAVIDSON, L. T., Amer. J. Dis. Childr. *54,* 1324, 1937. — 28. MONCRIEFF, A. and WHITBY, L. E. H., Arch. Dis. Childh. *12,* 263, 1937. — 29. GREENWALD, H. M., Amer. J. Dis. Childr. *33,* 900, 1927. — 30. MACFARLANE, R. G., The Lancet 1938 I, p. 309. — 31. GLANZMANN, E., STEINER, H. and KELLER, H., Schweiz. med. Wchschr. *70,* nr. 51, p. 1243 and nr. 52, p. 1261, 1940. — 32. CREVELD, S. VAN, Geneesk. Tydschr. v. Ned.-Indië *78,* 1154, 1938. — 33. SCHÖNHOLZER, G., D. Arch. Klin. Med. *184,* 496, 1939. — 34.

See a. o. PARSONS, L. G., HAWKSLEY, J. C. and GITTINS, R., Arch. Dis. Childh. *8*, 159, 1933. — 35. POHLE, F. J. and TAYLOR, F. H. L., J. Clin. Investig. *17*, 677, 1938. CREVELD, S. VAN and HAMER, R., Nederl. Tydschr. v. Tandheelk. *47*, 5, 1940. — 36. HANDLEY, R. S. and NUSSBRECHER, A. M., Quarterl. J. o. Medic. *4*, 165, 1935. — 37. See a. o. WILLEBRAND, E. A. v. and JÜRGENS, R., D. Arch. klin. Mediz. *175*, 453, 1933.

Experimental (osteo-dentino-)amelo-dystrophia hyperpara-thyreotica in rats.

By

PAUL E. SJÖQUIST.

Med. Lic. Dentist.

(Dental schoolclinic of the Falköping Board schools, Sweden).

In Acta Pædiatrica (april 1937) I published my results of a research on Enamel deformation in schoolchildren. I made a description of them and a theory of their evolution, that according to my meaning could explain the evolution of the deformations as well as the great variation in their form. As the provoking cause I held a retarding or stopping of the outgrowth of the *dentine* over the pulp-papilla in connection with the uninterrupted progress of the involution of the enamel organon, but only so long as it was the question of so called »rachitic» deformations, that are placed transversally in the tooth. I remarked that rachitic deformation was a nomination and that it might say nothing about the cause of the deformation. In children that had been spasmophil (nursed in hospitals for tetany) I showed other deformation. Where the hyperplasia and the hypoplasia were placed longitudinally in the tooth and where the deformation must be due to local destruction in the dentine outgrowth zone especially in the margin of this zone as a rule of disseminated spreading.

The retarding moment might be rickets, but it caused serious objection that rickets are very scarce at the age in which the deformation must develop to judge from the niveau in the tooth which it occupies. The prevailing skeleton malady at this age is osteodystrophia fibrosa. I thought it possible already then that this malady might be the cause of the retarded dentine outgrowth, and that it possibly might be a consequence of rachitis.

Two years before PERRAS of the Berlin University had published a record of an experiment on osteodystrophia fibrosa, which he had provoked by overcharging rats with the hormone of the Parathyreoid gland (Virchows Archiv Bd. 296 p. 218). He had divided his material in four groups with different supplies of D-vitamin and lime: rats on a very rich D-vitamin supply (my group H.), rats with ordinary D-vitamin supply (my group N.), rats without D-vitamin but with sufficient lime supply (my group R.) and rats on a ratio deficient both in D-vitamine and lime (my group S.). In all his animals he provoked osteodystrophia fibrosa, slighter dystrophia in group H. than in group N. grave dystrophia in group R. and very severe dystrophia in group S. He had paid no attention to eventual alterations in the teeth, as he used the kneejoint of the animals as test. As I had a suspicion that enamel deformation and osteodystrophia fibrosa might have the same cause as they develop at the same age, I thought it necessary to repeat his experiment with special attention to the teeth.

Karolinska Institutet granted a sum for the experiment and later on for the histologic examination of the material, for which I am very much indebted to the Institute. As my experiment is quite uniform with that of PERRAS, I refer to his publication for details of the arrangement. The only difference is that I have used considerably more parathormone than he administered to his rats. I continued the experiment during five weeks. Only one animal, the control of the group S, died three days before the end of the experiment, and one (of the N-group) just as I was conserving the material of that group. I held that every animal got 7 Collip units every day of parathormone, but there may be some uncertainty. I used Parke, Davis & Co's Paroidin and had got to know, that it was dosed in Hansen Units, but later on I was told, that it was dosed in the units of the U. S. A. pharmacopaea. I have held both these units to correspond to Collips Unit 5 to 1.

The principal intention with the experiment was to provoke enamel deformation in the rats. In the molars of the rats, teeth with closed pulp, I hold that in almost all molars, fissures are present in all mastication grooves. So is also the case in the four half jaws that I have skeletonized. In four of their 12 molars decay is present. In four more jaws, where ground sagittal cuts are laid, fissures are present in all mastication grooves but one and in many of the fissures enamel decay is observed under the microscope. In the many decalcified and dyed cuts all the enamel is dissolved, but in all »mastication grooves» of the dentine we find a parcel bordered in its bottom part and sides by a lining that strongly reminds of an enamel cuticula and often ends as free lashes and which contains in the bottom of the parcel a cellular detritus impossible to recognize and over the detritus desquamated mucosa epithelium. The lining is placed at a distance from the dentine, that seems just to correspond to the thickness of the dissolved enamel, only the bottom of the parcel reaches deeper or shallower into the dentine grooves and sometimes nearly gets forth to the bottom of the dentin furrow. Such parcels are never found in the interdental rooms between the teeth. The form, the position and the contents of these parcels make me consider them as mouldings of fissures in the dissolved enamel, the more as they can be pursued through many cuts of the same tooth. (Picture III).

To speak of enamel deformation of a similar type as in human incisors in the rat incisors is impossible, this deriving probably from the rat incisors being teeth with open pulps. Yet there is sometimes a step in the enamel thickness from a proximal thicker to an apical thinner enamel. The mature enamel in the proximal end of the rat incisor is from the edge, about a third of the length of the tooth brownish and hard, but in the apical two thirds it is blueish grey and soft, it can be carved by an ordinary pocket knife. This soft enamel must be considered as deformed and the further histologic examination will reveal a very serious alteration and immaturity of the enamel that must be held as the equivalent of enamel deformation. We must state that in the molars we have found typical deformation and in the incisors an alteration equivalent to enamel deformation, and as they both repeat themselves in every animal, the experiment has been successful in this respect.

Before we enter into a close examination of the enamel we must look a little at the tissues of the pulp, the dentine, the enamel organon and at the surrounding bone of the jaw. We observe then at first the exceedingly great blood supply, especially in the most apical part of the enamel organon and in the rootpart of the pulp. The bone of the jaw presents a very definite osteodystrophia fibrosa with the same variation between the different groups of experimental animals as in the experiment of PERRAS. The pulp tissue is not visibly alterated, the odontoblasts are of normal size and just as regularly arranged as usually. The dentinoid is always broadened most in the S.-group and decreasing more and more in the R., N. and H.-groups, but I consider the dentinoid layer broadened even in this last group. In the S.-group the dentinoid often shows vacuoles in its substance and a very irregular line of its contour both at the odontoblast margin and the limit against the dentine. In all groups the dentine shows interglobular dentine from the proximal to the apical end of the tooth, but in the H.-group the interglobular spheroids are more dispersed and discrete, they are more numerous in the N-group and they dominate the dentine in the groups R. and S. In the S.-group there are very often broad bands of interglobular dentine, where the spheroids are very diffuse and which remind of dentinoid rather than of interglobular spheroids. The dentinal tubules seem wider than normally and in the dentine close by the dentino enamel junction, the dentine seems more translucid possibly from the dentinal tubuliculi being wider than normally.

The jaws intended for histological examination were decalcified in 5 % trichloracetic acid or in 5 % nitric acid, in both, the jaws were as soft as other soft tissues in 24 hours and were embedded in paraffin and cut to 5 μ thickness and manipulated just as soft tissue cuts. In some cases I used 3 % trichloracetic acid for two to four days with good decalcification. All the mature enamel was completely dissolved i. e. all the enamel in the molars and all the proximal enamel in the incisors. In the area where this enamel had been (the enamel area) one cannot find any tissue debris,

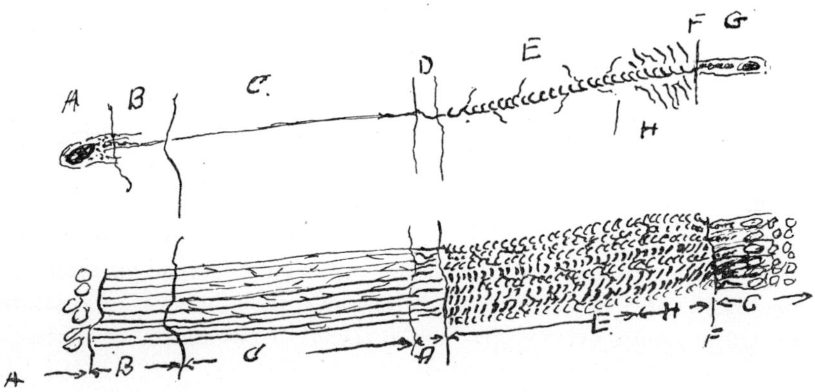

A Odontoblasts.
B Dentinoid.
C Dentine.
D Region of tubuliculi.
E Enamel inner region.
F Basal membr. of ameloblasts.
G Ameloblasts and Enamel organon.
H Enamel outer region.

Scheme of dentinal tubules tubuliculi, spiral structures of the enamel and central structure of ameloblasts as a unit.

Picture I.

it is completely empty. In the incisors the enamel area passes deep under the enamel organon, deeper close by the dentino enamel junction than along the ameloblast layer. In some animals of the group H. the enamel along the dentine border is dissolved, so that the enamel nowhere reaches the dentine layer. In the other groups there is always a space where the enamel is in contact with both the dentine and the ameloblast layer. In front of the ameloblast layer sometimes the enamel cuticula is to be seen as a free ending lash. The »enamel area» thus is the area of dissolved enamel and contains no enamel.

If we now look at the remaining enamel in a Laidlow-dyed (silverdyed) cut we shall immediatly observe that two different layers are to be discerned in the enamel, the outer (along the ameloblast layer) brighter by far than the inner (along the dentino enamel junction). The limit between them runs about in the middle of the enamel, in the middle between the dentine surface and the ameloblast row. Across both layers run structures of spiral formation, that begin with straight or curved structures of similar appearence as the lines in the spiral structures in the enamel, in the utmost brighter layer of the dentine and continue through the enamel across the basal membrane of the ameloblasts into them as a central structure in their exoplasm and are interrupted in the neighbourhood of their nucleus, but never reach it. The arrangement of these spiralstructures parallel to eachother and in quite regular distances from eachother remind of the enamel prisms. In the interval between the structures there is always a brighter field here and there traversed by anastomosing lines between the structures, but nowhere have I been able to find anything, that has a likeness with a prism-sheath between them. (If we compare the microphotos of intra vitam dyed enamel, that E. W. Fish has published: »A physiological survey of the nature of the enamel in carnivora and primates» we shall find in the pictures 2 and 4 that the prisms are bordered by the dyeing only on one side, just as it would look in a crosscut of a »prism» surrounded by such a spiralformed structure as the one here described). Such spiral formations have been observed before by Lams, Weidenreich, Loher, Marcus and Gustafsson, the latter in ground cuts of enamel, that were etched with concentrated acids). I will at last point out that the basal membrane of the ameloblast is very distinct in the Laidlow- dyed cuts and that the prismsheath seems very disputable, and I cannot see any interprismatic structure whose direction and position answers to the position of a sheathwall. I am most inclined to deny its existence.

I must add that the threads proximally from the outer remaining enamellayer dye with the Laidlow silver tinction but not as much as the spiral structures, and that the outer enamel layer can be followed to the apical end of the enamel as it is the youngest formation of the enamel.

If we follow the ameloblast layer from proximal to apical in a Bock-dyed cut, we find close to the ameloblast layer but deep under the enamel organon the first debris of enamel persisting in the form of threads or tufts in the enamel area, often free from the basal membrane, but as a rule in connection with it. The more we move apically the coarser and longer they grow and form a wide-meshed net that grows apically more and more fine until the threads lay themselves close together and form a layer where the threads can just be seen but where no meshes can be observed any longer. If we follow this layer in apical direction we shall find inward from it a layer that is easier to dye and where the spiralstructures are regularly repeated but when they reach the outer thready layer, the spirals disappear. More apically contourless shadows, often disappearing, cross the thready layer, but the more we advance in apical direction the shadows grow more manifest and reach the ameloblasts just as is described from the Laidlow cuts. Immediately afterwards the difference between the two layers of enamel disappears in the Bock-dyed cuts. In the silvercut the difference can be discerned to the apical end of the enamel.

In the inner layer, the spirals in the proximal part of it are dissolved in their inner end and thus end freely in the enamel area, but as we follow the layer in apical direction they grow longer and finally reach the dentino enamel junction. Even in the Bock-dyed cuts the spirals are discerned as spiral formations. The spirals seem to be limeholding but even the interspiral substance and the substance between the part structures of the spiral seem to be covered by a fine granulation that evidently is limeholding. In Bock-dyed cuts, no anastomoses between the spirals are to be observed, but the transgressions of the dentino enamel junction are often to be seen and often very evident. The continuations into the ameloblasts are very clear and may present themselves as a fringe

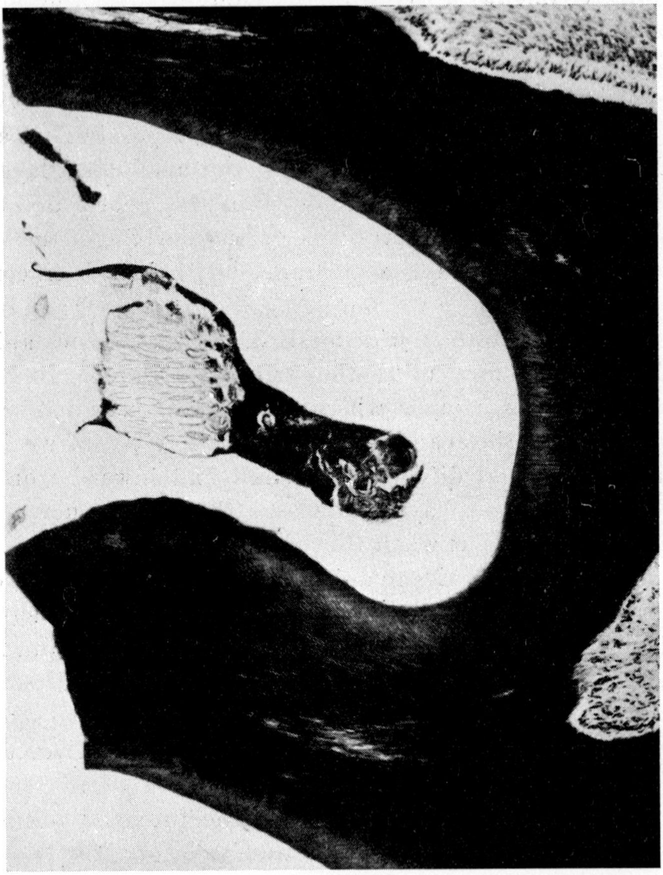

Picture III.

on the outer border of the enamel, when the continuity between enamel and ameloblast is interrupted in cutting, apparently drawn out from the ameloblasts (central structure of the ameloblast). In these cases the basal membrane of the ameloblasts seems to be intact.

It may be remarked that in cuts dyed with Hansen collagen

dying no collagen can be seen, neither elastin in cuts dyed for this purpose.

If we examine a Bock-dyed preparate of a molar from a newborn rat (age not exactly known, it may be from one to three days) that I took care of when conserving the other animals of the series, we see that at that age neither dentine nor enamel is developed. Odontoblasts and ameloblasts are arranged in a double row of cells round the pulp both kinds of normal size and arrangement. The odontoblasts are broken up in fine penecillike processes against the row of cells, but sometimes we find a thick process with the same dyeability as the spiral structures, that begins in the neighbourhood of the nucleus of the odontoblast and continues across the limit between the odontoblasts and the ameloblasts to the vicinity of the nucleus of the ameloblast. This structure may be broader than the spiral structure but its position corresponds fully with that of the spiral structure, and it seems certain to me that this band structure is the first stage of a developing spiral structure, and as it passes through the space where later on the dentinal tubules develop, it must also be looked upon as a Tomes process. Thus I conclude that the spiral structures have their origin in the odontoblasts. From their tincture in Bock-dyed cuts we see that the structures are limeholding and probably transport the lime from the odontoblasts to the enamel and that the calcifying of the enamel depends on the function of the odontoblasts. But the spiral structures are also continued into the ameloblasts across their basal membrane to the vicinity of their nucleus, apparently it has some task for the function of the ameloblasts.

We have hitherto demonstrated three different constituents of the enamel formation. One the spiral structure which is apparently the first beginning of the enamel evolution, the second the thread layer that is probably formed by a secretion from the ameloblasts or by a transformation of the ameloblast exoplasm, I will not decide the question though I am inclined to hold that it is a secretion, as the basal membrane of the ameloblasts always limits the threads against the ameloblasts, and the third element the granulation deposited both on the spiral structures and on the threads, that I hold to have been transported there by the spiral structures and thus to be the result of the vital action of the odontoblasts. As a fourth constituent we may remark the substance that makes the mature enamel optically homogeneous, but that I have not been able to demonstrate in this connection. It may be that this substance deprives the mature enamel of the power of resistance against the decalcifying acids used.

It seems as if the threads of the thread layer are bundled by the spiral structure and thus are tighter where the spiral structures run and poorer in the intervals between them.

If we consider the form of the enamel area and the form of the persisting enamel it is clear that the persisting enamel is younger than the enamel that once occupied the enamel area. The persisting enamel is immature enamel or an enamel whose maturation has been retarded apparently by the parathormone administered in vivo. But it may also be that mature enamel by the same hormone has been reduced to a more immature state. If it is so a dedifferentiation has taken place in the mature enamel. Retarded differentiation and dedifferentiation is well known in bone and dentine (HANSEN, HÄGGQVIST, WESTIN, WILTON), but hitherto not demonstrated in the enamel. But if a great part of the enamel evolution depends on the vital action of the odontoblasts, this retardation of enamel maturation and possibly dedifferentiation of mature enamel to a more immature stage lies very near at hand in animals treated in vivo with parathormone as these processes in dentine are provoked with parathormone in young tissue without difficulty. In our case the dentine is severely immature in all the groups of animals (the general spreading of interglobular dentine throughout all the dentine) and the great part of the persisting enamel must be considered as immature. Whether this state has developed by a retarded differentiation of immature enamel or by a dedifferentiation of mature plays no part. The chief point is that this state of the enamel is an analogon in the enamel to the osteo-dentino-dystrophia and a part of the same process.

These considerations remind of the pictures of the second zone of GOTTLIEB (and ERDHEIM) on the evolution of »Enamel hypoplasia». In their cuts the enamel from the dentino enamel junction is quite dissolved and also the ectoplasm of the ameloblasts, but the cytoplasm with their nucleus is conserved as an unbroken layer of the outer ends of the ameloblasts. Only poor debris of the enamel tissue and small lime particles remain in the area of the resorbed enamel. This evolution seems very easy to explain if we only accept that the odontoblasts are able to resorb the chalk by means of the spiral structures just as they have transported it there by means of them. I hold that the enamel hypoplasia of ERDHEIM and GOTTLIEB, my enamel deformation, is only a consequence of the dystrophia of the odontoblasts, the Tomes processes, the spiral structures and the central pillar of the ameloblasts and that this unity is the instrument of the resorption as I hold it to be the instrument of enamel evolution. Differentiation and dedifferentiation are known to be reversible processes.

As a first point in the discussion of the formations described in the previous part of my account I state that two factors have worked the decalcification of the material. One the decalcification by the acid used, the other the violent doses of the hormone of the parathyreoid gland administrated to the animals during the last five weeks of their life.

As there is no probability that the enamel should be transformed into new structures the described structures must be the regular structure of the enamel but reduced to a stage that better resists the decalcification than the normally maturated enamel does. Acids generally dissolve the enamel without remains, but in this case considerable remains persist, though they differ widely from the enamel that we are aquainted to see, the remains have lost their optic homogenity and the structures of the tissue appear instead of the homogenity that covered them. By this I have not intended to maintain that the acids have not been active in the area of the remaining enamel. On the contrary they have revealed the structure by destroying the homogenity. Also the acids would have dissolved more of the substance by a prolonged activity than they have done in this case, the decalcification being performed in only 24 hours until the tooth was soft as other soft tissues, such as muscles mucosa and the like. It must have been the parathormone administration during the life of the rats that has caused the structures to persist when the enamel was treated with acids.

Parathormone is known to be active especially in the youngest part of the tissue on which it works. In the incisor of the rat, the oldest part is the proximal part (near the edge of the tooth) and the enamel is younger the nearer we approach to the root end (apically). But we must also remember that the part of the enamel close by the dentino enamel junction is older than the enamel close by the ameloblast layer. Thus the enamel most apically in the teeth and the enamel nearest to the ameloblasts should be most resistant to decalcification by acids if the tissue has been treated by parathormone in vivo. In these rats it is so: the enamel that resists is placed far apically in the teeth and the acid dissolution continues farther in apical direction in the neighbourhood of the dentino enamel junction than close by the ameloblasts. Thus I hold that the parathormone activity in my animals is proved even if I omit the alterations of the bone tissue and the dentine where the activity is very pronounced and of well known appearance.

In my preparates we discern two layers of persisting enamel, one close to the ameloblast layer and one close to the dentino enamel junction which in the proximal part does not reach this junction but is limited a little apart from it, ending freely in the enamel area. The first of these layers begins most proximally by threads or tufts that emanate from the emeloblast border of the enamel and proceed inwards and forwards into the area of dissolved enamel, and end freely in this area forming an irregularly meshed net. Later on in apical direction the threads flow together to an unbroken layer, nearly homogeneous but with a somewhat thready structure. Somewhat apically from the beginning of the continuous layer, direct continuations from the spiral structures of the next layer cross it, first as contourless shadows, but more apically still well contoured and clear, the most characterizing quality of this layer being the thready groundsubstance that is difficult to dye fletching itself in the turns of and between the passing spiral structures.

The groundsubstance of the inner enamel layer is covered by a somewhat granular covering. Possibly the threads of the outer layer continue but it is not to be seen. In this groundsubstance, the spiral structures regularly return running from the dentino enamel junction almost in the same direction as the dentinal tubules in the corresponding dentine across both enamel layers to the ameloblasts, reminding by their arrangement of the enamel prisms. *But I have never found any structure that could make me believe in an enamel sheath, and thus I cannot speak of enamel prisms.* I don't deny that they may exist but then they must be covered by the above mentioned granular substance or be more exposed to the activity of the decalcifying acid than the rest of the enamel substance. Possibly the spiral structures themselves may have given the conception of an enamel sheath. I remind here of the experiment of E. W. Fish to dye enamel in vivo, where he described that the dye in the enamel follows the enamel sheath. His microphotos however show the dyening only on one side of the prisms »between the prism and the sheath» and I should rather accept that the dyening lies within the turns of the spiral structures.

The spiral structures pass the enamel from the dentino enamel junction to the ameloblasts at regular distances between the spirals. *Outward they seem to continue in the central structure of the ameloblasts through the exoplasm and are interrupted near the nucleus, but at the dentino enamel junction they also very visibly traverse the junction and seem to continue in the tubuliculi of the dentine in its utmost layer.* Even though not all transgressions are visible (They are often curved) this relation to the odontoblasts is extremely important and must be held in mind as it positively indicates that the odontoblasts partake in the evolution of the enamel and may represent the way of the metabolism of the enamel, when it has grown out from the surrounding soft tissues.

The spiral structures and the granulation seem to contain lime and the acid decalcification attacks their lime (the shadowy contours in the thready layer) and transforms the layer into a nearly homogeneous. But the circumstance that both these layers persist, indicates that the enamel has undergone a remarkable alteration already in vivo that makes these layers continuous when the decalcification by acids is used and makes the structures to be maintained.

The remaining enamel is placed under the apical region of the enamel organon and must be held to be developed during the time when the parathormone was administered to the animals. The maturation of this enamel (the calcification) has been retarded by it, and the organic matrix is more resistant by its immaturity. But the most proximal part of the enamel, that persists may be older than the beginning of the parthormone administering and then this part must have undergone a dedifferentiation intra vitam and regained the power to persist when exposed to acids.

Whether it is the question of a retarded differentiation or a dedifferentiation seems to me not to make any difference. The point is that the tissue on behalf of its maturity is younger than its place in the tooth indicates and remains coherent when other enamel will be fylly dissolved. This state of the incisor enamel of my rats should be held as a parallelism in the enamel to the tissue reactions before described in bone and dentine. (WILTON).

In a previous publication on »Enamel Deformation caused by rickets or spasmophilia» I held that the real cause of their evolution was a retardation or stopping of the *dentine* outgrowth over the pulp papilla and that »rachitic deformation» might prove to be a nomination saying nothing about

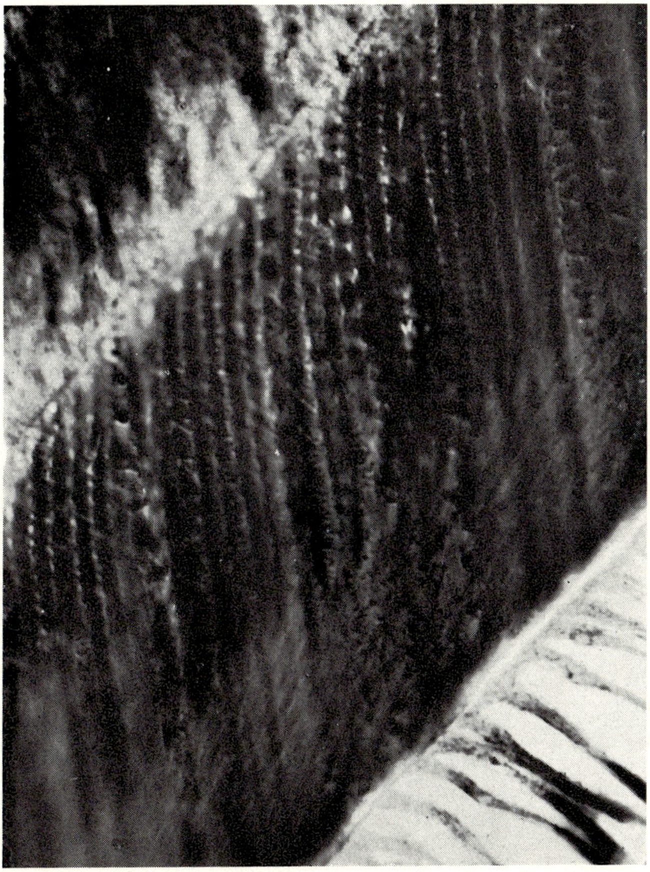

Picture II.
Boçk-dyed.

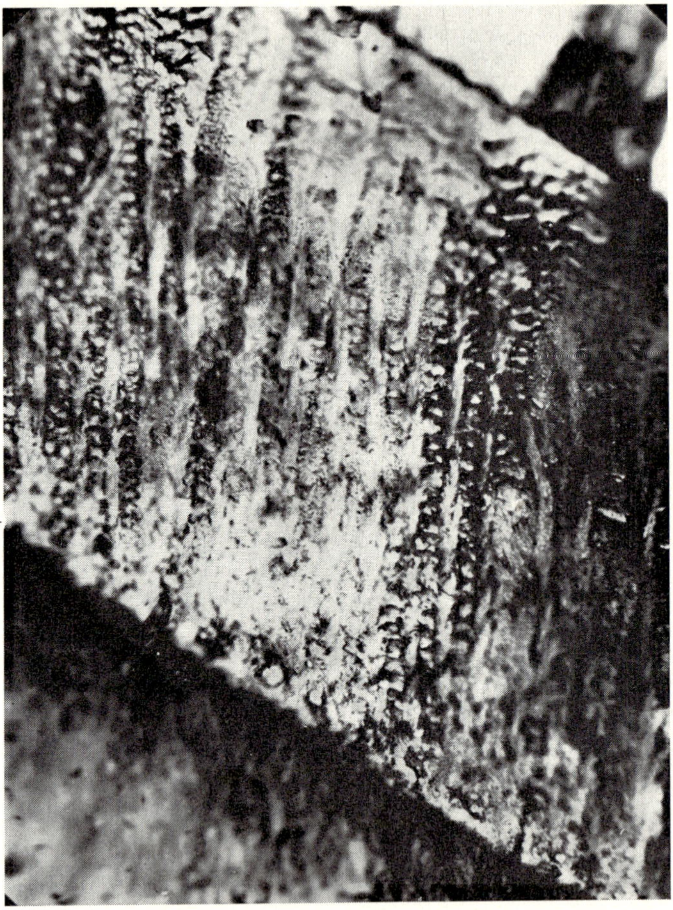

Dentine.

Dent. Enamel junct. Enamel.

Ameloblasts.

Enamel.

Picture IV.

Laidlow-dyed.

the real cause. If we accept rachitis to be a tendency to lower the lime supply in the blood and the parathyreoid gland is the regulating organon of the lime metabolism, the expression »caused by rickets» is not wholly incorrect. The hypersecretion of the parathyreoid gland may last longer than the clinical rickets and cause dystrophia. An antithesis »caused by hyperparathyreosis or hypoparathyreosis» will better correspond to my present meaning and be more clear. Both a rachitis and an hyperparathyreosis may retard the differentiation of the odontoblasts and cause a dystrophia of the dentine and consequently also of the enamel.

I can't omit here to point out that in human enamel deformation the interglobular dentine layer and the Retzius band in the enamel meet in the same point on the dentino enamel border just where the Zsigmondy interruption line attains the junction. All these three formations must then be contemporary in evolution and provoked by the same cause. They all represent the youngest parts in the tooth at their evolution time. This circumstance makes me accept that an hyperparathyreosis is the cause of enamel deformation, which always attacks the youngest parts.

Summary.

Even if we disregard the facts that the research has given about the microanatomy of the enamel, its connection with the odontoblasts and the hints on the normal evolution of the enamel, which follow as a consequence of these facts, I state the presence of enamel deformation in the form of fissures in almost every mastication groove of the molars and severe dystrophia of the enamel in the apical part of the incisors in all the experimental animals. The dystrophia of the incisor enamel must be considered as a more severe alteration than the fissure evolution.

In both cases a retarding factor (the parathormone) has been working, but as the dentine outgrowth in the incisors is greater than in the mastication grooves, where it is slow

(Zsigmondy) the retarding factor works more violently (Wilton) and the immaturity of the enamel will be greater.

I also remark the great frequency of decayed molar fissures in the skeletonized preparates, and the still greater frequence of decay in the fissures of the ground molar cuts, and although the number of observed fissures is too small to decide the question, the decay seems to be due to the influence of parathormone, that possibly is the cause of the incipient dental decay. But here further evidence must be collected.

The pictures II and IV are microphotographs intended to show the spiral structures of the enamel and their connection with the dentinal tubuliculi and by them with the odontoblasts and also their connection with the central structure in the exoplasm of the ameloblasts. The Pict. II is made from a Bockdyed cut and Pict. IV from a Laidlowdyed cut.

The pict. III demonstrates the described mouldings of molar fissures as they present themselves in almost all mastication grooves of the rat molars.

The Pict. I is a scheme of the totality of the connections between odontoblasts and ameloblasts. According to my interpretation of the material of cuts.

Diphtheria, Anatoxine and Tuberculosis.

By

Dr. G. J. HUËT.

Cases of diphtheria can be expected when susceptible persons come into contact with patients or with carriers of the bacilli. It is clear that diphtheria, resulting from this contact will be found oftener in closed milieux than in free society. As the susceptibility decreases with age, the greatest incidence of diphtheria will be found in children-homes, especially in those with much intercourse among the residents and with frequent contact to the outer world. At the head of the list will be found children-homes with a long nursing-time, such as sanatoria for tuberculous children and nursing-homes.

Ramon and Debré (1) noted in the Hôpital Maritime at Berck-Plage with a number of 1,000 occupied beds during 3 years 137 cases of diphtheria, that is 45 cases yearly. At Hoog-Blaricum with a number of 200 occupied beds I found during 5 1/2 years 26 cases, which means half the percentage of Berck-Plage, namely 22 cases per year on 1,000 patients.

What can be done against this nuisance?

As known we dispose of two means: firstly the spreading of the infection can be prevented by isolating the patient and the carriers; secondly the susceptibility of the contacts can be diminished by active immunisation.

But the effect of both of these measures is not unlimited. It is of interest to know these limits.

In diphtheria the contamination is spread from three sources:

1. the patients, of which some become
2. temporary carriers, some
3. permanent carriers.

The danger of temporary and that of permanent carriers are different. In the temporary carriers the danger lies in number, but as a rule they lose their bacilli before long. Permanent carriers on the contrary are much less numerous, but, though it is said that the bacilli lose their virulence within 6—8-weeks, danger may persist as long as the bacilli are present, and this may continue for years. A striking example is given in the Annual Report of the Medical Service of the city of Rotterdam (2): a boy of 6 years, who visited an infant-school suffered from diphtheria in 1936. In 1937 two cases of diphtheria occurred in his form, one of whom died. The original boy appeared to be a carrier, but after tonsillectomy the smears were negative (nose and throat). In the autumn another school-fellow died from diphtheria. Again the original boy was examined and proved still to be a carrier. From then he stayed at home, the smears being alternatively negative and positive. In the next year he was taken to relations elswhere: within five days two more cases of diphtheria followed, one of which died. Surely a warning not to trust the so-called avirulence of carriers after 6—8 weeks!

As to the measures to be taken, different views are held whether prevention is wanted in free society or in closed centres. Though a few authorities still plead for the isolation of diphtheria-carriers under all circumstances (Wieland, Hagen (3)) the majority (Degkwitz, de Rudder, Friedemann (3), Kleinschmidt (4)) have the conviction that efficient prevention will never be reached in this way and therefore does not justify the strain and the considerable expenses of the measure.

On the other hand for establishments with a population which is kept apart from the outer world, isolation of patients and carriers is still required by all authorities. It may be true that excellent results can be obtained by this measure, but this rule will not do as soon one has to deal with sanatoria, children-homes etc. where regular or periodical connections are kept up with the outer world by new-comers or visitors.

According to Seeligmann (3), who examined 100,000 healthy children in Berlin during a period of three years, the percentage of carriers varies between 0.4 and 1.3 %. But in times of epidemy this percentage can rise considerably. At Hoog-Blaricum we found from Oct. 1940 till March 1941, besides two new probationers, 9 out of 83 new-comers (10.8 %) carriers for diphtheria.

Which is the average term during which the bacilli persist? CLAUBERG (5) found as an average duration of the contagiousness among carriers of

the typus mitis: 18 days (1—191 days)
the typus gravis: 43 » (5—161 »).

In a number of ex-patients and mere carriers at Hoog-Blaricum we found the following data:

Diphth.-bacilli were present during:	Ex-patients			Carriers
	Immunized	Not immunized	Total	
0—4 weeks . . .	in 12 pat.-s	in — pat-.s	12	in 14 pat.-s
1—2 months . .	3	6	9	5
2—3 » . .	1	3	4	1
3—4 » . .	3	1	4	—
4—5 » . .	2	—	2	1
5—6 » . .	—	—	—	2
6—7 » . .	1	—	1	—
16 » . .	—	1	1	1
over 2 » . .	—	1	1	—
» 7 » . .	1	—	1	—
» 10 » . .	—	1	1	—
	23	13	36	24

This table shows that in about 50 %, of patients as well of mere carriers, the bacilli persist for more than 4 weeks. Therefore it is clear that normal accommodations will not be sufficient for the isolation of such numbers. But supposing this difficulty could be surmounted, there is still another one to overcome.

The examination of new-comers takes at least 3—4 days before an answer can be had and in this time, if not held in quarantaine, they may infect other patients in the same ward. It seems one that diphtheria-bacilli spread very easily. One day, when all the available boxes were occupied, we were obliged to place a new-comer directly in one of the wards. This child, a girl 6 years old, proved to be a carrier, sporadic bacilli being found in the nose. In a fortnight 6 out of 9 patients in the same ward, all at a distance of at least 1.50 M from each other, proved to have become carriers (nose). The same observation was made in a ward of 9 boys of 16—18 years, of whom 3 became carriers within 10 days. This draws our attention to the possibility that nurses also can contract the bacilli from this source and carry them further on. Thus, to face these different possibilities, it is necessary to dispose not only of numerous boxes, but also of a certain number of reserve-nurses.

The next difficulty lies in the fact that the bacteriological examination of the throat and nose is not always reliable. For instance: August 20 1938 a boy of 5 years was admitted to the sanatorium, and as he was known to be a carrier of diphtheria-bacilli, he was placed at once in the infectuous department. From 6—30 December his throat and nose proved 4 times in succession negative. Nevertheless on January 16 *virulent* bacilli again were present. From February 21 till March 9 nose and throat again were 3 times in succession negative, but then the bacilli reappeared and were still present at his dismission in May 1939.

These observations give evidence that the present system of quarantaine and isolation, even when applied with great accuracy, will not prevent spreading of the infection under all circumstances.

In order to invigorate this supposition, all cases of diphtheria, that occurred at Hoog-Blaricum from August 1929 till January 1940, were classed according date and ward. From 62 cases 45 originated in another ward as their preceding case, and only 17 in the same ward, mostly in groups of 2 or 3, and but once 4 at a time. In these 17 cases the interval between two cases amounted to:

1—11 days . . . . (10 cases)
3 weeks till 3 months . . . . (7 cases)

In the 45 discontinuous cases the interval amounted to:

less than 1 month . . . . (20 cases)
1—5 months . . . . (25 cases).

Discontinuous cases were seen as a rule in distant wards without direct connection.

All in all a strong indication to the fact that in most of these cases, the infection was carried in by new-comers, visitors or nurses, anyhow not by direct contact from one patient to another.

Here follows an enumeration of the cases of diphtheria seen at Hoog-Blaricum from 1925 till 1941, in relation to the effect of isolation and active immunisation.

	Not or insufficiently immunized	Immunized at H-Blaricum	Total	Average number of patients	Morbidity in Amsterdam per 10,000
1925	3	—	3	163	157.3
1926	3	—	3	203	121.7
1927	—	—	—	216	73.2
1928	1	—	1	227	62.8
1929	7	—	7	219	59.9
1930	5	—	5	222	85.1
1931	13	—	13	224	63.3
1932	3	—	3	227	80.2
1933	5	—	5	229	70.7
1934	2	1	3	209	43.8
1935	2	4	6	210	16.9
1936	—	—	—	226	10.6
1937	4	2	6	233	8.4
1938	6	—	6	232	16.2
1939	12	2	14	230	9.9
1940	7	—	7	192	?

Till June 1931 the prevention was limited to mere isolation of patient and carriers. At first the results were good:

sporadic and light cases. But in 1929 there was a reversal, the number of cases increased and in this year and the next one a patient died from toxic diphtheria, in spite of immediate serum-therapy.

This brought us to active immunisation, first of the youngest patients (0—6 years), then of the children under 10 years (April 1933), finally of all ages (October 1935). We used the anatoxine-Utrecht (40 AE in 3 injections) and from October 1935 the same anatoxine fortified (50 AE in 2 injections). Nurses and probationers were not immunized.

At present we dispose of a number of 631 patients; based on the data of these patients we intend to discuss the merits and drawbacks of the active immunisation, especially with regard to tuberculous children.

The great benefit of the method is that in duly immunized children — by which are meant children in the period from 2 till 12 months after the final injection — the morbidity and mortality are diminished.

Diphtheria-Morbidity and Mortality

	Beck-Plage		Hoog-Blaricum	
without anatoxine		died		died
per year				
per 1,000 patients	45	4	22	1.8
immunized by anatoxine				
per year				
per 1,000 patients	3.3	0.33	4.1	—

The same effect is shown by the following table:

Hoog-Blaricum			diphtheria
full immunisation	696	patients	9 = 1.5 %
not yet duly immunized .	11	»	11
no longer duly immunized	8	»	8
not immunized	1438	»	21
Total not immunized	1,457	patients	40 = 2.7 %.

On the other hand it is rather unsatisfactory that the anatoxine-treatment does not afford full protection. As is seen in the above mentioned table 9 among our patients contracted diphtheria notwith-standing their being immunized only 2—12 months before. With one exception all were children under 6 years. 5 out of them however suffered from a light form of diphtheria, the remaining 4 even from a very light one. This may be considered as another benefit of the anatoxine-treatment[1].

Has anatoxine-treatment any drawbacks?

Last year serious consequences were reported from Fribourg in Switserland (6). In an orphanage at Montrevers 11 children out of 26, who had been submitted to immunisation by anatoxine, died in consequence, evidently by an error at the preparation. As far as we know, no similar experiences have hitherto been reported.

But a more frequent danger lies in the fact that persons under treatment are brought into the so called negative phase, in which they are defenceless in case of diphtheria. The existence of a negative phase is fully denied by Ramon and Debré: »a negative phase does not exist; if someone under treatment does not show resistance in case of diphtheria, it means only that he is not yet sufficiently immunized and that he wants anti-serum».

But this opinion is not shared by other authorities. Herderschee (7) for instance reports the following case: a female carrier, 6 years old, already two days in observation, no membrane on the tonsils nor even an irritation in the throat, developes the day after a Schick-test had been performed, a typical diphtheria, that required several injections of anti-serum before to subside. This experience reminds the experiments of Hamburger, who found in consequence to a simple Schick-test, in many children a decline of the antitoxine-titer, that greatly surpassed the 1/50 AE, wanted to neutralize the small

[1] At Hoog-Blaricum we use to isolate at once any suspect case of angina till the bacteriological examination is finished. It is therefore quite possible that some of our cases of diphtheria may have been mere harmless anginae in carriers of diphtheria-bacilli. As discrimination is impossible, we prefer to take certainty for uncertainty. Perhaps the high number of diphtheria must partly be explained in this way.

amount of Schick-toxine. This negative phase is said to be of short duration, and not to surpass a weeks time.

In order to detect any influence of a negative phase, I examined our cases of diphtheria whether the number of cases occurring within two months after the anatoxine-treatment surpasses the ones that developed later on.

Diphtheria. Number of cases at Hoog-Blaricum between August 1931 and January 1940.

I.	Immunized patients			
	interval after immunis. less than 2 months	11	=	22.4 %
	» » » 3—12 months	9	=	18.4 %
	» » » more than 12 months	8	=	16.3 %
II.	not immunized patients	21	=	42.8 %
	Total	49	=	100 %.

There is indeed a small preponderance of cases occurring in the first two months after the immunisation. Considering the small difference between these percentages, it is questionable whether it points to an effect of a negative phase or not. Moreover in 10 out of these 11 patients the diphtheria was a very light one. On the other hand it is remarkable that the 11th patient of this series died from a toxic diphtheria in spite of immediate and large doses of antiserum[1]. It must

[1] Boy, 4 years old, diagnosis: tuberculosis of the ileocoecal glands:

7 Nov. 1931	Admission to the sanatorium.		
12 » »	Schick. test positive.		
18 » »	$^1/_2$ cc. anatoxine.		
2 Dec. »	diphtheric membrane on the R. tonsil	12,000	AE antiserum
3 » »		6,000	» »
4 » »	(albuminuria)	6,000	» »
5 » »		6,000	» »
6 » »		6,000	» »
	Total	36,000	AE antiserum
7 Dec. 1931	throat clear again.		
17 » »	paralysis of the palatum molle.		
12 Jan. 1932	paralysis of the pharynx, reflexes of the lower extremities abolished, urine normal again.		
21 » »	exitus by paralysis of the diaphragm.		

be admitted however, that the interval between the injection of anatoxine and the beginning of the diphtheria in this case was more than a week.

Further nuisance depends on the introduction of protein-substances proceeding from the body of the diphtheria-bacilli, out of which the anatoxine is prepared. Hence vigorous reactions may ensue in persons, who by previous natural contact became sensitive to this protein. To avoid misunderstanding the proper anatoxine-reactions are meant here and not the eventual activating of a preexisting tuberculosis, which subject will be discussed later on.

We had very little trouble from these proper anatoxine-reactions.

Reaction on the injection of anatoxine.

Number of patients . . .	631		Number of injections .	1,599	
No reaction	563	89.2 %	No reaction	1,510	94.9 %
Reaction < 38.5	32	5.0 %	Reaction < 38.5	42	2.6 %
Reaction > 38.5	36	5.7 %	Reaction > 38.5	39	2.4 %

Children 0—5 years number	415	
No reaction	366	88.2 %
Children 6—10 years number	144	
No reaction	134	93 %
Children 11—18 years number	72	
No reaction	63	87.5 %

Anatoxine Utrecht

No. 285 (3 injections = 40 AE)		
number of injections	972	
no reaction	927	95.4 %
No. 285 a (2 injections = 50 AE)		
number of injections	614	
no reaction	579	94.9 %

This table shows that, taken as a whole, the number of reactions was very small, and independent from the age of the children and from the kind of anatoxine used. Moreover, when present, half of the reactions was a light one.

These results are in striking contradiction to the high number of reactions observed by ETIENNE BERNARD and CHEVALLEY, who in the same way immunized tuberculous children. BERNARD (8) saw severe reactions in 36 %, CHEVALLEY (9) even in 66 % of the cases, accompanied in 1/5 of the cases by affections of the upper respiratory tract and even by pulmonar congestions. This can originate from the fact that in France stronger doses are used (at least 60 AE), while the anatoxine Utrecht contains only 40 AE (No. 285, in 3 injections) or 50 AE (No. 285 a, in 2 injections). Moreover CHEVALLEY made use of an anatoxine-mixte, immunizing against diphtheria and tetanus as well. One may ask whether these rather severe reactions in tuberculous children (affections of the respiratory tract, prolonged fever) should not be regarded as exacerbations of the preexisting tuberculosis. Such at least is the opinion of CHEVALLEY himself, because they were seen especially among the youngest children.

This would mean that anatoxine-treatment is not harmless in tuberculous children. Some even go further and charge this treatment with unevitable and irreparable damage to healthy people.

Now it is most remarkable that, although the medical literature at one hand affords ten thousands of anatoxine-immunisations, in which, in spite of careful follow-up, no accident ever was seen[1], a small number of casuistic communications is published, in which, even by critical reading, it can't be denied that damage was done by the anatoxine-treatment. It is CHAVANON (10) who in this respect goes farthest, pretending on account of a not quite impartial study of literature, that even deafness and idiocy can be the consequences of an anatoxine-injection. Even anginae with septic lethal course are

[1] f. i. LESNÉ (Hôp. Trousseau, Paris) 51,000 children.
LEREBOULLET (Hôp. des Enf. Ass., Paris) 40,000 children.
M:lle G. DREYFUSZ-SÉE, Paris 1,162,891 scholars.
TUNTLER Med. Serv. of the city of Amsterdam 384,000 children.

imputed by him to the anatoxine. But on the other hand he reports haematuria, haemorrhagic nephritis, purpura and urticaria in immediate connection to the injection of anatoxine, and, as to transient haematuria, the same is reported by LEREBOULLET (11), as well as intestinal haemorrhague following in that case the third injection. Similar cases are seen by VAN WESTRIENEN (12): 4 years old boy developed in connection to anatoxine-treatment allergic purpura and strophulus; another boy suffered hence from rebellious attacks of urticaria with persisting sensitiveness towards all proteins.

As to our 600 patients with nearly 1,600 injections nothing of the kind was seen.

There remains the question in how far anatoxine-injections may produce exacerbations of a preexisting tuberculosis.

This was examined by collecting the cases with arrested or inactive tuberculosis, in which, no other cause being present, an exacerbation developed in immediate connection to anatoxine-treatment. The determination of the conditions under which an exacerbation should be considered to be the effect of anatoxine-treatment or not, is not easy. As startingpoint served the experience that the fever indicating the exacerbation of a tuberculosis in consequence to intercurrent infections, follows the latter immediately or after a short interval (as a rule we found in our cases 2—19 days). Therefore it is obvious to require a similar interval to prove the connection of an exacerbation to the injection of anatoxine.

I was able to collect a few cases that answer to this demand. The interval between the injection of the anatoxine and the exacerbation of the tuberculosis amounts to

1 day	(3 cases)	7 days	(1 case)
2 days	(2 »)	9 »	(1 »)
3 »	(1 case)	15 »	(1 »)
5 »	(1 »)	3 weeks . . .	(1 »)

On a total of 631 children we saw in connection to anatoxine-injection:

pleural effusion	6	cases	
focal reactions (pointed out by X-ray)	6	»	
prolonged fever	3	»	
Total	15	cases	= 2.3 %
probable but not quite certain cases	16	cases	
Total	31	cases	= 4.9 %

Thus the proper percentage of post-anatoxine exacerbations lies between 2.3 and 4.9 %.

Among the control-group without anatoxine, numbering 488 patients, the following number of spontaneous exacerbations and of exacerbations in connection to some intercurrent infection were seen:

pleural effusion	3	cases	
peritoneal effusion	3	»	
focal reaction (pointed out by X-ray)	6	»	
prolonged fever	3	»	
Total	15	cases	= 3 %
of these spontaneous	5	»	= 1 %
in connection to a preceding intercurrent infection	10	»	= 2 %

Thus the amount of exacerbations in connection to anatoxine (2.3—4.9 %) is more than 2 times the percentage of spontaneous exacerbations. Therefore it is likely that anatoxine-treatment may lead to exacerbations in tuberculous children.

In order to get an insight into the mechanism to which this effect is due, I examined the changes of the sedimentation rate of the red bloodcells (WESTERGREN) in consequence to the anatoxine-treatment.

750 cases were ranged according to activity in:

1. arrested and inactive cases: sedimentation rate . . . . 0— 5 mM
2. doubtful activity: sedimentation rate 6—10 »
3. active cases: sedimentation rate . . 11 » and more

The effect of anatoxine-treatment on the sedimentation rate was compared to that of intercurrent infection by noting its modification at the next determination. As to these modifications 3 possibilities were distinguished, namely

1. equal = lowered, equal or not more increased than 2 mM
2. uncertain = rise of 3—4 mM
3. increased = rise of more than 5 mM

The following table gives the results in percentages. The regularity in the increase of the percentage for: »*increased*» according to the administration of anatoxine or the occurrence of an intercurrent infection, or both of these factors, points out that anatoxine, as well as intercurrent infections are able to modify the proteinspectrum of the plasma, as far as this is shown by the sedimentation-test, and in consequence probably also the immunisatory relations.

anatoxine	—	+	—	+	
interc. infection	—	—	+	+	
total number of cases	302	176	154	118	total 750
I. Patients with an initial sedimentation-rate to an amount of *0—5 mM.*					
number of cases	64	58	32	39	
out of these the percentage in which at the next determination the sedimentation-rate was found:					
equal (0—2 mM)	84.3	60.4	53.1	46.2 %	
uncertain (3—4 mM)	6.2	14.4	6.2	23.1 %	
increased (5 mM or more)	9.4	25.2	40.6	30.8 %	
II. Patients with an initial sedimentation-rate to an amount of *6—10 mM*					
number of cases	76	47	40	36	
out of these the percentage in which at the next determination the sedimentation-rate was found:					
equal (0—2 mM)	85.4	74.4	60.0	63.7 %	
uncertain (3—4 mM)	6.5	10.6	15.0	8.0 %	
increased (5 mM or more)	7.8	14.9	25.0	27.8 %	
III. Patients with an initial sedimentation-rate to an amount of more than 10 mM					
number of cases	162	71	82	43	

out of these the percentage in which at the next determination the sedimentation-rate was found:

equal (0—2 mM)	77.9	77.4	73.1	81.4 %
uncertain (3—4 mM)	6.2	5.6	7.4	2.3 %
increased (5 mM or more) .	16.0	16.8	19.5	16.3 %

We draw attention to the fact that among group I the effect of the cooperation of anatoxine and intercurrent infection is smaller than we expected and smaller than the effect of infection alone. This depends most probably on the exceptional high number »*uncertain*» (rise of 3—4 mM) in which column several cases in which the increase was apparently a real one, happened to have been placed.

It is not to be wondered at, that group III does not answer to the rule, if one realizes, that an already considerably increased sedimentation will not easily be augmented by a new factor.

Apparently we must assume that some tuberculous affections, in spite of normal temperature and rather normal sedimentation of the red bloodcells, may stay as well in unstable condition so that, besides other causes, also the injection of anatoxine may start an exacerbation of the process. Any cause at that time would have had the same effect.

Unfortunately it is not possible to avoid this danger by selecting the children, who are to undergo the anatoxine-treatment, unless one should exclude such a number that the immunisation as a whole would lose its value. Though some of the children, who got an exacerbation, had a raised sedimentation rate (23 mM, 50 mM, 70 mM), in as many others temperature and sedimentation rate were quite normal (5 mM, 6 mM, 8 mM, 10 mM). One could indeed restrain the number of candidates by submitting them to Schicks test before and exclude the negative ones.

Chevalley (see above) reports that many children suffered from affections of the upper respiratory tract in connection to the anatoxine-treatment. Independently we too got the impression that the susceptibility to intercurrent infections was augmented by the injection of anatoxine.

I tried to prove this suggestion by statistics.

The first difficulty to overcome was to select two equivalent groups, one treated with anatoxine and the other not, for it happened that some of the children had been immunized immediately after admission, while others had got the anatoxine later on, and had suffered in the meantime from intercurrent infections. Another difficulty was offered by the different ages of the children: the older a child, the more his susceptibility of infections decreases. Therefore for the comparison were chosen an anatoxine-group and a control-group, each composed of equivalent children as to number and age. Care was taken that the anatoxine-group contained merely children, who had been immunized immediately after admission. An enumeration was made of the infections during the first three months, among the immunized children from the day of the first anatoxine-injection, among the controls from the day of admission.[1]

The result was:

Anatoxine-group 176 infections among 232 children
i. e. 75.8 infections per 100 children

Control-group 142 infections among 232 children
i. e. 61.2 infections per 100 children

The difference is 14.6; the average deviation $\pm$ 4.3.

Much value is often attached to the fact whether a difference surpasses or not 3 times the average deviation. But this rule is not tenable under all circumstances, as Dr. NEURDENBURG explained to me. Therefore on his advice the problem was again examined by the chi-quadrate-method, of which a description is given by Bradford Hill in »Principles of Medical Statitistics» (published by the Lancet 1937).

[1] As to this part of the enquiry I am much indebted to Dr. M. G. NEURDENBURG, statistical officer to the Medical Service of the city of Amsterdam, to whom I want to express my best thanks. But for his advice I was able to master the special statistical difficulties of this material.

The startingpoint of this method is to suppose, that no special factors — in casu: the anatoxine — have influenced one of the groups, that are to be compared. In that case the distribution of the data must agree with such distribution as would belong to the procentual relation between the totals of each group. Now it is the purpose of the chi-quadrate-method to examine whether this is so or not. In the last case it is probable that some special factor has had its influence on the composition of one of the groups. The practical application of the chi-quadrate-method is this one: the children of each group are classed in one of the following columns:

children with 0 infections
» » 1 infection
» » 2 infections and so on.

The total of these columns is determined by addition (*observed value*). Then for each column a calculation is made which value would correspond to the procentual relation of the groups in comparison (*expected value*). The differences between the observed and the expected values are raised to the second power and divided each by its belonging expected value. The addition of these quotients is *chi-quadrate*. To each number of terms, by addition of which chi-quadrate is determined, belongs a table, which gives for each given value of chi-quadrate the value of the *probability P*, that the observed distribution of the data agrees with their procentual composition.

It is assumed that, for a value P = 0.05 or more, the observed distribution agrees with the one, that can be expected under mere casual circumstances. On the other hand, for values P = less than 0.05, it is assumed that the observed distribution deviates so much from the »casual» distribution, that there must have been a special factor at work. This can be easily understood if one realizes that the *greater* P the smaller chi-quadrate — this is learnt from the tables — and the smaller chi-quadrate the *smaller* the differences between the observed and the expected values, by the addition of which chi-quadrate was found.

In order to keep account with the different frequencies of intercurrent infections at various ages, the children were classed in groups of 0—5 years, 6—10 years and 11—18 years, which were separately examined.

The result was that in all separate groups as in the combined groups as well, the value of P was above 0.05. This means that the differences between the observed and the expected distribution were too small to invoke the necessity of the influence of a special factor (in our case: the anatoxine). See appendix.

Therefore by this inquiry susceptibility in connection to anatoxine-treatment has neither been demonstrated nor excluded. Such a supposition however does not give the most probable explication of the significant difference we found in the number of infections among both groups.

Above we have shown why it is impossible to keep semi-closed children-homes free from diphtheria by mere isolation of the carriers.

Active immunisation is therefore indicated, though this method has many draw-backs.

As a conclusion the best method to prevent complications would be as far as we can see:

1. to limit the active immunisation to Schick-positive children.
2. to isolate the patients as long as they are under anatoxine-treatment.
3. to isolate as a rule:
   a. all patients with diphtheria positive angina
   b. permanent carriers
   c. temporary carriers in case of positive virulence-test.

Settling the immunisation before admission would exempt the sanatorium of some of its troubles, but this would not prevent the patients from exacerbations.

Summary.

An account is given of a ten years experience in preventing diphtheria in a sanatorium for tuberculous children. It is shown why mere isolation can not suffice in semi-closed children-homes. Merits and draw-backs of the active immunisation are discussed. An elaborate report is given of a statistical inquiry about the influence of anatoxine-injections on the susceptibility to intercurrent infections of the throat and the upper respiratory tract. Finally, in connection to the advantages, failures and dangers of the different methods of prevention, conclusions are drawn about the best rules to be followed in practice.

Résumé.

L'auteur donne ses expériences sur l'effet des mesures pour prévenir la diphthérie dans un sanatorium pour enfants tuberculeux pendant une période de dix ans. Il démontre pourquoi l'isolation à elle seule ne puisse donner des résultats satisfaisants dans un milieux demi-clos. Ensuite un exposé est donné des avantages et des inconvénients de l'immunisation active à l'anatoxine. Des recherches statistiques detaillées sont rapportées sur la question si l'anatoxine puisse augmenter la susceptibilité pour les infections banales des amygdales et des voies respiratoires supérieures. En se basant sur ses expériences et ses recherches l'auteur finit par formuler des règles à suivre en pratique pour la prévention de la diphthérie dans les centres demi-closes.

Zusammenfassung.

Es wird über eine 10-jährige Erfahrung berichtet bei der Vorbeugung von Diphtherie in einem Kindersanatorium. Die Massnahmen über die man verfügt werden besprochen. Es wird gezeigt warum man unter normalen Verhältnissen in halb-geschlossenen Anstalten mit blossen Isolationsmassnahmen nicht zum Ziel kommen kann. Vor- und Nachteile der aktiven Immunisation werden als dann besprochen. Es wird berichtet über eine ausgedehnte statistische Untersuchung über die Frage ob die Einspritzung von Diphtherie-anatoxin die Empfänglichkeit für banale Infektionen des Pharynx und der oberen Luftwege erhöht. Zum Schluss werden auf Grund der erwähnten Erfahrungen und Untersuchungen Vorschläge gemacht für Vorbeugungsmassnahmen in halb-geschlossenen Kinder-Heilstätten.

Litterature.

1. RAMON et DEBRÉ, Presse Médicale 1932, Nrs 29 & 32. — 2. Annual Report of the Med. Serv. of the city of Rotterdam, 1938. — 3. WIELAND, Kinderärztliche Praxis 1932, Hft. 1—4. HAGEN, ibid. FRIEDEMANN, ibid. SELIGMANN, ibid. — 4. KLEINSCHMIDT, Monatschr. f. Kinderheilk. 1938, Bnd 75, Hft. 4—6. — 5. CLAUBERG, Münch. Med Woch. 1935, p. 944. — 6. Ned. Tydschr. v. Geneesk. 1941, Nr. 7 p. 679 (ref. from Policlinico). — 7. HERDERSCHEE, Tydschr. v. Soc. Geneesk. 1930, p. 173. — 8. BERNARD, Bull. et Mém. d. l. Soc. des Hôp. de Paris 1939, Nr. 5. — 9. CHEVALLEY et ZIVY, Bull. d. l. Soc. d. Péd. de Paris 1939, Nr. 1. — 10. CHAVANON, »On peut tuer son enfant» Ed. Médicis, Paris 1938. — 11. LEREBOULLET, Bull. d. l. Soc. d. Péd. d. Paris l. c. (discussion). — 12. VAN WESTRIENEN, Maandschr. v. Kindergeneesk. 1938, p. 297.

Appendix.

Calculations by the chi-quadrate-method.

A+ = Anatoxine-group. A— = Control-group.

	Number of children with	0 inf.	1 inf.	2 inf.	3 inf.	4 & more inf.	Total
	Children 0—5 years old.						
A+	Observ. value . .	39	35	25	8	3	111
50 %	Expect. value . .	43	36	21 1/2	7	3 1/2	
	Difference . . .	— 4	— 1	+ 3 1/2	+1	+ 1/2	
	Quadr. differ. . .	16	1	12 1/4	1	1/4	
	Quadr./exp. val.	0.37	0.027	0.57	0.14	0.07	
A—	Observ. value . .	47	37	18	6	3	111
50 %	Expect. value . .	43	36	21 1/2	7	3 1/2	
	Difference . . .	+ 4	+ 1	— 3 1/2	—1	+ 1/2	
	Quadr. differ. . .	16	1	12 1/4	1	1/4	
	Quadr./exp. val.	0.37	0.027	0.57	0.14	0.07	

Chi-quadrate = 2.354 n (= amount of marginal numbers) = 4 P = ± 0.70.

	Number of children with	0 inf.	1 inf.	2 inf.	3 & more inf.	Total
	Children 6—10 years.					
A+	Observ. value . .	49	23	6	1	79
50 %	Expect. value . .	$53^1/_2$	19	$5^1/_2$	1	
	Difference . . .	$-\ 4^1/_2$	$+\ 4$	$+\ ^1/_2$	—	
	Quadr. differ. . .	$20^1/_4$	16	$^1/_4$	—	
	Quadr./exp. val.	0.37	0.84	0.045	—	
A—	Observ. value . .	58	15	5	1	79
50 %	Expect. value . .	$53^1/_2$	19	$5^1/_2$	1	
	Difference . . .	$+\ 4^1/_2$	$-\ 4$	$-\ ^1/_2$	—	
	Quadr. differ. . .	$20^1/_4$	16	$^1/_4$	—	
	Quadr./exp. val.	0.37	0.84	0.045	—	

Chi-quadrate = 2.51 n = 3 P = ± 0.50.

	Number of children with	0 inf.	1 inf.	2 & more inf.	Total
	Children 11—18 years.				
A+	Observ. value . .	31	10	1	42
50 %	Expect. value . .	$31^1/_2$	$8^1/_2$	1	
	Difference . . .	$-\ 1^1/_2$	$+\ 1^1/_2$	—	
	Quadr. differ. . .	$2^1/_4$	$2^1/_4$	—	
	Quadr./exp. val.	0.069	0.26	—	
A—	Observ. value . .	34	7	1	42
50 %	Expect. value . .	$32^1/_2$	$8^1/_2$	1	
	Difference . . .	$+\ 1^1/_2$	$-\ 1^1/_2$	—	
	Quadr. differ. . .	$2^1/_4$	$2^1/_4$	—	
	Quadr./exp. val.	0.069	0.26	—	

Chi-quadrate = 0.658 n = 2 P = 0.70—0.80.

	Number of children with	0 inf.	1 inf.	2 inf.	3 & more inf.	Total
	Children 0—10 years.					
A+	Observ. value . .	88	58	31	13	190
50 %	Expect. value . .	96 1/2	55	27	11 1/2	
	Difference . . .	− 8 1/2	+ 3	+ 4	+ 1 1/2	
	Quadr. differ. . .	72 1/4	9	16	2 1/4	
	Quadr./exp. val.	0.74	0.18	0.59	0.19	
A−	Observ. value . .	105	52	23	10	190
50 %	Expect. value . .	96 1/2	55	27	11 1/2	
	Difference . . .	+ 8 1/2	− 3	− 4	− 1 1/2	
	Quadr. differ. . .	72 1/4	9	16	2 1/4	
	Quadr./exp. val.	0.74	0.18	0.59	0.19	

Chi-quadrate = 3.40 n = 3 P = ± 0.30.

	Number of children with	0 inf.	1 inf.	2 inf.	3 inf.	4 & more inf.	Total
	All children together (0—18 years)						
A+	Observ. value . .	119	68	31	10	4	232
50 %	Expect. value . .	129	63 1/2	27 1/2	8 1/2	3 1/2	
	Difference . . .	−10	+ 4 1/2	+ 3 1/2	+ 1 1/2	+ 1/2	
	Quadr. differ. . .	100	20 1/4	12 1/4	2 1/4	1/4	
	Quadr./exp. val.	0.77	0.31	0.44	0.26	0.07	
A−	Observ. value . .	139	59	24	7	3	232
50 %	Expect. value . .	129	63 1/2	27 1/2	8 1/2	3 1/2	
	Difference . . .	+10	− 4 1/2	− 3 1/2	− 1 1/2	− 1/2	
	Quadr. differ. . .	100	20 1/4	12 1/4	2 1/4	1/4	
	Quadr./exp. val.	0.77	0.31	0.44	0.26	0.07	

Chi-quadrate = 3.7 n = 4 P = 0.30—0.50.

Über Scharlach und Diphtherie in Finnland und Schweden während der letzten Dezennien.

Von

BERTIL SOURANDER, Åbo.

Ehem. Chefarzt am Epidemiekrankenhaus Wiborg, Finnland.

De Rudder hat in der Epidemiologie die Bezeichnung Zivilisationsseuchen eingeführt. Unter diesem Ausdruck versteht er solche epidemischen Krankheiten, die immer noch in den hochstehenden Kulturländern konstant endemisch sind. Im Gegensatz zu dem, was bei anderen Seuchen, wie Pocken, Cholera und Pest, erreicht worden ist, ist es der modernen Zivilisation nicht gelungen diese Epidemien auszurotten. Die Seuchen, die von alters her vom Gemeinwesen als besonders verhängnisvoll für die Volksgesundheit betrachtet worden sind und die daher auch gesetzliche Massregeln mit Isolierung der Krankheitsfälle erheischt haben, haben bekanntlich im Verlaufe des letzten Jahrhunderts an Anzahl bedeutend abgenommen. Die Epidemiekrankenhäuser des Nordens haben seit der Jahrhundertwende nur ausnahmsweise Fälle von Pocken und Fleckfieber beherbergen müssen. Nur einzelne Fälle von Cholera sind vorgekommen.

Scharlach und Diphtherie, einzelne Fälle von epidemischer Genickstarre, Kinderlähmung und, durch örtliche Umstände der Krankenhäuser bedingt, auch Typhus, Paratyphus und einige andere, mehr seltene, epidemische Krankheiten, haben die hauptsächliche Belegung der Epidemiekrankenhäuser ausgemacht. Die epidemischen Krankheiten, die dem Isolierungszwang nicht unterworfen sind, wie die Masern, der Keuchhusten und die Influenza, sind wohl nur in den geräumigen Epidemiekrankenhäusern der grösseren Städte als Belegung in Frage gekommen. Die Rolle der epidemischen Krankheiten im Kulturstaat hat ohne Zweifel in hohem Grade abgenommen, teils weil einige schwere, epidemische Krankheiten verschwunden sind, teils weil die übrigbleibenden, vor allem der Scharlach und die Diphtherie, sowohl hinsichtlich der Ausbreitung wie der Beschaffenheit der Fälle, einen milderen Charakter angenommen haben.

Da die Frage von der Prophylaxe des Scharlachs und der Diphtherie, besonders in Amerika im letzten Jahrzehnt stark in den Vordergrund getreten ist und auch zu ausgebreiteter Impfung gegen diese beiden Seuchen geführt hat, muss die Zeit als geeignet betrachtet werden, im Norden, wo keine Immunisierungsversuche in grossem Masstabe unternommen worden sind, die Frage von der Einwirkung der natürlichen Immunität auf das Auftreten der erwähnten Krankheiten zu diskutieren.

Die Klarlegung, die hier gemacht werden soll, ist insofern mangelhaft als die offizielle finnische Statistik nur seit dem Jahre 1927 brauchbar ist. Früher wurden die Zahlen der Erkrankten zum Teil nur annähernd angegeben, und die Anzahl der in epidemischen Krankheiten Gestorbenen wird erst seit dem Jahre 1927 regelmässig angegeben.

Noch im Jahre 1915 war der Scharlach in Finnland eine sehr gefürchtete Krankheit. Im Berichte der Medizinalverwaltung über dieses Jahr wird nämlich gesagt: »Der Scharlach ist eine von unseren verheerendsten Seuchen. Die Anzahl der Todesfälle erreichte nach den Angaben der geistlichen Behörden die Zahl 458, welche 14,9 % von den Erkrankten ausmachte.»

Über die Sterblichkeit in der Diphtherie gibt es keine offiziellen Angaben. Aus dem Obenerwähnten erhellt indessen, dass der Scharlach wenigstens im Jahre 1915 eine Krankheit mit einer Letalität von 15 % war und desgleichen, dass er bis zum Jahre 1918 (finnisches Kriegsjahr), als die Zahl der Erkrankten mit über 100 % zunahm, verhältnismässig spärlich vorkam. Die Fälle von Diphtherie erreichten ungefähr die selbe Anzahl wie die Scharlachfälle, überstiegen sogar in den Jahren 1919—1922 bedeutend die letzteren. Die offizielle finnische Statistik gibt besonders die Fälle von Krupp für die Jahre 1915—1917 an; von sämtlichen Diphtheriefällen machte der Krupp etwa ein Viertel aus.

Ein Vergleich mit der offiziellen schwedischen Statistik zeigt:

Sowohl der Scharlach als die Diphtherie traten bedeutend zahlreicher auf in Schweden als in Finnland in den Jahren 1915—1917. Die Letalität bei Scharlach schwankte in Schweden zwischen 5 % und 1 % in der Periode 1915—1926. Die Vermehrung der Diphtheriefälle verläuft ziemlich gleichartig, erreicht sein Maximum in den beiden Ländern im Jahre 1919, nimmt dann allmählich ab. Die Letalität bei Diphtherie schwankte in Schweden zwischen 7 % und 4 %.

Für die Periode 1927—1937 ist die Statistik der beiden Länder völlig vergleichbar.

Dass die Sterblichkeit während der Periode 1927—1936 von 1 bis 5 auf 100 000 Einwohner gewachsen ist hängt keineswegs von einer Steigerung der Bösartigkeit des Scharlachs ab; die Anzahl der Erkrankten hat im selben Masse wie die Sterblichkeit zugenommen. Diese Vermehrung kann auf einer grösseren Ausbreitung des Virus beruhen, aber kann auch analog mit der üblichen Auffassung vom pandemischen Charakter der Kinderlähmung, als eine Folge der veränderten Immunitätsverhältnisse in der Bevölkerung betrachtet werden. Im Gegensatz zu dem Verhältnis beim Scharlach wird im Jahre 1929 eine Steigerung der Bösartigkeit der Diphtherie an einem Minimum von diagnostizierten Diphtheriefällen beobachtet. Bei Ausbreitung der Diphtherie nimmt die Bösartigkeit ab. (Die Letalität des Jahres 1929: 24 % > im Jahre 1936 9 %.)

Die folgenden Tabellen zeigen die Verhältnisse in Schweden:

In Schweden sehen wir eine ähnliche Zunahme der Scharlachfälle wie in Finnland. Auch dort entspricht ihr keine deutliche Vermehrung der Bösartigkeit. Die Steigerung der Bösartigkeit der Diphtherie in Finnland, die mit einem Mi-

Tabelle 1.

Der Scharlach in Finnland.

Jahr	Erkrankte im ganzen Lande	Erkrankte auf 100 000 Einw.	Gestorbene im ganzen Lande	Letalität	Mortalität
				(Die Gestorbenen von den Erkrankten.)	(Gestorbene auf 100 000 Einw.)
1915	3 068	94	458	15 %	14
1916	3 566	108			
1917	3 147	95			
1918	7 917	237			
1919	7 335	220			
1920	1 969	59			
1921	1 359	40			
1922	972	29			
1923	1 150	33			
1924	1 842	53			
1925	1 691	48			
1926	2 221	63			

Tabelle 2.

Die Diphtherie in Finnland.

Jahr	Erkrankte im ganzen Lande	Erkrankte auf 100 000 Einw.	Gestorbene im ganzen Lande	Letalität	Mortalität
				(Die Gestorbenen von den Erkrankten.)	(Gestorbene auf 100 000 Einw.)
1915	3 354	103			
1916	3 433	104			
1917	3 452	104			
1918	5 112	153			
1919	8 761	263			
1920	6 348	190			
1921	3 918	116			
1922	1 947	57			
1923	1 803	52			
1924	1 306	38			
1925	1 230	35			
1926	1 153	33			

Tabelle 3.

Der Scharlach in Schweden.

Jahr	Erkrankte im ganzen Lande	Erkrankte auf 100 000 Einw.	Gestorbene im ganzen Lande	Letalität	Mortalität
				(Die Gestorbenen von den Erkrankten.)	(Gestorbene auf 100 000 Einw.)
1915	13 086	230	330	3 %	13
1916	10 482	183	418	4 »	11
1917	9 490	165	456	5 »	16
1918	7 769	134	284	4 »	31
1919	9 310	160	267	3 »	35
1920	9 750	167	188	2 »	23
1921	9 264	157	109	1 »	12
1922	10 718	180	74	1 »	6
1923	10 829	181	101	1 »	4
1924	10 882	181	81	1 »	3
1925	10 613	176	63	1 »	3
1926	8 513	141	65	1 »	3
			Im Durchschnitte	2 %	Durchschnittszahl 13

Tabelle 4.

Die Diphtherie in Schweden.

Jahr	Erkrankte im ganzen Lande	Erkrankte auf 100 000 Einw.	Gestorbene im ganzen Lande	Letalität	Mortalität
				(Die Gestorbenen von den Erkrankten.)	(Gestorbene auf 100 000 Einw.)
1915	11 471	202	733	6 %	6
1916	12 385	217	648	5 »	7
1917	14 674	255	900	6 »	8
1918	27 645	477	1 785	7 »	5
1919	40 514	697	2 035	5 »	5
1920	26 446	452	1 246	5 »	3
1921	15 133	256	695	5 »	2
1922	6 610	111	381	6 »	1
1923	4 840	81	214	4 »	2
1924	4 240	71	195	5 »	1
1925	3 820	63	181	5 »	1
1926	3 561	59	183	5 »	1
			Im Durchschnitte	5 %	Durchschnittszahl 4

Tabelle 5.

Der Scharlach in Finnland.

Jahr	Erkrankte im ganzen Lande	Erkrankte auf 100 000 Einw.	Gestorbene im ganzen Lande	Letalität	Mortalität
				(Die Gestorbenen von den Erkrankten.)	(Gestorbene auf 100 000 Einw.)
1927	1 966	55	49	3 %	1
1928	2 380	66	51	2 »	1
1929	4 943	137	114	2 »	3
1930	3 861	106	71	2 »	2
1931	4 010	109	58	1 »	2
1932	3 910	106	68	2 »	2
1933	3 942	106	80	2 »	2
1934	4 654	124	95	2 »	3
1935	6 310	168	73	1 »	2
1936	11 420	302	206	2 »	5
1937	10 976	288	177	2 »	
				Im Durchschnitte 2 %	Durchschnittszahl 2

Tabelle 6.

Die Diphtherie in Finnland.

Jahr	Erkrankte im ganzen Lande	Erkrankte auf 100 000 Einw.	Gestorbene im ganzen Lande	Letalität	Mortalität
				(Die Gestorbenen von den Erkrankten.)	(Gestorbene auf 100 000 Einw.)
1927	876	22	186	21 %	5
1928	984	27	156	16 »	4
1929	702	19	171	24 »	5
1930	967	27	155	16 »	4
1931	1 170	32	203	17 »	6
1932	1 613	44	247	15 »	7
1933	1 993	54	300	15 »	8
1934	3 137	84	348	11 »	9
1935	3 903	104	383	10 »	10
1936	4 535	120	391	9 »	10
1937	4 339	114	356	8 »	9
				Im Durchschnitte 15 %	Durchschnittszahl 7

Tabelle 7.

Der Scharlach in Schweden.

Jahr	Erkrankte im ganzen Lande	Erkrankte auf 100 000 Einw.	Gestorbene im ganzen Lande	Letalität	Mortalität
				(Die Gestorbenen von den Erkrankten.)	(Gestorbene auf 100 000 Einw.)
1927	5 289	87	59	1 %	1
1928	6 017	99	52	1 »	1
1929	8 533	140	101	1 »	2
1930	8 046	131	59	1 »	1
1931	5 922	96	42	1 »	1
1932	5 241	85	32	1 »	1
1933	7 428	120	45	1 »	1
1934	10 912	176	68	1 »	1
1935	8 081	130	66	1 »	1
1936	7 567	122	59	1 »	1
1937	14 572	233	152	1 »	2
			Im Durchschnitte	1 %	Durchschnittszahl 1

Tabelle 8.

Die Diphtherie in Schweden.

Jahr	Erkrankte im ganzen Lande	Erkrankte auf 100 000 Einw.	Gestorbene im ganzen Lande	Letalität	Mortalität
				(Die Gestorbenen von den Erkrankten.)	(Gestorbene auf 100 000 Einw.)
1927	3 776	62	206	6 %	3
1928	2 820	46	145	5 »	2
1929	2 630	43	144	6 »	2
1930	4 178	68	143	3 »	2
1931	2 576	42	93	4 »	2
1932	1 933	31	55	3 »	1
1933	1 705	28	54	3 »	1
1934	935	15	46	5 »	1
1935	916	15	24	3 »	0—0,5
1936	781	12	26	3 »	0—0,5
1937	299	5	12	4 »	0—0,5
			Im Durchschnitte	4 %	Durchschnittszahl 1

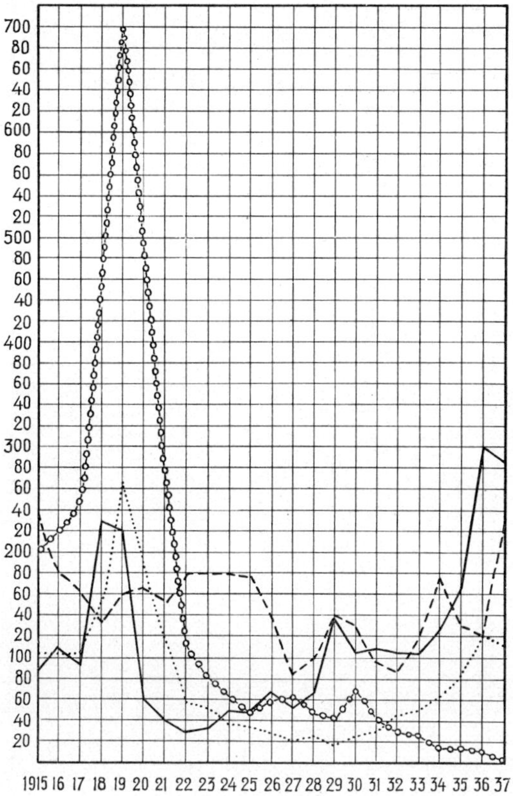

Abb. 1. Verlauf der Scharlach- und Diphtheriemorbidität in Finnland und Schweden auf je 100 000 Einwohner.

——— Scharlach in Finnland
- - - - - » » Schweden
·········· Diphtherie in Finnland
o-o-o-o-o-o » » Schweden

nimum von den in Finnland im Jahre 1929 diagnostizierten Fällen zusammenfällt, kann als ein Beleg dafür aufgefasst werden, dass die Diphtheriewelle, die 1926 in Mitteleuropa seinen Anfang nahm, auch Finnland[1] erreicht hat. Schweden dürfte dagegen kaum die bösartige mitteleuropäische Diph-

[1] SOURANDER: Acta pædiatr. 1939, XXIV, 266.

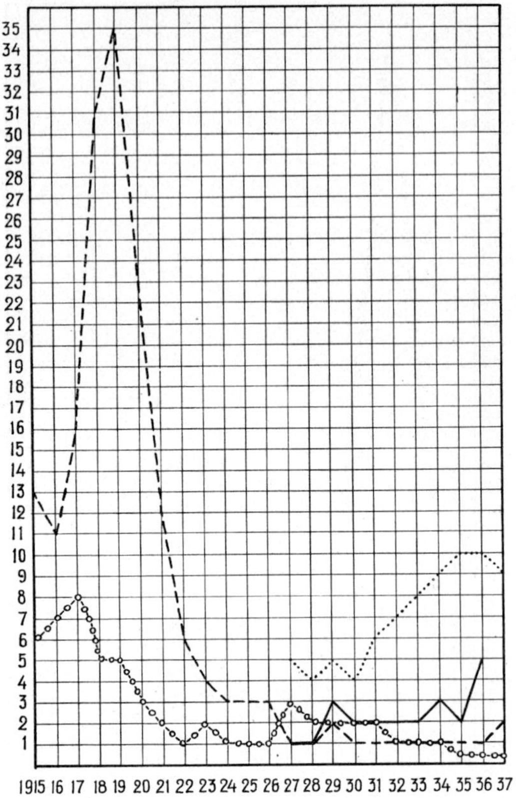

Abb. 2. Scharlach- und Diphtheriesterblichkeit in Finnland und Schweden pro Hunderttausend Lebender.

——— Scharlach in Finnland
- - - - - » » Schweden
.... Diphtherie in Finnland
o-o-o-o-o-o-o » » Schwedan

therie verspürt haben. Da die Anzahl der Ärzte in Schweden verhältnismässig grösser gewesen ist als in Finnland, ist es wahrscheinlich, dass die gelinderen Fälle von sowohl Scharlach als Diphtherie in Schweden häufiger gemeldet worden sind als in Finnland, wo das Landvolk bei leichter Erkrankung nicht immer den Arzt ruft. Dieser Umstand kann doch kaum

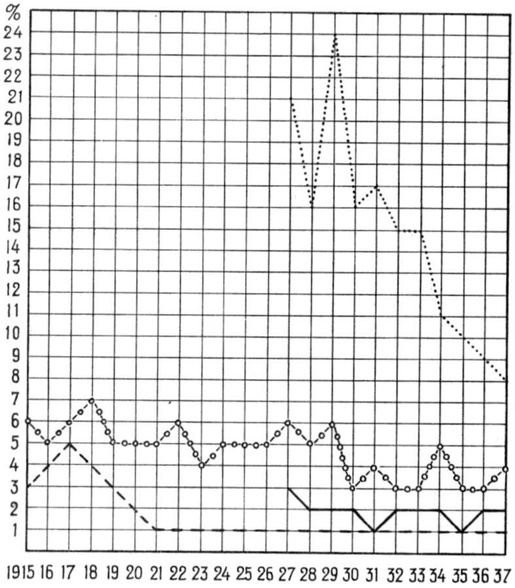

Abb. 3. Verlauf der Scharlach- und Diphtherieletalität in Finnland und Schweden.

———————	Scharlachletalität in Finnland
- - - - - -	» » Schweden
··················	Diphtherieletalität in Finnland
o-o-o-o-o-o-o	» » Schweden

die Krankheitsstatistik in so hohem Grade beeinflussen, dass die Ziffern nicht vergleichbar wären.

Als Zusammenfassung der oben tabellarisch und graphisch dargestellten offiziellen Ziffern werden folgende Schlüsse gezogen:

1) Der Scharlach hat während der letzten Dezennien sowohl in Finnland als in Schweden einen pandemischen Charakter aufgewiesen mit besonders starker Ausbreitung in Finnland im Kriegsjahr 1918. Gleichzeitig hat der Scharlach in den beiden Ländern, in Schweden jedoch in höherem Grade, seinen schweren Charakter verloren, was sich in der Mortalität, aber ganz besonders deutlich in der Letalität abspiegelt.

2) Die Diphtherie zeigt grosse Verschiedenheiten in den beiden Ländern. Nach dem Jahre 1919, als die Diphtherie in Finnland und besonders in Schweden eine pandemische Ausbreitung hatte, nimmt die Seuche in Schweden sukzessiv ab, und wird dann eine Krankheit, die seit vielen Jahren seinen seuchenartigen Charakter verloren zu haben scheint. In Finnland dagegen, vielleicht in Verbindung mit einer beträchtlichen Ausbreitung von bösartiger Diphtherie in Mitteleuropa am Ende der zwanziger Jahre, nimmt die Diphtherie bei einem Minimum von diagnostizierten Fällen einen äusserst bösartigen Charakter an, der jedoch durch Ausbreitung der Seuche sukzessiv vermildert wird.

3) Die geringe Sterblichkeit in Schweden während des letzten Dezenniums, sowohl bei Scharlach als bei Diphtherie, kann, nach der heutigen Auffassung von der Bedeutung undiagnostizierter, leichter Scharlachfälle und Diphtheriebazillenträger für die Entstehung von Epidemien, auf keine andere Weise, als durch eine bedeutend gesteigerte natürliche Immunität der Bevölkerung, erklärt werden. Der Grund dazu liegt nahe. Ein hoher materieller und allgemeinhygienischer Lebensstandard in einem verhältnismässig spärlich bevölkerten, nördlichen Lande muss die wichtigste Ursache zur Abnahme der Verheerungen der hier behandelten Zivilizationsseuchen sein, ein Gesetz, das in der Geschichte aller jetzt schon im Norden ausgestorbenen epidemischen Krankheiten verspürt wird.

AUS DER GEBURTSHILFLICHEN KLINIK DES KAROLINISCHEN INSTITUTS IN DER ALLGEMEINEN ENTBINDUNGSANSTALT DER STADT STOCKHOLM (VORSTAND: PROF. OLOW; DAMALIGER KINDERARZT DER KLINIK UND VORSTAND IHRER ABTEILUNG FÜR FRÜHGEBORENE KINDER: DOZENT C. GYLLENSWÄRD).

Physiologische Temperaturerhöhung bei Neugeborenen.

Von

CURT GYLLENSWÄRD.

Seit über einem Jahrhundert ist die Säuglingssterblichkeit in Schweden — wie auch in den meisten anderen Kulturstaaten — mehr und mehr zurückgegangen. Diese Abnahme beruht indessen relativ mehr auf einem Senkung derselben während der letzten 11 Monate des ersten Lebensjahres als während des ersten Monats. Die Mortalität im ersten Lebensmonat hat sich mehr konstant gehalten, oder ist während der letzten Zeit ehestens sogar gestiegen. Auf diese Weise ist es zu einer relativen Verschiebung der Mortalität gekommen. Diese Verschiebung wird beim Studium des Verhaltens der Säuglingssterblichkeit in den grösseren Städten besonders deutlich. In Stockholm entfiel noch vor einigen Jahrzehnten etwa die Hälfte der Säuglingssterblichkeit auf den ersten Lebensmonat und die Hälfte auf die letzten 11 Monate des ersten Lebensjahres, während heutzutage fast drei Viertel dieser Mortalität in den ersten Lebensmonat fallen. Diese Entwicklung scheint noch nicht abgeschlossen zu sein. Die Säuglingssterblichkeit in Stockholm sank von durchschnittlich 40,22 ‰ während der Fünfjahrsperiode 1931—35 auf 33,39 ‰ während der Jahre 1936—40. Die Differenz beträgt 6,83 ± 1,34 ‰ (dreifache mittlere Abweichung = 4,02). Die Mortalität im ersten Lebensmonat ging während derselben Zeit von

27,82 ‰ auf 23,95 ‰ zurück. Die Differenz ist 3,87 ± 1,29 ‰ (dreifache mittlere Abweichung = 3,87). Wir finden also einen Rückgang der Mortalität sowohl während des ersten Lebensmonats als während des ersten Lebensjahres, aber die Sterblichkeit während des ersten Lebensmonats nahm verhältnismässig weniger ab als die des ganzen ersten Lebensjahres. Der Anteil des ersten Lebensmonats an der gesamten Säuglingssterblichkeit stieg demnach von 69,03 % in den Jahren 1931—35 auf 72,26 % 1936—40. Während der Jahre 1937—40 ist die Mortalität im ersten Lebensmonat nicht weiter gesunken. Dieselbe weist im Gegenteil — gleichzeitig mit einer absolut und relativ wesentlich erhöhten Geburtenzahl — eine steigende Tendenz auf (siehe Tab. 1).

Die Mehrzahl der Todesfälle während des ersten Lebensmonats trifft schon in der ersten Lebenswoche ein.

Die Bekämpfung der Frühsterblichkeit ist also eine besonders wichtige Aufgabe der vorbeugenden Mütter- und Kinderfürsorge geworden. Eine Reihe von Todesfällen in dieser allerersten Lebenszeit beruhen mehr oder weniger direkt auf Ursachen in der Neugeborenenperiode und während der Schwangerschaft. Für den Ausbau der vorbeugenden Mütter- und Kinderfürsorge nach sich auf Tatsachen gründenden Richtlinien sind demzufolge Untersuchungen über die Ursachen von Gesundheitsstörungen in der Neugeborenenperiode von besonderer sozialpädagogischer Bedeutung.

Eine vielfach erörterte, ihrem Wesen nach aber noch nicht völlig geklärte Erscheinung während dieser Zeit sind ziemlich oft wiederkommende Fieberzustände, die im Schrifttum meistens als »Durstfieber» bezeichnet werden. Über Ursache und Bedeutung dieser Zustände gehen die Ansichten noch weit auseinander.

In dem Namen »Durstfieber» liegt, dass die meisten Autoren dafür halten, dass der Fieberzustand durch Flüssigkeitsmangel verursacht ist. Letzterer sollte zu einer Austrocknung führen, welche dann ihrerseits Fieber entstehen lasse. Auch unter den Anhängern dieser Theorie herrscht indessen keine Einigkeit über die Rolle des Flüssigkeitsmangels.

Tab. 1.

In verschiedenen Lebensmonaten während des ersten Lebensjahrs Verstorbene etc. in Stockholm 1931—40.

Jahr	Verstorbene während Lebensmonat			Verstorbene während des 1. Monats in % der im Alter 0—1 Jahr Verstorbenen	Im Alter von 0—1 Jahr Verstorbene pro 1 000 Lebendgeborene	Im Alter von 0—1 Monat Verstorbene pro 1 000 Lebendgeborene	Lebendgeborene	Volksmenge am Jahresende
	1	2—12	1—12					
1931	132	93	225	58,67	41,96	24,62	5 362	514 333
1932	168	84	252	66,67	43,60	29,07	5 780	519 711
1933	148	48	196	75,51	37,25	28,13	5 262	521 618
1934	156	48	204	76,47	39,91	30,52	5 111	526 027
1935	145	63	208	69,71	38,36	26,74	5 423	533 884
1931—1935	749	336	1 085	69,03 ± 1,40	40,22 ± 0,94	27,82 ± 1,00	26 938	
1936	114	55	169	67,46	28,19	19,01	5 996	543 785
1937	157	81	238	65,97	37,85	24,97	6 288	556 954
1938	175	76	251	69,72	35,07	24,45	7 158	570 771
1939	200	48	248	80,65	32,10	25,89	7 725	583 621
1940	203	66	269	75,46	33,72	25,44	7 978	590 543
1936—1940	849	326	1 175	72,26 ± 1,31	33,39 ± 0,96	23,95 ± 0,82	35 154	

So halten einige diesen für die alleinige Ursache, während andere demselben nur eine sekundäre Wirkung zuschreiben.

Man begegnet jedoch im Schrifttum noch ganz anderen Anschauungen über die Genese. Eine Richtung will die Ursache des Fiebers in mangelnder Nahrungszufuhr erblicken, einem Mangel, welcher infolge der in diesem Alter rein flüssigen Kost automatisch eine Flüssigkeitsverarmung nach sich zieht, sofern nicht Flüssigkeit besonders zugeführt wird. Andere suchen die Ursache in einer erhöhten Salzkonzentration noch andere in schwerer Entbindung.

Das Bild wird durch eine Ansicht vervollständigt, nach der bestritten wird, dass irgendeine Temperatursteigerung normalerweise während der ersten Lebenstage vorkommt.

Eröss (1886) vertrat, auf ein Material von 100 Neugeborenen gestützt, den Standpunkt, am 2. Lebenstage trete eine leichte Temperatursteigerung (37,31°) mit Rückgang am 3. und 4. Tage ein. Das Kind, welches die höchste Temperatur hatte, wies eine erhebliche Gewichtsabnahme auf. Für die Temperatursteigerung werden »Krankheitszustände minderer Bedeutung», wie Dyspepsien, von der Nabelwunde ausgehende Störungen usw. verantwortlich gemacht.

Die Frequenz des Fiebers wird von Holt (1895, 1909) mit 10 % sämtlicher Neugeborenen, die Höhe desselben mit 39° und 40° und die Gewichtsabnahme bei diesen Kindern mit dem Dreifachen des Gewichtsverlusts bei nicht fiebernden angegeben. Sobald die Kinder zuzunehmen beginnen, sinkt die Temperatur. Holt glaubt, dass Hunger und Durst zusammen das Fieber verursachen, Christopher (nach Rietschel) hält nur Hunger für die Ursache.

Von Reuss (1912) findet ein Fieber, welches am 3. oder 4., seltener am 5. Tage einsetzt. Dasselbe dauert gewöhnlich 2—3, niemals mehr als 5 Tage. Als Ursachen werden Übergang von der Meconium- zur Mischflora im Darm mit Resorption von Zerfallsprodukten als Folge, Flüssigkeitsmangel, Austrocknung und mangelhafte Funktion des Wärmeregulierungsmechanismus erwähnt.

Heller (1912), der Fieber bei 17 % der Neugeborenen

fand, unterstreicht den Zusammenhang mit der Gewichtsabnahme. Wenn der Gewichtsverlust 500 g überschritt, fieberten 55 % der Kinder. Bei einer Abnahme von 200—300 g fieberten nur 5,4 %. Eine Konzentrationsstörung im Organismus durch Wasserverlust wird für die Ursache gehalten. Es wird jedoch auch eine Intoxikation durch pyrogen wirkende Eiweissabbauprodukte in Betracht gezogen.

Adair und Stewart legen das Fieber teils Nahrungs- und Flüssigkeitsmangel und teils dem Einfluss der Aussentemperatur zur Last. In den Monaten Mai—September war die Fieberfrequenz 17,4—34,0 %, Januar—April 0—8,2 % und Oktober—Januar 2,4—7,0 % der Neugeborenen.

Nach Rietschel (1934) hat man keine Veranlassung, zu bezweifeln, dass das Fieber des Neugeborenenalters ein Durstfieber ist, wenn auch Zerfallsprodukte aus dem Blut oder den Körpergeweben das Zustandekommen desselben fördern können. Das Fieber, welches rasch in Intoxikationserscheinungen übergehen kann, sei dem echten Konzentrationsfieber gleichzusetzen.

Abt behauptet, das Auftreten transitorischen Fiebers lasse sich durch Zufuhr von Nahrung nach den ersten 24 St. nach der Geburt verhindern. Nachdem man begonnen hatte, die Nahrungszufuhr beim Stillen zu kontrollieren, und nachdem die Kinder abgespritzte Muttermilch oder Milchmischung erhielten, wenn die Milchsekretion noch nicht in Gang gekommen war, verschwanden die Fälle von »transitorischem Fieber» in einer angegebenen Entbindungsanstalt. Vor der Kontrolle der Nahrungszufuhr war ein derartiges Fieber bei 5 % der Neugeborenen aufgetreten. Aus der verhältnismässig geringen Frequenz sollte hervorgehen, dass das Fieber nicht infektiösen oder kontagiösen Ursprungs wäre. Als Behandlung werden kalte Packungen und forcierte Nahrungs- und Flüssigkeitszufuhr, evtl. mittels Sonde, empfohlen.

Wollstein (1934) fand Temperatursteigerung bei 40 % der Neugeborenen. Die Hauptursache erblickt er in dem Verlauf der Gewichtskurve, aber auch andere Faktoren wären zu beachten, wie Art der Nahrung, operative Entbindung, Fieber der Mutter, Geschlecht des Kindes, Ikterus, Dauer der Entbindung u. a. m.

Salmi (1934) fand, dass unter 225 normal sowie 54 mittels Kaiserschnitts und 45 mittels Zange geborenen Kindern »das sog. transitorische Fieber» bei $^1/_5$ der normal geborenen, bei $^1/_4$ der mittels Kaiserschnitts und bei $^1/_2$ der mittels Zange zur Welt gebrachten Kinder auftrat. In der Gruppe der normal geborenen hatte die Entbindung bei den fiebernden Kindern viel länger gedauert als bei den nicht fiebernden. Bei $^1/_3$ der fiebernden Kinder hatte sich das Austreibungsstadium über mehr als 24 st hingezogen, während dies nur bei $^1/_{10}$ der nicht fiebernden der Fall gewesen war. Beim Kaiserschnitt waren die entsprechenden Zahlen $^1/_2$ bzw. $^1/_3$, bei der Zangenentbindung $^2/_3$ bzw. $^1/_2$. Salmi vermutet, dass die gesteigerten Möglichkeiten einer Infektion und eines Entbindungstraumas im Anschluss an schwere, langdauernde und komplizierte Entbindungen beim Zustandekommen des transitorischen Fiebers die Hauptrolle spielen.

Die Anschauungen über sowohl Vorkommen wie Ursachen der Fieberzustände bei Neugeborenen gehen also sehr auseinander, und diese Meinungsverschiedenheiten haben auch in den zahlreichen Namen Ausdruck gefunden, unter welchen man derartigen Fieberzuständen im Schrifttum begegnet: neben »Durstfieber» (E. Müller) finden wir die Bezeichnung »Inanitionsfieber» (Holt), »Salzfieber» (Heim und John), »Übergangsfieber» (Lindig), »Austrocknungsfieber» (Peteri), »transitorisches Fieber» (von Reuss) u. a. m.

Problemstellung.

Es handelt sich hier also einerseits darum, ob eine Temperatursteigerung während der ersten Lebenstage mehr allgemein vorkommt, und andererseits darum, ob sie in diesem Falle durch Mangel an Flüssigkeit oder Nahrung verursacht wird, oder ob sie vielleicht eine ganz andere Ursache hat.

Es ist vorauszusetzen, dass die Zufuhr von Flüssigkeit und Nahrung die Gewichtsveränderungen bei den Kindern beeinflussen muss. Falls ein Zusammenhang zwischen einem Fieberzustand und Flüssigkeitsmangel oder einem gleichzeitigen Nahrungs- und Flüssigkeitsmangel beim Neugeborenen bestände, müsste sich diese Beziehung in einem Zusammenhang zwischen dem Fieberzustand und den Gewichtsveränderungen widerspiegeln. Es muss also von grundlegender Bedeutung sein, an Hand eines grösseren Untersuchungsmaterials Temperatur und Gewichtsveränderungen bei Kindern während der ersten Lebenstage systematisch zu untersuchen und festzustellen, ob irgendeine Wechselbeziehung zwischen diesen Faktoren existiert. Ein derartiges Material als Grundlage einer zuverlässigeren Beurteilung steht indessen bisher noch aus.

Mit der vorliegenden Untersuchung wird in erster Linie beabsichtigt, diese Lücke auszufüllen. Das Material wurde während Verf.s Tätigkeit als Kinderarzt an der Allgemeinen Entbindungsanstalt der Stadt Stockholm zusammengestellt.

Untersuchungsplan.

Es ist eine bekannte Tatsache, dass praktisch sämtliche Neugeborenen zunächst abnehmen. Die Gewichtsabnahme pflegt schon während des 1. Lebenstages einzusetzen und am 2., 3., evtl. auch 4. Tage und manchmal noch länger anzuhalten.

Als ein wesentliches Charakteristikum des sog. Durstfiebers» wird gewöhnlich angegeben, dass der Zeitpunkt des Eintretens der Temperatursteigerung mit dem Maximum des Untergewichts des Kindes im Verhältnis zum Geburtsgewicht zusammenfällt.

Dieses Maximum soll meistens am 3., bisweilen am 2. oder 4. Tage erreicht sein. Diese Tage sind also die wichtigsten für die Behandlung der vorliegenden Frage.

Wenn ein ursächlicher Zusammenhang zwischen einer Gewichtsabnahme, insbesondere einem erheblicheren Untergewicht, und einem Fieberzustand besteht, würde sich dies in einer Temperatursteigerung äussern, welche man prinzipiell bei sämtlichen Kindern wiederfindet, welche abnehmen. Man kann dagegen annehmen, dass die Höhe der Temperatursteigerung in Beziehung zur Grösse des Gewichtsverlusts variiert. Kann der Gewichtsfall zum Wechseln gebracht werden, so würden folglich entsprechende Variationen in der Temperatursteigerung ausgelöst werden. Verschiedenheiten in der Gewichtsabnahme sollten sich durch Variationen der Nahrungs- und Flüssigkeitszufuhr erzielen lassen.

Praktische Gründe veranlassen uns dazu, diese Einschränkung so kurz wie möglich zu gestalten. Die Unterlassung, dem Kinde während des ersten Lebenstages Nahrung und Flüssigkeit zuzuführen, lässt sich voll und ganz verantworten. Namentlich seitens französischer Geburtshelfer ist geltend gemacht worden, dass eine derartige Abstinenz dem Kinde und in zweiter Linie der Mutter eine wohlverdiente und nützliche Ruhe verschaffe. Untersuchungen, welche einer solchen Anschauung eine faktische Unterlage verleihen, scheinen jedoch nicht vorzuliegen. Für Fasten und Nahrungsmangel von längerer Dauer lassen sich entsprechende Gründe jedenfalls nicht anführen.

Dass fiebernde Kinder abnehmen, ist eine gewöhnliche Erscheinung. Wenn man studieren will, inwiefern Flüssigkeits- und Nahrungsmangel und die damit zusammenhängende Gewichtsabnahme zu einer Temperatursteigerung führen, muss es daher wichtig sein, dass fiebernde Kinder aus dem Material ausgeschlossen werden, deren Fieber a priori anderer, und da in erster Linie infektiöser Genese gewesen ist, oder wo man einen begründeten Verdacht in dieser Richtung hegen konnte. Ansteckend kranke Mütter sowie deren Kinder werden in der Allgemeinen Entbindungsanstalt auf eine besondere Abteilung aufgenommen bzw. auf diese verlegt, wenn die Mütter im Wochenbett erkranken. In dieser Abteilung behandelte Kinder und Mütter sind bei der vorliegenden Untersuchung nicht berücksichtigt worden. Wäre etwa das Fieber bei Kindern dieser Mütter nicht durch Infektion, sondern durch Flüssigkeits- oder Nahrungsmangel verursacht, so stört der Ausschluss derselben doch das Resultat nicht. Die besagten Fieberfälle sind in diesem Falle extreme Varianten. Ihr Ausschluss be-wirkt lediglich, dass der Gradunterschied zwischen Gruppen von Kindern mit verschiedener Flüssigkeits- und Nahrungszufuhr in Wirklichkeit noch höhere Werte erreichen können würde, als es sich aus dem Untersuchungsmaterial ergibt.

Eine Folge des Ausschlusses ansteckend kranker Mütter ist, dass Mütter mit einer Temperatur über 38,5° im Material praktisch nicht vorkommen.

Untersuchungsmaterial.

Das Untersuchungsmaterial besteht aus auf 2 grossen allgemeinen »reinen» Abteilungen der Entbindungsanstalt betreuten Kindern. Diese wurden in 2 Gruppen eingeteilt. Ein Unterschied in der Nahrungszufuhr wurde dadurch zustande gebracht, dass die Kinder in der einen Gruppe im Prinzip schon 12 St. nach der Geburt an die Brust gelegt wurden (Abt. I), während die Kinder in der anderen Gruppe erst nach 24 St. die Brust erhielten (Abt. II). Der Unterschied in der Nahrungsabstinenz beträgt folglich 12 St. Um Flüssigkeitsmangel gleichzeitig mit Nahrungsmangel zu vermeiden, erhielten zunächst sämtliche Kinder auf Abt. II Ringersche Lösung per os, 10 g pro Mahlzeit, und zwar mit Beginn an demselben Zeitpunkt, wo die Kinder auf Abt. I an die Brust gelegt wurden, und dann an den Brustmahlzeiten entsprechenden Zeiten. Ringersche Lösung statt Wasser wurde mit Rücksicht auf einen eventuellen Einfluss der Salzzufuhr gewählt. Ausserdem trinken die Neugeborenen diese Lösung meist mit besserem Appetit als Wasser, woraus sich grössere Sicherheit ergibt, dass die Flüssigkeit auch wirklich von den Kindern aufgenommen wird.

Nachdem sich gezeigt hatte, dass die Grösse des Materials eine weitere Teilung ohne Gefährdung des Beweiswertes gestattete, wurde eine weitere Gruppe aufgestellt, in der die Kinder während des ersten Lebenstages weder Nahrung noch Flüssigkeit erhielten. Zu diesem Zwecke wurde Abt. II in zwei Gruppen geteilt. Den Kindern in der einen wurde wie zuvor Ringersche Lösung zugeführt (Abt. II Ringer), während die Kinder in der anderen während des ersten Lebenstages weder an die Brust gelegt wurden, noch Nahrung oder Flüssigkeit erhielten (Abt. II 0 Ringer). Auf diese Weise gelangte man zu drei vergleichbaren Gruppen von Kindern: eine, in der die Kinder schon nach 12 St. sowohl Nahrung wie Flüssigkeit bekamen (Muttermilch, Abt. I), eine, wo sie nach 12 St. nur Flüssigkeit — Ringersche Lösung —, aber erst nach 24 St. Muttermilch erhielten (Abt. II Ringer) und eine, in welcher ihnen während 24 St. weder Nahrung noch Flüssigkeit zugeführt wurde (Abt. II 0 Ringer).

Wo die Muttermilch bis zu der Zeit, wo die Kinder mit Rücksicht auf das Ziel der Untersuchung Nahrung erhalten sollten, noch nicht eingeschossen war, wurde zur Zusatzfütterung mit abgespritzter Muttermilch gegriffen. Während des zweiten Tages wurden 10 g pro Mahl zugeführt bzw. auf diese Menge ergänzt, während des dritten Tages 20 g pro Mahl usw. Eine Begrenzung der Milchmenge, welche die Kinder selbst an der Brust tranken, wurde nicht vorgenommen.

Um die Einflüsse verschiedener Aussentemperatur, verschiedener Infektionszustände in der Umgebung od. dgl. während der einzelnen Jahreszeiten in allen Abteilungen nach Möglichkeit auszugleichen, wurden in das Hauptmaterial sämtliche während eines ganzen Jahres betreute Kinder aufgenommen. Bei der Vierteljahrseinteilung wurden, namentlich mit Rücksicht auf die behauptete höhere Frequenz des »Durstfiebers» während des Sommers, im Juni, Juli und August, geborene Kinder zu einer Dreimonatsgruppe vereinigt. Die im März—April—Mai, September—Oktober—November und Dezember—Januar—Februar geborenen Kinder bilden die übrigen drei.

Die Einteilung der Abt. II in »Ringer» und »0 Ringer» wurde vorgenommen, nachdem die Untersuchung zwei Vierteljahre lang im Gange gewesen war. Während der Vierteljahre März—Mai und Juni—August gehören daher alle Kinder in Abt. II zur Gruppe Abt. II Ringer, während sie sich in den Vierteljahren September—November und Dezember—Februar auf Abt. II Ringer und Abt. II 0 Ringer verteilen. Um Material vom Typ »0 Ringer» auch während der beiden ersteren Vierteljahre zu erhalten, wurde die Untersuchung ein weiteres Halbjahr (Vierteljahr März—Mai und Juni—August) für diese Abteilung fortgesetzt. Da dieses Extramaterial »Extra-Abt. II 0 Ringer» nicht gleichlaufend mit dem Hauptmaterial beobachtet worden war, wird besonders angegeben, wenn dasselbe mitberücksichtigt ist.

Das Geburtsgewicht wurde auf der Entbindungsabteilung unmittelbar nach der Geburt bestimmt. Die später folgenden Wägungen und Temperaturmessungen exakt 24 St. danach vorzunehmen, lässt sich aus praktischen Gründen nicht durchführen. Ebensowenig ist es möglich, in der Folgezeit das 24-St.-Intervall ganz genau einzuhalten. Auf einer grossen Abteilung ist es selbstverständlich unmöglich, sämtliche Kinder auf einmal zu wiegen, zu messen oder zu füttern. Der Wert eines solchen Vorgehens wäre ausserdem fraglich. Die Beobachtungen verteilen sich nicht gleichmässig über Tag und Nacht, sondern häufen sich am Tage. Namentlich die Mahlzeiten müssen auf den Tag verlegt werden und lassen sich in der Folge nicht nach gewissen, bestimmten Zeitpunkten im Verhältnis zum Augenblick der Geburt anordnen. Der Einfluss eines möglichen 24Stundenrhythmus lässt sich ausserdem nicht ausschalten.

Es wurde daher ein festerer Zeitpunkt für die erste Wägung und Temperaturmessung nach der Bestimmung des Geburtsgewichts gewählt, nämlich die Messung nach der Aufnahme auf die Pflegeabteilung, nachdem das Kind von der Entbindungsabteilung verlegt worden war. Die Beobachtungen der ersten Tage haben also diese Zeit als Ausgangspunkt. Vor dieser haben die Kinder in keiner Abteilung Flüssigkeit oder Nahrung erhalten. Der »erste Tag» in den Tabellen wird auf diese Weise eine Kontrolle der Vergleichbarkeit des Materials in den verschiedenen Abteilungen. Ein Unterschied zwischen den einzelnen Abteilungen in bezug auf Nahrungs- und Flüssigkeitszufuhr tritt erst während des Tages ein, welcher in den Tabellen als 2. Tag bezeichnet wird.

Die Länge des 1. Tages muss aus verschiedenen Gründen in den einzelnen Abteilungen einmal innerhalb gewisser Grenzen schwanken und ferner 24 St. nicht erreichen. Sämtliche Kinder bleiben zur Beobachtung eine gewisse Zeit auf der Entbindungsabteilung. Platzmangel auf den Abteilungen kann eine Verlängerung dieser Zeit erforderlich machen. In der Nacht geborene Kinder werden bis zum nächsten Morgen zurückgehalten, um Störungen in den Pflegeabteilungen zu vermeiden. Der Wechsel dieser Ursachen trifft indessen alle Abteilungen gleichmässig. Im grossen ganzen wurden die Beobachtungen des 1. Tages 12 St. nach der Geburt des Kindes vorgenommen. Die Veränderungen gegenüber dem Zustand bei der Geburt, welche bis zum Ablauf des 1. Tages eingetreten sind, brauchten demnach etwa 12 St. zu ihrer Entstehung. Die Intervalle zwischen den folgenden Tagen betragen dagegen 24 St.

Auf den Pflegeabteilungen erfolgten die Wägungen zwischen 6 und 8 Uhr. Die Temperaturmessungen wurden zweimal täglich vorgenommen. Die Morgentemperatur wurde bei Gelegenheit der Wägung gemessen, die Abendtemperatur zwischen 14 und 15,30 Uhr.

Die Mahlzeiten wurden auf 6, 10, 14, 18 und 22 Uhr verlegt, ausser bei Kindern mit einem Geburtsgewicht unter 3 000 g. Diese erhielten 6 Mahlzeiten um 6, 9,30, 12,30, 16, 19 und 22 Uhr. Die erste Nahrungs- oder Flüssigkeitszufuhr (Brust, Ringersche Lösung, evtl. Zusatzfütterung) wurde auf den Zeitpunkt für diejenige Mahlzeit verlegt, welche am nächsten nach 12 St. [Abt. I (Brust), Abt. II Ringer (Flüssigkeit)] bzw. 24 St. [Abt. II Ringer (Brust), Abt. II 0 Ringer (Brust)] nach der Geburt eintraf.

In Abt. I fällt der Zeitpunkt der ersten Nahrungszufuhr im wesentlichen mit dem Beginn des 2. Tages zusammen. In Abt. II Ringer wird mit der Zufuhr von Ringerscher Lösung an demselben Zeitpunkt begonnen, mit der Nahrungszufuhr aber erst 12 St. später, während in Abt. II 0 Ringer weder Nahrungs- noch Flüssigkeitszufuhr vor Ablauf des halben zweiten Tages erfolgt.

Im Hinblick auf das verschiedene Geburtsgewicht und damit zusammenhängende denkbare Verschiedenheiten in bezug auf Temperatur- und Gewichtsveränderungen wurden die Kinder in drei Gewichtsgruppen eingeteilt, nämlich Kinder mit einem Geburtsgewicht von 2 200—3 099 g, Kinder mit einem Geburtsgewicht von 3 100—3 699 g und Kinder mit einem höheren Geburtsgewicht als 3 700 g. Auf Grund einer Untersuchung von LINDERS über das Geburtsgewicht von ungefähr 80 700 in vier Entbindungsanstalten in Schweden während der Jahre 1911—1920 geborenen Kindern wurde angenommen, dass die Mittelgruppe bei dieser Einteilung etwa die Hälfte der Kinder enthalten würde, während sich der Rest ungefähr gleich auf die beiden Seitengruppen verteilen würde.

Kinder mit einem Geburtsgewicht unter 2 200 g, welche in der Allg. Entbindungsanst. in einer besonderen Abteilung für schwächliche Kinder untergebracht sind, wurden nicht mitberücksichtigt. Ihr Ausschluss hat seinen Grund in der bekannten Schwierigkeit, schon bei gewöhnlicher Zimmertemperatur die Körperwärme aufrechtzuerhalten. Für Kinder mit extrem hohem Geburtsgewicht gilt das Entsprechende nicht. Eine obere Grenze hinsichtlich des Geburtsgewichts wurde daher für die Aufnahme der Kinder in das Material nicht festgesetzt.

Knaben und Mädchen wurden gesondert. Ein Unterschied nach der Ordnungszahl der Geburt wurde nicht gemacht.

Auch die Temperatur der Mütter wurde verzeichnet.

Aus dem Material sind zwar ansteckend kranke und damit bis auf wenige Ausnahmen auch alle fiebernden Mütter mit ihren Kindern ausgeschlossen worden. Die Temperatur der Mutter kann aber aus verschiedenen Gründen von Interesse sein. Man kann sich vorstellen, dass eine Infektion der Mutter das Kind ansteckt und bei letzterem Fieber verursacht, während diese Infektion bei der Mutter selbst nur eine leichte Temperatursteigerung auslöst, deren infektiöse Genese nicht diagnostiziert wird. An Hand eines grossen Materials kann sich ein Zusammenhang auch bei kleinen Unterschieden feststellen lassen.

Ta

Verteilung des Materials nach Geburtsgewicht, Abteilung, Jahre

Geburtsgewicht der Kinder	Abteilung		März—April—Mai							Juni—Juli—August						
			♂			♀			♂+♀	♂			♀			♂+
			Morg.	Abd.	Sa.	Morg.	Abd.	Sa.	Sa.	Morg.	Abd.	Sa.	Morg.	Abd.	Sa.	Sa.
2 200—3 099	Abt. I. Erste Mahlzeit 12 St. nach der Geburt		16	16	32	20	15	35	67	14	13	27	18	8	26	53
	Abt. II. Erste Mahlzeit 24 St. nach der Geburt	Ringer	20	14	34	26	26	52	86	9		9	23	10	33	42
		0 Ringer														
	Summe		36	30	66	46	41	87	153	23	13	36	41	18	59	95
3 100—3 699	Abt. I. Erste Mahlzeit 12 St. nach der Geburt		46	23	69	32	36	68	137	36	18	54	24	28	52	10[illegible]
	Abt. II. Erste Mahlzeit 24 St. nach der Geburt	Ringer	41	29	70	36	27	63	133	38	20	58	42	20	62	12[illegible]
		0 Ringer														
	Summe		87	52	139	68	63	131	270	74	38	112	66	48	114	22[illegible]
> 3 700	Abt. I. Erste Mahlzeit 12 St. nach der Geburt		31	29	60	18	18	36	96	37	16	53	27	19	46	9[illegible]
	Abt. II. Erste Mahlzeit 24 St. nach der Geburt	Ringer	27	21	48	28		28	76	18	18	36	19	11	30	6[illegible]
		0 Ringer														
	Summe		58	50	108	46	18	64	172	55	34	89	46	30	76	16[illegible]
Zusammenlegung 2 200—>3 700	Abteilung I		93	68	161	70	69	139	300	87	47	134	69	55	124	25[illegible]
	Abteilung II.	Ringer	88	64	152	90	53	143	295	65	38	103	84	41	125	22[illegible]
		0 Ringer														
	Summe		181	132	313	160	122	282	**595**	152	85	237	153	96	249	**48[illegible]**

Der behauptete Zusammenhang zwischen »schwerer Entbindung» und »Durstfieber» lässt eine Beziehung zwischen der Temperatur der Mutter sowie möglicherweise auch dem Geburtsgewicht des Kindes und der Dauer der Entbindung möglich erscheinen.

eit, Morgen- oder Abendobservation. Ohne Extra-Abt. II 0 Ringer.

Sept.—Okt.—Nov.							Dez.—Jan.—Febr.							*Zusammenlegung*		
♂			♀			♂+♀	♂			♀			♂+♀			
Morg.	Abd.	Sa.	Morg.	Abd.	Sa.	Sa.	Morg.	Abd.	Sa.	Morg.	Abd.	Sa.	Sa.	Sa. ♂	Sa. ♀	Sa. ♂+♀
13	19	32	18	16	34	66	15	19	34	36	37	73	107	125	168	293
			10	10	20	20		14	14		13	13	27	57	118	175
	14	14	10		10	24					16	16	16	14	26	40
13	33	46	38	26	64	110	15	33	48	36	66	102	150	196	312	**508**
34	23	57	38	34	72	129	42	35	77	64	49	113	190	257	305	562
29	13	42	18	16	34	76		31	31		21	21	52	201	180	381
19	16	35	19	15	34	69		25	25		28	28	53	60	62	122
…2	52	134	75	65	140	274	42	91	133	64	98	162	295	518	547	**1 065**
…2	17	49	13	23	36	85	44	29	73	35	21	56	129	235	174	409
…5		15	11		11	26		22	22				22	121	69	190
…0		20				20		22	22		16	16	38	42	16	58
…7	17	84	24	23	47	131	44	73	117	35	37	72	189	398	259	**657**
79	59	138	69	73	142	280	101	83	184	135	107	242	426	617	647	1 264
44	13	57	39	26	65	122		67	67		34	34	101	379	367	746
39	30	69	29	15	44	113		47	47		60	60	107	116	104	220
…2	102	264	137	114	251	**515**	101	197	298	135	201	336	**634**	**1 112**	**1 118**	**2 230**

Aus dem letztgenannten Grunde wurde auch die Dauer der Entbindung verzeichnet. Diese wurde nach der Länge der Wehenzeit bestimmt, in Stunden von dem Zeitpunkt an gerechnet, wo die Mutter das Einsetzen starker und anhaltender Wehen angab. Diese Angabe ist selbstverständlich subjektiv. Offenbar sinnlose oder zweifelhafte Angaben wurden nicht mitberücksichtigt.

Die Beobachtungszeit umfasst 6 Tage. Die starke Belegung der Entbindungsanstalt gestattete in der Regel keine längere Behandlungszeit als eine knappe Woche.

Die statistischen Berechnungen gründen sich auf nur eine Temperaturmessung pro Tag, und diese war stets dieselbe wie bei der ersten Messungsgelegenheit. Die Kinder wurden daher in »Morgen-» und »Abendkinder» eingeteilt, und zwar je nach dem Zeitpunkt der Geburt des Kindes, am Morgen oder am Abend. Für die Mütter der »Morgenkinder» wurden die Berechnungen auf Grund der Morgentemperatur der Mütter ausgeführt, für die Mütter der »Abendkinder» auf Grund der Abendtemperatur derselben.

Die Korrelationsberechnung wurde fast ganz, die übrige statistische Bearbeitung zum kleineren Teil in der Staatlichen rassenbiologischen Anstalt unter Kontrolle von Herrn Professor Gunnar Dahlberg bewerkstelligt. Bei der Bearbeitung des Materials wurde jede Unterabteilung für sich behandelt. Beobachtungen an weniger als 10 Individuen wurden statistischen Berechnungen nicht zugrunde gelegt. Namentlich während der ersten Lebenstage kam es vor, dass Beobachtungen verabsäumt wurden oder nicht rechtzeitig stattfanden. Die Anzahl Kinder, auf welche sich die Berechnungen gründen, variiert folglich an den einzelnen Lebenstagen und bei verschiedenen Arten von Beobachtungen.

Das Hauptmaterial besteht aus 2 230 Kindern und ihren Müttern. Hierzu kommen 251 Kinder in der Extra-Abt. II 0 Ringer während der Vierteljahre März—Mai und Juni—August. Insgesamt sind also 2 481 (2 230 + 251) Kinder beobachtet worden.

Das ganze Material, mit Ausnahme des Extramaterials in Abt. II 0 Ringer, ist in Tab. 2 zusammengestellt, und zwar nach Geburtsgewicht, Jahreszeit der Geburt, Geschlecht des Kindes und Zeitpunkt der ersten Temperaturmessung eingeteilt.

Die Verteilung auf verschiedene Jahreszeiten zeigt die niedrigste Kinderanzahl während des Vierteljahrs Juni—August und die höchste während Dezember—Februar, sehr dicht gefolgt von März—Mai. Die Anzahl der Geburten pflegt in Schweden in der Zeit März—Mai am höchsten und in der Zeit Oktober—Dezember am niedrigsten zu sein, mit einem kleineren Gipfel im September.

Die Verteilung auf Knaben und Mädchen ist fast die gleiche, nämlich 1 112 Knaben und 1 118 Mädchen. Würde sich die Geschlechtsverteilung bei der Geburt ganz genau widerspiegeln, so sollten statt dessen die Knaben etwas überwiegen. 1931—1940 wurden in Stockholm 1 065 Knaben pro 1 000 Mädchen geboren.

Die Morgenkinder bestehen aus 596 Knaben und 585 Mädchen oder insgesamt 1 181 Kindern. Die Abendkinder sind 516 Knaben und 533 Mädchen, zusammen 1 049 Kinder.

Was das Geburtsgewicht betrifft, so entfällt fast die halbe Anzahl Kinder (1 065) auf die Mittelgruppe (Geburtsgewicht zwischen 3 100 und 3 699 g). Bei den insgesamt 1 165 Kindern der beiden übrigen Gruppen überwiegt die Gruppe mit höherem Geburtsgewicht (657 Kinder mit Geburtsgewicht $>$ 3 700 g gegen 508 mit Geburtsgewicht 3 099—2 200 g). Kinder mit einem Geburtsgewicht $<$ 2 200 g wurden, wie bereits erwähnt, nicht mitberücksichtigt.

Die Gruppe Abt. II 0 Ringer fehlt während der Zeit März—August in der Tabelle. Abt. II wurde, wie oben angegeben ist, erst mit dem Beginn des Vierteljahrs September—November in Untergruppen geteilt. Während der Vierteljahre März—Mai und Juni—August gehören daher sämtliche Kinder in Abt. II zur Gruppe Abt. II Ringer. Diese ist folglich während der besagten Vierteljahre ungefähr ebenso gross wie Abt. I. Während der Vierteljahre September—November und Dezember—Februar nimmt sie um die Hälfte ab, und gleichzeitig kommt die Abt. II 0 Ringer hinzu.

Temperatur des Kindes.

Die Temperatur des Kindes beträgt am ersten Lebenstage 36,54°. Am zweiten Tage steigt sie auf 36,86° und am dritten

Tab. 3.

Temperatur des Kindes in den verschiedenen Abteilungen.
Gesamtmaterial ohne Extra-Abt. II 0 Ringer.

Tag	Gesamtmaterial			Abt. I			Abt. II. Ringer + 0 Ringer			Abt. II. Ringer			Abt. II. 0 Ringer		
	n	$M \pm \varepsilon(M)$	σ	n	$M \pm \varepsilon(M)$	σ	n	$M \pm \varepsilon(M)$	σ	n	$M \pm \varepsilon(M)$	σ	n	$M \pm \varepsilon(M)$	σ
1	1 736	36,54 ± 0,01	± 0,46	776	36,54 ± 0,02	± 0,53	960	36,54 ± 0,01	± 0,39	741	36,50 ± 0,01	± 0,37	219	36,55 ± 0,03	± 0,41
2	1 737	36,86 ± 0,01	± 0,44	775	36,94 ± 0,02	± 0,52	962	36,79 ± 0,01	± 0,35	743	36,78 ± 0,01	± 0,36	219	36,83 ± 0,02	± 0,30
3	2 173	36,90 ± 0,01	± 0,54	1 208	36,91 ± 0,02	± 0,59	965	36,88 ± 0,01	± 0,46	745	36,87 ± 0,02	± 0,49	220	36,91 ± 0,02	± 0,37
4	2 201	36,83 ± 0,01	± 0,57	1 236	36,82 ± 0,02	± 0,62	965	36,85 ± 0,02	± 0,50	745	36,84 ± 0,02	± 0,51	220	36,89 ± 0,03	± 0,43
5	2 195	36,66 ± 0,01	± 0,43	1 232	36,62 ± 0,01	± 0,47	963	36,72 ± 0,01	± 0,39	745	36,69 ± 0,01	± 0,39	218	36,83 ± 0,03	± 0,37
6	2 170	36,64 ± 0,01	± 0,35	1 222	36,60 ± 0,01	± 0,38	948	36,69 ± 0,01	± 0,34	732	36,67 ± 0,01	± 0,32	216	36,75 ± 0,02	± 0,31

Tab. 4.

Differenz in der Temperatur der Kinder von Tag zu Tag. Alle Abteilungen mit und ohne Extra-Abt. II 0 Ringer zusammengelegt.

Differenz zwischen Tag	Alle Abteilungen zusammengelegt ohne Extra-Abt. II 0 Ringer		Alle Abteilungen zusammengelegt mit Extra-Abt. II 0 Ringer	
1—2	+0,32 ± 0,014	* = 0,042	+0,28 ± 0,014	* = 0,042
2—3	+0,04 ± 0,014	* = 0,042	+0,10 ± 0,014	* = 0,042
3—4	−0,07 ± 0,014	* = 0,042	−0,14 ± 0,014	* = 0,042
4—5	−0,17 ± 0,014	* = 0,042	−0,16 ± 0,014	* = 0,042
5—6	−0,02 ± 0,014	* = 0,042	−0,01 ± 0,014	* = 0,042
1—3	+0,36 ± 0,014	* = 0,042	+0,38 ± 0,014	* = 0,042

* Dreif. mittl. Abw.

auf 36,90°. Dann sinkt die Temperatur wieder am 4. Tage auf 36,83°, um sich am 5. und 6. Tage bei etwa 36,65° zu stabilisieren.

Die Differenzen sind in Tab. 4 angegeben. Es wurde auch eine Berechnung angestellt, bei der das Extramaterial in Abt. II 0 Ringer mitberücksichtigt wurde (siehe Tab. 7).

Der Unterschied in der Körpertemperatur zwischen 1. und 2. Lebenstage beträgt 0,32 ± 0,014 und ist also gesichert. Der Unterschied zwischen 2. und 3. Tage macht im Hauptmaterial 0,04 ± 0,014 (dreifache mittlere Abweichung = 0,042) aus. Wird das Material mit der Extra-Abt. II 0 Ringer, Material von März —August, erweitert, so wird die Differenz zwischen 2. und 3. Tage 0,10 ± 0,014 (dreif. mittl. Abw. = 0,042). Sie ist also sicher. Die Temperatursenkung vom 3. zum 4. und vom 4. zum 5. Tage ist ebenfalls gesichert. Die Temperaturen am 5. und 6. Tage sind identisch. Die Temperatur stabilisiert sich. Dies spiegelt sich auch in dem während der letzteren Tage in sämtlichen Abteilungen niedrigen σ-Wert wider (Tab. 3).

Die Temperatursteigerung vom 1. zum 2. Tage ist erheblich, vom 2. zum 3. Tage ist sie bedeutend geringer. Die

Rückkehr zu niedrigeren Temperaturen ist umgekehrt vom 3. zum 4. Tage etwas weniger deutlich und vom 4. zum 5. Tage ausgesprochener.

Die Temperatur des Kindes ist also am 1. Tage niedrig. Sie weist dann eine rasche Steigerung zum 2. Lebenstage sowie eine weitere, aber geringere solche zum 3. Tage auf. Darauf sinkt die Temperatur mässig bis zum 4. Tage und steiler zum 5., um sich am 5. und 6. Lebenstage bei einem Niveau zu stabilisieren, welches etwas höher liegt als das Temperaturniveau des Geburtstages. Es besteht also eine Temperatursteigerung während der Zeit 2.—4. Lebenstag. Die gesamte Steigerung beträgt ungefähr 0,4°. Während des 1. Tages (bis 12 St. nach der Geburt) liegt ein gewisser Grad von Untertemperatur vor.

Die Variationsbreite hält sich während aller dieser 5 ersten Lebenstage bei ungefähr 0,5°. Die Temperatur erreicht also in der Regel kaum eine Höhe, welche man als Fieber bezeichnen könnte. Bei $^{2}/_{3}$ der Kinder überschreitet die Temperatur nämlich 37,5° nicht (am 3. Tage, wo sie höchstens $36{,}90 \pm 0{,}54$ beträgt). Sie kann jedoch 38,5° erreichen.

Temperatur des Kindes bei frühzeitiger Zufuhr von Nahrung und Flüssigkeit oder von Flüssigkeit allein sowie bei Nahrungs- und Flüssigkeitsabstinenz.

Wenn das Material in Abteilungen mit verschiedener Nahrungs- und Flüssigkeitszufuhr eingeteilt wird (Tab. 3), findet man in sämtlichen denselben prinzipiellen Verlauf. Die einzelnen Abteilungen untereinander weisen dagegen in bezug auf die Entwicklung dieses Verlaufs Unterschiede auf.

In Tab. 5 sind die Differenzen *innerhalb* jeder Abteilung von Tag zu Tag berechnet. Am 1. Tage ist die Temperatur, wie zu erwarten stand, in allen identisch. Während dieses »Tages» lag keinerlei Unterschied in bezug auf Nahrungs- und Flüssigkeitszufuhr vor. Der Kontrolltag zeigt also die Homogenität des Materials.

In Abt. I steigt dann die Temperatur rasch und erreicht

Tab. 5.

Differenz in der Temperatur der Kinder von Tag zu Tag *innerhalb* der verschiedenen Abteilungen ohne Extra-Abt. II 0 Ringer.

Differenz zwischen Tag	Abt. I		Abt. II Ringer + 0 Ringer		Abt. II Ringer		Abt. II 0 Ringer	
1—2	+ 0,40 ± 0,028	* = 0,084	+ 0,25 ± 0,014	* = 0,042	+ 0,28 ± 0,014	* = 0,042	+ 0,28 ± 0,036	* = 0,108
2—3	− 0,03 ± 0,028	* = 0,084	+ 0,09 ± 0,014	* = 0,042	+ 0,09 ± 0,022	* = 0,066	+ 0,08 ± 0,028	* = 0,084
3—4	− 0,09 ± 0,028	* = 0,084	− 0,03 ± 0,022	* = 0,066	− 0,03 ± 0,028	* = 0,084	− 0,02 ± 0,036	* = 0,108
4—5	− 0,20 ± 0,022	* = 0,066	− 0,13 ± 0,022	* = 0,066	− 0,15 ± 0,022	* = 0,066	− 0,06 ± 0,042	* = 0,126
5—6	− 0,02 ± 0,014	* = 0,042	− 0,03 ± 0,014	* = 0,042	− 0,02 ± 0,014	* = 0,042	− 0,08 ± 0,036	* = 0,108
1—3	+ 0,37 ± 0,028	* = 0,084	+ 0,34 ± 0,014	* = 0,042	+ 0,37 ± 0,022	* = 0,066	+ 0,36 ± 0,036	* = 0,108

* Dreif. mittl. Abw.

bereits während des 2. Lebenstages ihr Maximum. In dem zusammengelegten Material sowie in Abt. II ist dies erst während des 3. Tages der Fall. Andererseits sinkt die Temperatur in Abt. I wieder rascher als in Abt. II (Abb. 1).

Abb. 1 veranschaulicht den Verlauf der Temperaturkurve.

Die Temperaturdifferenz zwischen 2. und 3. Tage in Abt. I ist zu klein, als dass man sich darüber äussern könnte, ob

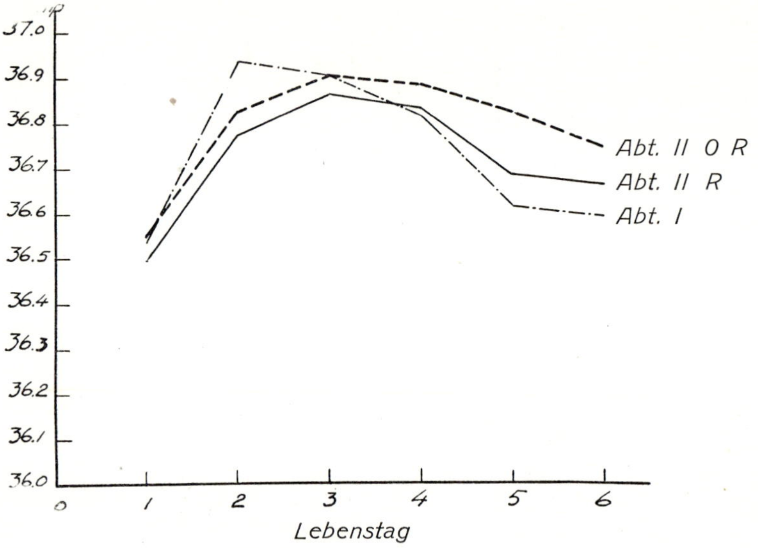

Abb. 1. Temperatur während der ersten 6 Lebenstage bei verschiedener Nahrungs- und Flüssigkeitszufuhr.

ein wirklicher Unterschied vorliegt. Die Differenz ist 0,03 ± 0,028. Dagegen sind die Differenzen zwischen 2. und 3. Tage in Abt. II, sowohl zusammengelegt wie in der Gruppe Abt. II Ringer, wenn diese für sich betrachtet wird, sicher. Die Differenz für Abt. II (Ringer + 0 Ringer) zwischen 2. und 3. Tage beträgt 0,09 ± 0,014 (dreif. mittl. Abw. = 0,042). Die Differenz für Abt. II Ringer zwischen 2. und 3. Tage macht 0,09 ± 0,022 (dreif. mittl. Abw. = 0,066) aus.

In der kleinsten Abteilung, Abt. II 0 Ringer, ist die Differenz zwischen 2. und 3. Tage 0,08 ± 0,028 (dreif. mitt. Abw.

Tab. 6.

Differenz in der Temperatur der Kinder zwischen verschiedenen Abteilungen Tag für Tag ohne Abt. II 0 Ringer.

Tag	Differenz zwischen							
	Abt. I—Abt. II Ringer + 0 Ringer		Abt. I.—Abt. II Ringer		Abt. I—Abt. II 0 Ringer		Abt. II Ringer—Abt. II 0 Ringer	
1	0 ± 0,022	* = 0,066	−0,04 ± 0,022	* = 0,066	+0,01 ± 0,036	* = 0,108	+0,05 ± 0,032	* = 0,096
2	−0,15 ± 0,022	* = 0,066	−0,16 ± 0,022	* = 0,066	−0,11 ± 0,028	* = 0,084	+0,05 ± 0,022	* = 0,066
3	−0,03 ± 0,022	* = 0,066	−0,04 ± 0,028	* = 0,084	0 ± 0,028	* = 0,084	+0,04 ± 0,028	* = 0,084
4	+0,03 ± 0,028	* = 0,084	+0,02 ± 0,028	* = 0,084	+0,07 ± 0,036	* = 0,108	+0,05 ± 0,028	* = 0 084
5	+0,10 ± 0,014	* = 0,042	+0,07 ± 0,014	* = 0,042	+0,21 ± 0,032	* = 0,096	+0,14 ± 0,032	* = 0,096
6	+0,09 ± 0,014	* = 0,042	+0,07 ± 0,014	* = 0,042	+0,15 ± 0,022	* = 0,066	+0,08 ± 0,032	* = 0,096

* Dreif. mittl. Abw.

= 0,084) und demnach praktisch gleich der dreifachen mittleren Abweichung.

In Tab. 6 sind die Differenzen *zwischen* den verschiedenen Abteilungen Tag für Tag angegeben.

Die Differenzen der Temperatur während des 2. Tages zwischen den Kindern in Abt. I und in beiden Gruppen der Abt. II sind gesichert. Die Differenz zwischen Abt. I und Abt. II (Ringer + 0 Ringer) beträgt 0,15 ± 0,022 (dreif. mittl. Abw. = 0,066), zwischen Abt. I und Abt. II Ringer 0,16 ± 0,022 (dreif. mittl. Abw. = 0,066) und zwischen Abt. I und Abt. II 0 Ringer 0,11 ± 0,028 (dreif. mittl. Abw. = 0,084).

Ein Vergleich zwischen Abt. II Ringer und Abt. II 0 Ringer ergibt, dass die Temperaturkurve während der ganzen Zeit bei derjenigen Gruppe, welche nicht eher als 24 St. nach der Geburt Nahrung oder Flüssigkeit erhalten hatte, ungefähr ½ Zehntelgrad höher liegt als bei der Gruppe, der schon nach 12 St. Ringersche Lösung zugeführt worden war. Die Gleichmässigkeit, mit welcher dies der Fall ist, fällt unleugbar in die Augen. Der Unterschied ist indessen bereits während des 1. Tages vorhanden, wo noch keine Verschiedenheit in bezug auf Nahrungs- oder Flüssigkeitszufuhr obwaltet. Statistisch liegt auch kein Unterschied vor. Die Differenz zwischen Abt. II Ringer und Abt. II 0 Ringer übersteigt praktisch nie die doppelte mittlere Abweichung. Dies ändert sich übrigens nicht, wenn das Extramaterial in Abt. II 0 Ringer mitberücksichtigt wird. Die Temperatur während des 3. Tages in der zusammengelegten Abt. II 0 Ringer wird 36,85° ± 0,02 und also numerisch etwas niedriger als in Abt. II Ringer.

Die Untersuchung liefert demnach das vielleicht etwas verblüffende Resultat, dass die Temperatursteigerung rascher bei Kindern eintritt, welche zuerst Nahrung und Flüssigkeit erhalten haben (Abt. I), und weniger rasch bei Nahrungs- und Flüssigkeitsabstinenz (Abt. II 0 Ringer). Flüssigkeitszufuhr allein verhindert das Einsetzen der Temperatursteigerung nicht und verringert auch nicht die Höhe derselben (Abt. II Ringer),

Es ist möglich, dass die Temperatur schon am 3. Tage zu sinken beginnt, wenn das Kind frühzeitig Nahrung erhält.

Bei Nahrungsabstinenz während der ganzen ersten 24 St. steigt die Temperatur dagegen auch während des 3. Tages und tut dies auch, wenn (lediglich) Flüssigkeit zugeführt wird.

Beim Temperaturfall ordnen sich die Abteilungen so, dass diejenige, in welcher am zeitigsten sowohl Flüssigkeit wie Nahrung gegeben wurde (Abt. I), den raschesten und ausgiebigsten Temperaturfall aufweist. Dann kommt die Abteilung mit nur Flüssigkeit (Abt. II Ringer), und die, in der weder Nahrung noch Flüssigkeit verabreicht wurde (Abt. II 0 Ringer), zeigt die langsamste Temperatursenkung und hat am 6. Tage noch die höchste Temperatur. Ob ein wirklicher Unterschied zwischen den beiden letzteren Abteilungen vorliegt, ist indessen aus denselben Gründen, wie sie oben hinsichtlich der Temperatursteigerung angeführt worden sind, ungewiss. Flüssigkeitszufuhr allein hat jedenfalls im Vergleich zur Zufuhr von Nahrung keinerlei Einfluss auf den Temperaturfall gehabt, ebensowenig wie auf die Temperatursteigerung.

Die Unterschiede in Temperatursteigerung und Temperaturfall *zwischen* den Abteilungen sind indessen viel kleiner als Steigerung und Fall von Tag zu Tag *innerhalb* der Abteilungen.

Temperatur des Kindes während verschiedener Jahreszeiten.

Eine Einteilung des Materials nach der Jahreszeit findet man in Tab. 7 und Abb. 2.

Die Temperaturkurven für die zusammengelegten verschiedenen Abteilungen weisen für jedes Vierteljahr für sich prinzipiell denselben Verlauf auf, wie wir ihn oben für das ganze Jahr kennengelernt haben. Der 1. Tag zeigt einen gewissen Grad von Untertemperatur, der 2. und 3. eine fortschreitende Temperatursteigerung. Zum 4. Tage sinkt die Temperatur, mit weiterem Fall auch bis zum 5. Tage. Am 5. und 6. Tage finden wir ungefähr dieselbe Temperatur; diese hat sich also stabilisiert.

Untereinander weisen indessen die verschiedenen Vierteljahre Unterschiede betreffs der Temperatur auf. Die Untertemperatur des 1. Tages ist während der Sommermonate geringer als während der übrigen Vierteljahre. Die Differenz

Tab.

Temperatur des Kindes während

Jahreszeit	Lebens- 1			2			3		
	n	$M \pm \varepsilon(M)$	σ	n	$M \pm \varepsilon(M)$	σ	n	$M \pm \varepsilon(M)$	σ
							Gesamtmaterial ohne		
März–Mai	405	36,53 ± 0,02	± 0,42	404	36,77 ± 0,02	± 0,43	582	36,85 ± 0,02	± 0,53
Juni–Aug.	326	36,60 ± 0,02	± 0,44	328	36,82 ± 0,02	± 0,40	453	36,86 ± 0,02	± 0,52
Sept.–Nov.	462	30,53 ± 0,02	± 0,46	461	36,92 ± 0,02	± 0,41	509	36,99 ± 0,02	± 0,56
Dez.–Febr.	543	36,51 ± 0,02	± 0,48	544	36,89 ± 0,02	± 0,49	629	36,89 ± 0,02	± 0,53
									Abt.
März–Mai	112	36,74 ± 0,04	± 0,42	110	36,86 ± 0,05	± 0,51	288	36,82 ± 0,05	± 0,53
Juni–Aug.	101	36,86 ± 0,06	± 0,55	101	36,88 ± 0,05	± 0,50	225	36,89 ± 0,04	± 0,57
Sept.–Nov.	227	36,48 ± 0,03	± 0,50	227	36,96 ± 0,03	± 0,46	274	37,01 ± 0,04	± 0,65
Dez.–Febr.	336	36,41 ± 0,03	± 0,52	337	36,97 ± 0,03	± 0,57	421	36,92 ± 0,03	± 0,59
						Abt. II Ringer + 0 Ringer			
März–Mai	293	36,45 ± 0,02	± 0,39	294	36,74 ± 0,02	± 0,38	294	36,88 ± 0,03	± 0,53
Juni–Aug.	225	36,49 ± 0,02	± 0,32	227	36,80 ± 0,02	± 0,34	228	36,83 ± 0,03	± 0,47
Sept.–Nov.	235	36,58 ± 0,03	± 0,42	234	36,89 ± 0,02	± 0,34	235	36,98 ± 0,03	± 0,43
Dez.–Febr.	207	36,68 ± 0,02	± 0,36	207	36,76 ± 0,02	± 0,27	208	36,83 ± 0,02	± 0,36
									Abt. II
März–Mai	293	36,45 ± 0,02	± 0,39	294	36,74 ± 0,02	± 0,38	294	36,88 ± 0,03	± 0,53
Juni–Aug.	225	36,49 ± 0,02	± 0,32	227	36,80 ± 0,02	± 0,34	228	36,83 ± 0,03	± 0,47
Sept.–Nov.	122	36,57 ± 0,04	± 0,42	121	36,90 ± 0,03	± 0,36	122	36,98 ± 0,04	± 0,48
Dez.–Febr.	101	36,63 ± 0,03	± 0,30	101	36,74 ± 0,03	± 0,27	101	36,83 ± 0,04	± 0,38
					Abt. II 0 Ringer.		*Während März—Mai*		
März–Mai*	132	36,72 ± 0,03	± 0,36	133	36,81 ± 0,02	± 0,28	132	36,80 ± 0,04	± 0,42
Juni–Aug.*	109	36,89 ± 0,04	± 0,40	114	36,72 ± 0,03	± 0,28	115	36,84 ± 0,03	± 0,37
Sept.–Nov.	113	36,58 ± 0,04	± 0,42	113	36,88 ± 0,03	± 0,32	113	36,99 ± 0,04	± 0,38
Dez.–Febr.	106	36,73 ± 0,04	± 0,39	106	36,77 ± 0,03	± 0,27	107	36,83 ± 0,03	± 0,33

* Extramaterial.

7.

verschiedener Jahreszeiten.

t a g								
4			5			6		
n	$M \pm \varepsilon(M)$	σ	n	$M \pm \varepsilon(M)$	σ	n	$M \pm \varepsilon(M)$	σ
Extra-Abt. II 0 Ringer.								
590	36,76 ± 0,02	± 0,52	587	36,61 ± 0,02	± 0,42	575	36,60 ± 0,02	± 0,37
468	36,79 ± 0,03	± 0,57	470	36,59 ± 0,02	± 0,38	468	36,60 ± 0,02	± 0,33
511	36,92 ± 0,03	± 0,58	511	36,78 ± 0,02	± 0,43	508	36,72 ± 0,02	± 0,39
632	36,86 ± 0,03	± 0,69	627	36,68 ± 0,02	± 0,46	619	36,64 ± 0,02	± 0,36
I.								
296	36,72 ± 0,03	± 0,50	293	36,57 ± 0,02	± 0,42	285	36,55 ± 0,02	± 0,35
240	36,75 ± 0,04	± 0,58	242	36,53 ± 0,03	± 0,41	242	36,54 ± 0,02	± 0,33
276	36,90 ± 0,04	± 0,66	276	36,72 ± 0,03	± 0,47	276	36,69 ± 0,03	± 0,45
424	36,89 ± 0,04	± 0,77	421	36,65 ± 0,02	± 0,50	419	36,62 ± 0,02	± 0,40
(ohne Extra-Abt. II 0 Ringer).								
294	36,80 ± 0,03	± 0,53	294	36,65 ± 0,02	± 0,42	290	36,65 ± 0,02	± 0,39
228	36,84 ± 0,04	± 0,55	228	36,66 ± 0,02	± 0,34	226	36,66 ± 0,02	± 0,32
235	36,95 ± 0,03	± 0,46	235	36,85 ± 0,02	± 0,37	232	36,77 ± 0,02	± 0,35
208	36,81 ± 0,03	± 0,38	206	36,74 ± 0,03	± 0,36	200	36,68 ± 0,02	± 0,24
Ringer.								
294	36,80 ± 0,03	± 0,53	294	36,65 ± 0,02	± 0,42	290	36,65 ± 0,02	± 0,39
228	36,84 ± 0,04	± 0,55	228	36,66 ± 0,02	± 0,34	226	36,66 ± 0,02	± 0,39
122	36,97 ± 0,05	± 0,51	122	36,84 ± 0,03	± 0,37	119	36,75 ± 0,03	± 0,36
101	36,77 ± 0,03	± 0,33	101	36,69 ± 0,03	± 0,32	97	36,65 ± 0,02	± 0,23
und Juni—Aug. »Extramaterial».								
130	36,72 ± 0,02	± 0,28	130	36,66 ± 0,02	± 0,26	130	36,65 ± 0,02	± 0,28
115	36,72 ± 0,03	± 0,27	115	36,66 ± 0,03	± 0,29	112	36,68 ± 0,02	± 0,23
113	36,93 ± 0,04	± 0,43	113	36,86 ± 0,03	± 0,35	113	36,78 ± 0,03	± 0,35
107	36,84 ± 0,04	± 0,43	105	36,79 ± 0,04	± 0,39	103	36,71 ± 0,03	± 0,26

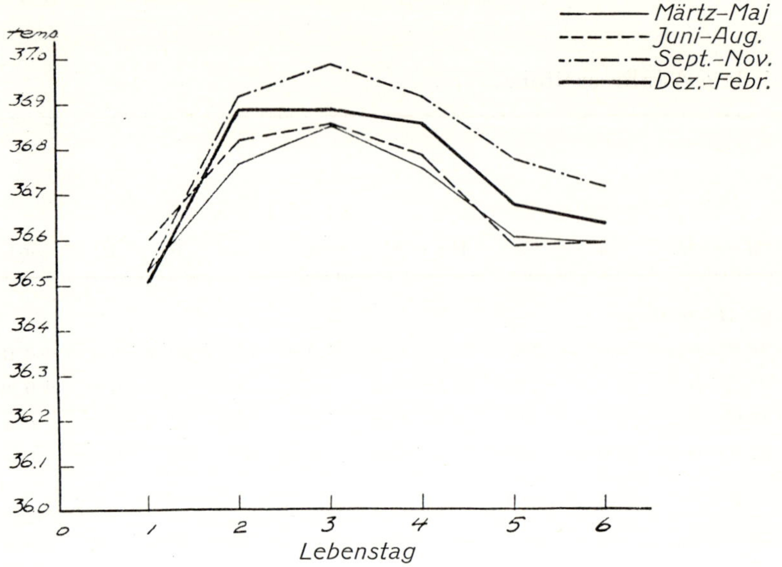

Abb. 2. Temperatur während der ersten 6 Lebenstage während verschiedener Jahreszeiten.

zwischen dem Vierteljahr Juni—August und dem eigentlichen Wintervierteljahr Dezember—Februar beträgt 0,09 ± 0,028 (dreif. mittl. Abw. = 0,084) und ist also gesichert. Während des folgenden Tages ist die Temperatur dagegen während des Herbstes, September—November, durchweg am höchsten. Später ist sie am höchsten während Dezember—Februar, niedriger während Juni—August und am allerniedrigsten während März —Mai (mit einer einzigen numerischen Ausnahme, nämlich

Tab.

Differenz in der Temperatur zwischen während März, April und Mai
(ohne Extra-Abt.

Lebens-					
1		2		3	
0 ± 0,028	* = 0,084	+ 0,15 ± 0,028	* = 0,084	+ 0,14 ± 0,028	* = 0,084

* Dreif. mittl. Abw.

dem 5. Tage, wo Juni—August numerisch einen niedrigeren Wert hat als März—Mai).

Die Temperatur ist also bis auf den 1. Tag während des Frühjahrs und Sommers niedriger als während des Herbstes und Winters.

Die Differenzen zwischen denjenigen Vierteljahren, welche die grössten Unterschiede aufweisen, nämlich September—November und März—Mai, sind gesichert (Tab. 8).

Die Temperatur liegt durchweg während des Herbstes ungefähr 0,15° höher als während des Frühjahrs.

Wenn das Material nach den entsprechenden Abteilungen eingeteilt wird, findet man in jeder Abteilung für sich das gleiche Verhalten, bis auf einzelne Tage, an welchen die Ordnung zufällig durchbrochen werden kann.

In Abt. II 0 Ringer, welche im Hauptmaterial während der Vierteljahre März—Mai und Juni—August fehlt, ist für die besagten beiden Vierteljahre das später gesammelte Material berücksichtigt worden. Besonders bemerkenswert ist, dass auch diese beiden Vierteljahre ebenso an die rechte Stelle kommen, als ob das Material in demselben Jahre wie das Hauptmaterial beobachtet worden wäre.

Es ist hervorzuheben, dass die Kinder in Abt. I vom 2. Tage an während sämtlicher Jahreszeiten eine höhere Temperatur haben als die Kinder in den übrigen Abteilungen. Der Faktor, welcher die in dieser Abteilung gegenüber den anderen höhere Temperatur verursacht, wirkt also unabhängig von der Jahreszeit.

8.

sowie während September, Oktober und November geborenen Kindern
II 0 Ringer).

tag					
4		5		6	
$+0{,}16 \pm 0{,}036$	$* = 0{,}108$	$+0{,}17 \pm 0{,}028$	$* = 0{,}084$	$+0{,}12 \pm 0{,}028$	$* = 0{,}084$

Tab.

Morgen- und Abendtemperatur des Kindes.

Material	Beobachtungszeit	Lebens- 1 $M \pm \varepsilon(M)$	1 σ	2 $M \pm \varepsilon(M)$	2 σ	3 $M \pm \varepsilon(M)$	3 σ
Sämtliche Gewichtsgruppen	Morgen	36,58 ± 0,015	± 0,47	36,87 ± 0,014	± 0,47	37,03 ± 0,015	± 0,51
	Abend	36,48 ± 0,015	± 0,42	36,84 ± 0,016	± 0,42	36,89 ± 0,013	± 0,41
	Differenz	−0,10 ± 0,021	* = 0,063	−0,03 ± 0,021	* = 0,063	−0,14 ± 0,020	* = 0,060

* Dreif. mittl. Abw.

Temperatur des Kindes bei Morgenbeobachtung und bei Abendbeobachtung.

»Morgenkinder» haben während der ersten 5 Lebenstage eine etwas höhere Temperatur als »Abendkinder». Der Unterschied erreicht an den meisten Tagen ungefähr 0,15°. Am 6. Tage erscheint der Unterschied ausgeglichen.

Temperatur des Kindes bei verschiedenem Geburtsgewicht.

Die Untersuchung wurde sowohl am Gesamtmaterial mit und ohne Extra-Abt. II 0 Ringer wie an Abt. I für sich ausgeführt (Tab. 10).

Die Temperatur ist an jedem einzelnen der 6 Beobachtungstage für sich durchweg um so höher, je grösser das Geburtsgewicht gewesen ist. Die Differenzen zwischen den Gruppen mit verschiedenem Geburtsgewicht sind überall gesichert (Tab. 11). Während des 6. Tages beträgt die Differenz zwischen den beiden Gruppen mit höchstem Geburtsgewicht (3 100—3 699 g und > 3 700 g) ganz unerheblich weniger als das Dreifache der mittleren Abweichung. Sonst sind die Differenzen stets grösser als die dreifache mittlere Abweichung. Eine Untersuchung der Kinder in Abt. I für sich ergibt ganz dasselbe Verhalten. Die Differenzen sind während früherer

9.

Gesamtmaterial ohne Extra-Abt. II 0 Ringer.

t a g					
4		5		6	
$M \pm \varepsilon (M)$	σ	$M \pm \varepsilon (M)$	σ	$M \pm \varepsilon (M)$	σ
36,90 ± 0,017	± 0,59	36,79 ± 0,011	± 0,39	36,65 ± 0,011	± 0,39
36,76 ± 0,017	± 0,53	36,64 ± 0,013	± 0,41	36,66 ± 0,010	± 0,33
− 0,14 ± 0,024	* = 0,072	− 0,15 ± 0,017	* = 0,051	+ 0,01 ± 0,015	* = 0,045

Lebenstage noch auffälliger und stärker hervortretend, wenn frühzeitig Nahrung zugeführt wird und also die Temperatursteigerung stark und zeitig eintritt, als in dem zusammengelegten Material.

Je grösser das Geburtsgewicht des Kindes ist, desto höher ist also die Temperatur desselben Tag für Tag während der ersten Lebenswoche, und je »normaler» die Verhältnisse sind, unter welchen es in bezug auf die Nahrungszufuhr lebt, desto ausgeprägter tritt der Unterschied hervor.

Dementsprechend könnte man erwarten, dass die Temperatursteigerung ihr Maximum um so rascher erreichen würde, je grösser das Geburtsgewicht des Kindes gewesen wäre. Eine gewisse Tendenz in dieser Richtung dürfte auch zu bemerken sein (Tab. 12). Die Differenzen sind aber zu klein, um eine bestimmte Schlussfolgerung zu gestatten.

Temperatur bei Knaben im Vergleich zu der bei Mädchen.

Knaben haben gewöhnlich ein höheres Geburtsgewicht als Mädchen. Dies ist auch im vorliegenden Material der Fall. Die Knaben sind prozentual in der niedrigsten, die Mädchen in der höchsten Geburtsgewichtsklasse am spärlichsten vertreten (Tab. 13).

Tab.

Temperatur des Kindes bei ver-

	Gewichtsgruppe	Lebens-								
		1			2			3		
		n	$M \pm \varepsilon(M)$	σ	n	$M \pm \varepsilon(M)$	σ	n	$M \pm \varepsilon(M)$	σ
Gesamtmaterial + Extra-Abt. II 0 Ringer	2200–3099	469	36,45 ± 0,02	± 0,48	472	36,67 ± 0,02	± 0,39	556	36,78 ± 0,02	± 0,36
	3100–3699	935	36,55 ± 0,01	± 0,42	938	36,85 ± 0,01	± 0,27	1158	36,92 ± 0,01	± 0,43
	3700 –>	573	36,69 ± 0,02	± 0,46	574	37,01 ± 0,02	± 0,44	706	37,11 ± 0,02	± 0,56
Gesamtmaterial ohne Extra-Abt. II 0 Ringer	2200–3099	406	36,41 ± 0,02	± 0,48	408	36,66 ± 0,02	± 0,41	492	36,80 ± 0,02	± 0,36
	3100–3699	826	36,52 ± 0,01	± 0,42	826	36,86 ± 0,01	± 0,41	1045	36,94 ± 0,01	± 0,43
	3700 –>	504	36,67 ± 0,02	± 0,46	503	37,02 ± 0,02	± 0,45	636	37,13 ± 0,02	± 0,55
Abt. I	2200–3099	194	36,39 ± 0,04	± 0,59	195	36,70 ± 0,04	± 0,51	277	36,91 ± 0,02	± 0,28
	3100–3699	326	36,51 ± 0,03	± 0,48	325	36,95 ± 0,03	± 0,50	543	37,01 ± 0,03	± 0,45
	3700 –>	256	36,69 ± 0,03	± 0,51	255	37,11 ± 0,03	± 0,49	388	37,14 ± 0,03	± 0,57

Das mittlere Gewicht beträgt für Knaben 3 532 ± 14 ($\sigma =$ 479) g, für Mädchen 3 370 ± 14 ($\sigma = 453$) g.

Der Unterschied ist 162 ± 20 g und demnach zugunsten der Knaben gesichert.

Da Kinder mit grösserem Geburtsgewicht höhere Temperatur haben als Kinder mit kleinerem, ist also zu erwarten, dass Knaben eine verhältnismässig etwas höhere Temperatur haben würden als Mädchen. Dies ist auch während sämtlicher Tage der Fall (Tab. 14).

10.

schiedenen Geburtsgewichten.

t a g								
4			5			6		
n	$M \pm \varepsilon(M)$	σ	n	$M \pm \varepsilon(M)$	σ	n	$M \pm \varepsilon(M)$	σ
558	36,61 ± 0,02	± 0,41	556	36,54 ± 0,01	± 0,34	554	36,56 ± 0,01	± 0,32
1171	36,80 ± 0,01	± 0,49	1171	36,65 ± 0,01	± 0,40	1154	36,67 ± 0,01	± 0,33
717	37,03 ± 0,02	± 0,65	713	36,79 ± 0,02	± 0,47	704	36,71 ± 0,01	± 0,39
496	36,62 ± 0,02	± 0,43	494	36,55 ± 0,02	± 0,36	493	36,55 ± 0,02	± 0,32
1058	36,81 ± 0,02	± 0,51	1059	36,65 ± 0,01	± 0,41	1043	36,68 ± 0,01	± 0,34
647	37,04 ± 0,03	± 0,68	642	36,79 ± 0,02	± 0,48	634	36,70 ± 0,02	± 0,40
281	36,61 ± 0,03	± 0,49	281	36,50 ± 0,02	± 0,37	281	36,53 ± 0,02	± 0,34
555	36,76 ± 0,03	± 0,56	556	36,59 ± 0,02	± 0,41	546	36,60 ± 0,02	± 0,42
400	37,02 ± 0,04	± 0,71	395	36,74 ± 0,03	± 0,50	395	36,65 ± 0,02	± 0,36

Der Unterschied ist überall gesichert, mit Ausnahme des ersten Tages (Tab. 15).

Um zu untersuchen ob irgendeine Geschlechtsdifferenz vorliegt, wurde auch an einer Gruppe mit *demselben* Geburtsgewicht eine Berechnung vorgenommen. Hierzu wurde die individuenreichste Gruppe mit dem Geburtsgewicht 3 100—3 699 g gewählt. Das Resultat war ganz dasselbe wie bei Zusammenlegung des gesamten Materials: die Knaben haben eine höhere Temperatur als die Mädchen. Die Tendenz ist

Tab.

Differenz in der Temperatur der Kinder während desselben

Gewichtsgruppe		Lebens- 1		2	
		Differenz	Dreif. mittl. Abw.	Differenz	Dreif. mittl. Abw.
Gesamtmaterial + Extra-Abt. II 0 Ringer	2200/3099= =3100/3699	+0,10 ± 0,022	0,066	+0,18 ± 0,022	0,066
	3100/3699= =3700/—>	+0,14 ± 0,022	0,066	+0,16 ± 0,022	0,066
	2200/3099= =3700/—>	+0,24 ± 0,028	0,084	+0,34 ± 0,028	0,084
Gesamtmaterial ohne Extra-Abt. II 0 Ringer	2200/3099= =3100/3699	+0,11 ± 0,028	0,084	+0,20 ± 0,024	0,072
	3100/3699= =3700/—>	+0,15 ± 0,028	0,075	+0,16 ± 0,024	0,072
	2200/3099= =3700/—>	+0,26 ± 0,032	0,096	+0,36 ± 0,028	0,084
Abt. I	2200/3099= =3100/3699	+0,12 ± 0,050	0,150	+0,25 ± 0,050	0,150
	3100/3699= =3700/—>	+0,18 ± 0,042	0,126	+0,16 ± 0,042	0,126
	2200/3099= =3700/—>	+0,30 ± 0,050	0,150	+0,41 ± 0,050	0,150

11.

Tages zwischen Gruppen mit verschiedenem Geburtsgewicht.

a g							
3		4		5		6	
Differenz	Dreif. mittl. Abw.	Differenz	Dreif. mittl. Abw.	Differenz	Dreif. mittl. Abw.	Differenz	Dreif. mittl. Abw.
+ 0,14 ± 0,022	0,066	+ 0,19 ± 0,022	0,066	+ 0,11 ± 0,014	0,042	+ 0,11 ± 0,014	0,042
+ 0,19 ± 0,022	0,066	+ 0,23 ± 0,022	0,066	+ 0,14 ± 0,022	0,066	+ 0,04 ± 0,014	0,042
+ 0,33 ± 0,028	0,084	+ 0,42 ± 0,028	0,084	+ 0,25 ± 0,022	0,066	+ 0,15 ± 0,014	0,042
+ 0,14 ± 0,021	0,063	+ 0,19 ± 0,025	0,075	+ 0,10 ± 0,021	0,063	+ 0,13 ± 0,019	0,057
+ 0,19 ± 0,026	0,078	+ 0,23 ± 0,031	0,093	+ 0,14 ± 0,023	0,069	+ 0,02 ± 0,019	0,057
+ 0,33 ± 0,027	0,081	+ 0,42 ± 0,033	0,099	+ 0,24 ± 0,025	0,075	+ 0,15 ± 0,021	0,063
+ 0,10 ± 0,036	0,108	+ 0,18 ± 0,042	0,126	+ 0,09 ± 0,028	0,084	+ 0,07 ± 0,028	0,084
+ 0,13 ± 0,042	0,126	+ 0,23 ± 0,050	0,150	+ 0,13 ± 0,036	0,108	+ 0,05 ± 0,028	0,084
+ 0,23 ± 0,036	0,108	+ 0,41 ± 0,050	0,150	+ 0,24 ± 0,036	0,108	+ 0,12 ± 0,028	0,084

Tab. 12.

Differenz in der Temperatur der Kinder zwischen verschiedenen Tagen innerhalb Gruppen mit demselben Geburtsgewicht. Gesamtmaterial mit Extra-Abt. II 0 Ringer.

Gewichts-gruppen	Differenz zwischen Lebenstag									
	1—2		2—3		3—4		4—5		5—6	
	Differenz	Dreif. mittl. Abw.	Differenz	Dreif. mittl. Abw.	Differenz	Dreif. mittl. Abw.	Differenz	Dreif. mittl. Abw.	Differenz	Dreif. mittl. Abw.
2200—3099	+0,22 ± 0,028	0,084	+0,11 ± 0,028	0,084	−0,17 ± 0,028	0,084	−0,07 ± 0,022	0,066	+0,02 ± 0,014	0,042
3100—3699	+0,30 ± 0,014	0,042	+0,07 ± 0,014	0,042	−0,12 ± 0,014	0,042	−0,15 ± 0,014	0,042	+0,02 ± 0,014	0,042
3700—>	+0,32 ± 0,028	0,084	+0,10 ± 0,028	0,084	−0,08 ± 0,028	0,084	−0,24 ± 0,028	0,084	−0,08 ± 0,022	0,066

Tab. 13.

Verteilung auf Geschlechter nach dem Geburtsgewicht ohne Extra-Abt. II 0 Ringer.

Geburtsgewicht	Anzahl		%		Mittl. Gewicht		Differenz ♂—♀
	♂	♀	♂	♀	♂	♀	
2200—3099	196	312	17,6	27,9	2 845,5 ± 17,5	2 839,2 ± 15,8	− 6,3 ± 23,6
3100—3699	518	547	46,6	48,9	3 409,0 ± 7,5	3 383,4 ± 7,0	−25,6 ± 10,3
3700—>	398	259	35,8	**23,2**	4 028,9 ± 14,2	3 983,1 ± 15,5	−45,8 ± 21,0
Gesamtmaterial	1 112	1 118	100,0	100,0	3 531,6 ± 14,2	3 370,5 ± 13,6	−161,1 ± 19,7

nicht zu verkennen. Am 3. Tage, wo der Temperaturunterschied am grössten ist, ist die Differenz auch in dem begrenzten Material, welches diese Gruppe darstellt, gesichert. Es könnte also den Anschein erwecken, als ob eine geschlechtsbedingte Differenz vorläge. Eine Untersuchung des Geburtsgewichts der Knaben und Mädchen in der Gruppe ergibt jedoch, dass sich die Mädchen vorzugsweise in der unteren und die Knaben in der oberen Klassenhälfte gruppieren. Das mittlere Gewicht beträgt in der Gruppe der Knaben $3\,409 \pm 7{,}5$ ($\sigma = 171$) g, in der der Mädchen $3\,383 \pm 7{,}0$ ($\sigma = 172$) g (siehe Tab. 13). Die Differenz ist 26 ± 10 g (= 2,6fache mittl. Abw.).

Die Abweichung in der Temperatur geht in dieselbe Richtung, wie es der Unterschied im Geburtsgewicht verursachen muss. Es ist also anzunehmen, dass die höhere Temperatur der Knaben mit dem höheren Geburtsgewicht derselben zusammenhängt und nicht auf einer geschlechtsbedingten Verschiedenheit beruht.

Das Geburtsgewicht der Knaben ist in jeder Gewichtsgruppe für sich durchweg höher. Der Unterschied wird um so grösser, je schwerere Kinder die Gewichtsgruppe enthält. Knaben mit extrem hohem Geburtsgewicht sind also häufiger als Mädchen mit ungewöhnlich hohem Geburtsgewicht.

Verteilung der Kinder nach dem Geburtsgewicht während verschiedener Jahreszeiten.

Die Beziehung zwischen Geburtsgewicht und Temperatursteigerung macht eine Untersuchung über das Geburtsgewicht der Kinder während verschiedener Jahreszeiten erforderlich, um zu ergründen, ob der nachgewiesenen höheren Temperatur während des Vierteljahrs September—November ein grösseres Geburtsgewicht bei während dieses Vierteljahrs geborenen Kindern entspricht.

Eine Berechnung der prozentualen Verteilung des Materials auf die betreffenden Vierteljahre mit Rücksicht auf das Geburtsgewicht (Tab. 16) spricht nicht dafür, dass das Geburts-

Tab

Temperatur bei Knaben im Vergleich zu Mädchen. Gesamtmateria
Extra-Abt. I

Abt.	Geschlecht	L e b e n s								
		1			2			3		
		n	$M \pm \varepsilon(M)$	σ	n	$M \pm \varepsilon(M)$	σ	n	$M \pm \varepsilon(M)$	σ
Gesamt-material	♂	886	36,55 ± 0,015	± 0,45	884	36,91 ± 0,015	± 0,43	1 090	37,04 ± 0,014	± 0,46
	♀	850	36,53 ± 0,016	± 0,46	853	36,80 ± 0,015	± 0,45	1 083	36,89 ± 0,015	± 0,49
Geburts-gewicht 3 100—3 699	♂	415	36,52 ± 0,019	± 0,38	414	36,89 ± 0,021	± 0,42	511	37,06 ± 0,025	± 0,57
	♀	411	36,52 ± 0,022	± 0,45	412	36,83 ± 0,020	± 0,40	534	36,82 ± 0,021	± 0,48

Tab

Differenz in der Temperatur zwischen Knaben und Mädchen währen
gewicht 3 100—3 699 ohn

Abt.	Geschlecht	L e b e n s					
		1		2		3	
		$M \pm \varepsilon(M)$	Dreif. mittl. Abw.	$M \pm \varepsilon(M)$	Dreif. mittl. Abw.	$M \pm \varepsilon(M)$	Dreif. mittl. Abw.
Gesamt-material	Diff. ♂—♀	−0,02 ± 0,022	0,066	−0,11 ± 0,021	0,063	−0,15 ± 0,021	0,063
Geburtsgewicht 3 100—3 699	Diff. ♂—♀	0 ± 0,029	0,087	−0,06 ± 0,029	0,087	−0,24 ± 0,032	0,096

gewicht während des Vierteljahrs September—November höher wäre als in anderen.

Die Berechnung des mittleren Gewichts bei der Geburt während verschiedener Jahreszeiten führt zu demselben Resultat (Tab. 17).

Der Unterschied im Geburtsgewicht während verschiedener

14.

sowie Kinder mit Geburtsgewicht 3 100—3 699 für sich ohne 0 Ringer.

t a g								
4			5			6		
n	$M \pm \varepsilon(M)$	σ	n	$M \pm \varepsilon(M)$	σ	n	$M \pm \varepsilon(M)$	σ
1 103	36,89 ± 0,018	± 0,59	1 100	36,71 — 0,014	± 0,45	1 086	36,70 ± 0,011	± 0,37
1 098	36,78 ± 0,016	± 0,54	1 095	36,62 ± 0,012	± 0,41	1 084	36,61 ± 0,011	± 0,35
517	36,85 ± 0,022	± 0,51	518	36,68 ± 0,019	± 0,43	510	36,72 ± 0,017	± 0,38
541	36,78 ± 0,021	± 0,50	541	36,61 ± 0,017	± 0,40	533	36,63 ± 0,015	± 0,35

15.

verschiedener Tage. Gesamtmaterial sowie Kinder mit Geburts- Extra-Abt. II 0 Ringer.

t a g					
4		5		6	
$M \pm \varepsilon(M)$	Dreif. mittl. Abw.	$M \pm \varepsilon(M)$	Dreif. mittl. Abw.	$M \pm \varepsilon(M)$	Dreif. mittl. Abw.
—0,11 ± 0,024	0,072	—0,09 ± 0,018	0,054	—0,09 ± 0,016	0,048
—0,07 ± 0,030	0,090	—0,07 ± 0,026	0,078	—0,09 ± 0,023	0,069

Vierteljahre ist nicht grösser, als dass er zufallsbedingt sein könnte.

Der Unterschied zwischen dem Geburtsgewicht der Kinder im Vierteljahr März—Mai, wo dasselbe am niedrigsten, und Juni—August, wo es am höchsten ist, beträgt 64 ± 29 g und ist also nicht gesichert. Numerisch ist das Geburtsgewicht

Tab. 16.

Prozentuale Verteilung der Kinder nach dem Geburtsgewicht auf verschiedene Jahreszeiten ohne Extra-Abt. II 0 Ringer.

Jahreszeit	Geburtsgewicht					
	2 200—3 099		3 100—3 699		3 700—>	
	n	%	n	%	n	%
März—Mai	153	25,71	270	45,38	172	28,91
Juni—August	95	19,55	226	46,50	165	33,95
September—November	110	21,36	274	53,20	131	25,44
Dezember—Februar	150	23,66	295	46,53	189	29,81

Tab. 17.

Geburtsgewicht der Kinder während verschiedener Jahreszeiten ohne Extra-Abt. II 0 Ringer. Knaben und Mädchen.

Jahreszeit	$M \pm \varepsilon(M)$	σ
März—Mai	3 429 ± 19	± 471
Juni—August	3 493 ± 22	± 477
September—November	3 440 ± 20	± 451
Dezember—Februar	3 448 ± 19	± 488

am nächstniedrigsten während September—November. Die höhere Temperatur während dieses Vierteljahrs wird also nicht von einem höheren Geburtsgewicht erklärt.

Änderungen im Gewicht des Kindes.

Die Gewichtsveränderungen, welche das Kind durchmacht, werden selbstverständlich von mehreren Faktoren bedingt, wie u. a. Abgang von Mekonium, Stuhl, Flüssigkeitsverlust und umgekehrt vom Wachstum. Man kann natürlich erwägen, ob

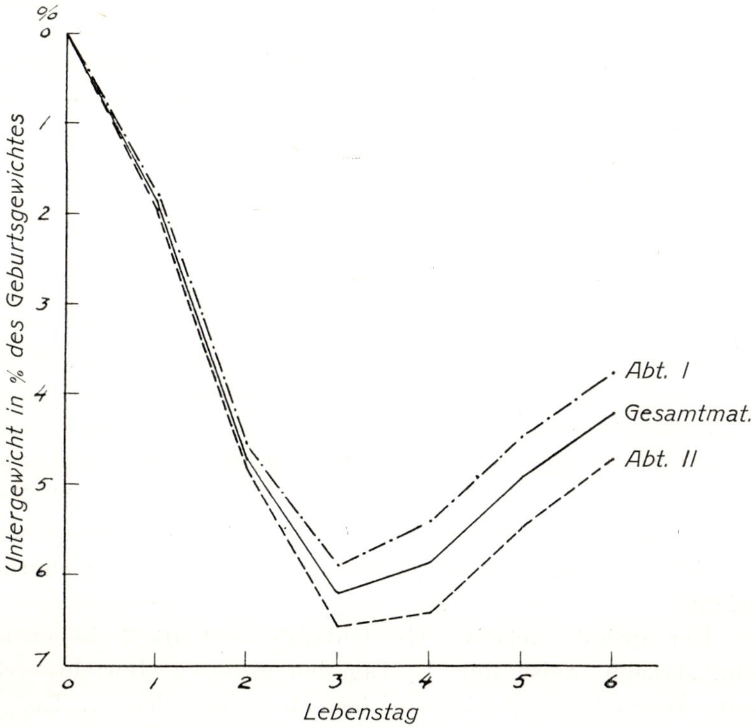

Abb. 3 a. Untergewicht in % des Geburtsgewichts (Gewichtsfall und Gewichtszunahme) während der ersten 6 Lebenstage bei verschiedener Nahrungs- und Flüssigkeitszufuhr.

und bis zu welchem Grade diese Faktoren von dem Geburtsgewicht des Kindes abhängig sind. Eine Berechnung des Gewichtsverlusts bezogen auf das Geburtsgewicht gibt jedenfalls einen plausiblen Ausgangspunkt. Die Änderungen des Gewichts sind daher in % des Geburtsgewichts berechnet worden.

Während der 3 ersten Lebenstage sinkt das Gewicht Tag für Tag (Tab. 18). Am 4. Tage beginnt es allmählich wieder zu steigen, und dieser Anstieg setzt sich während der beiden weiteren Tage der Beobachtungszeit fort. Insgesamt büsst das Kind etwa 6 % seines Geburtsgewichts ein. Die Steigerung ist langsamer als der Gewichtsfall, so dass noch am 6. Tage

T

Gewichtsveränderungen des Kindes in % des Geburtsgewic

Tag	Gesamtmaterial				Abt. I			
	Gewichtsveränderung			Untergewicht	Gewichtsveränderung			Unter gewic
	n	$M \pm \varepsilon(M)$	σ		n	$M \pm \varepsilon(M)$	σ	
1	1 736	−1,86 ± 0,04	± 1,71	1,86 ± 0,04	776	−1,78 ± 0,07	± 1,90	1,78 ± 0,
2	1 737	−2,82 ± 0,04	± 1,60	4,68 ± 0,06	775	−2,77 ± 0,06	± 1,78	4,55 ± 0
3	2 173	−1,53 ± 0,04	± 1,65	6,21 ± 0,07	1 208	−1,35 ± 0,05	± 1,68	5,90 ± 0
4	2 201	+0,35 ± 0,03	± 1,56	5,86	1 236	+0,48 ± 0,05	± 1,61	5,42
5	2 195	+0,94 ± 0,03	± 1,60	4,92	1 232	+0,95 ± 0,04	± 1,44	4,47
6	2 170	+0,75 ± 0,03	± 1,49	4,17	1 222	+0,74 ± 0,04	± 1,40	3,73

erst $^1/_3$ desselben eingeholt ist (Abb. 3 a). Das Untergewicht beträgt m. a. W. noch am 6. Tage ungefähr 4 % des Geburtsgewichts.

Der grösste relative Gewichtsfall tritt am 2. Lebenstage ein, danach weist der 1. Tag den grössten Gewichtsverlust auf. Hierbei ist jedoch zu beachten, dass der »1. Tag» im Material in Wirklichkeit durchschnittlich nur etwa 12 St. umfasst. Während des 3. Tages sinkt das Gewicht am wenigsten. Das Wiedereinholen des Gewichts ist am 4. Tage am kleinsten und am 5. am grössten. Am 6. Tage ist dasselbe kleiner als am 5., aber wesentlich grösser als am 4.

Bei einer Einteilung nach Abteilungen findet man denselben prinzipiellen Verlauf in bezug auf die Gewichtsveränderungen wieder (Tab. 18). Aus der Tabelle werden teils die Gewichtsveränderungen und teils das Untergewicht des Kindes im Verhältnis zum Geburtsgewicht Tag für Tag ersichtlich.

Die Gewichtsabnahme ist in allen Abteilungen während des 2. Tages am grössten, dann folgt der 1. Tag, und am 3. ist sie am kleinsten. Die Differenzen sind überall gesichert (Tab. 19).

Innerhalb der verschiedenen Abteilungen erfolgt indessen

8.

esamtmaterial ohne Extra-Abt. II 0 Ringer.

Abt. II Ringer + 0 Ringer				Abt. II Ringer				Abt. II 0 Ringer			
ewichtsveränderung			Untergewicht	Gewichtsveränderung			Untergewicht	Gewichtsveränderung			Untergewicht
n	$M \pm \varepsilon(M)$	σ		n	$M \pm \varepsilon(M)$	σ		n	$M \pm \varepsilon(M)$	σ	
60	$-1,93 \pm 0,05$	$\pm 1,54$	$1,93 \pm 0,05$	741	$-1,88 \pm 0,06$	$\pm 1,51$	$1,88 \pm 0,06$	219	$-2,09 \pm 0,11$	$\pm 1,63$	$2,09 \pm 0,11$
62	$-2,87 \pm 0,05$	$\pm 1,44$	$4,80 \pm 0,07$	743	$-2,84 \pm 0,05$	$\pm 1,40$	$4,72 \pm 0,08$	219	$-2,97 \pm 0,11$	$\pm 1,57$	$5,06 \pm 0,16$
65	$-1,75 \pm 0,05$	$\pm 1,57$	$6,55 \pm 0,09$	745	$-1,66 \pm 0,06$	$\pm 1,56$	$6,38 \pm 0,10$	220	$-2,05 \pm 0,10$	$\pm 1,55$	$7,11 \pm 0,18$
65	$+0,17 \pm 0,05$	$\pm 1,55$	6,38	745	$+0,19 \pm 0,06$	$\pm 1,55$	6,19	220	$+0,13 \pm 0,10$	$\pm 1,48$	6,98
63	$+0,94 \pm 0,04$	$\pm 1,30$	5,44	745	$+0,97 \pm 0,05$	$\pm 1,25$	5,22	218	$+0,84 \pm 0,10$	$\pm 1,44$	6,14
48	$+0,76 \pm 0,04$	$\pm 1,25$	4,68	732	$+0,75 \pm 0,04$	$\pm 1,21$	4,47	216	$+0,79 \pm 0,09$	$\pm 1,28$	5,35

weder die Abnahme noch die Wiederherstellung des Gewichts in gleichem Umfang oder mit derselben Geschwindigkeit.

Am deutlichsten geht dies aus Abb. 3 b und Tab. 20 hervor.

In der Tabelle wird das Untergewicht während der verschiedenen Tage bei Kindern in den einzelnen Abteilungen vergleichsweise dargestellt.

Während des Kontrolltages (1. Tag) ist, ebenso wie es betreffs der Temperatur der Fall war, die Gewichtsabnahme

Tab. 19.

Differenz im prozentualen Gewichtsfall während verschiedener Tage in den einzelnen Abteilungen. Ohne Extra-Abt. II 0 Ringer.

Differenz zwischen Tag	Gesamtmaterial	Abt. I	Abt. II Ringer + 0 Ringer	Abt. II Ringer	Abt. II 0 Ringer
1—2	$+0,96 \pm 0,06$	$+0,99 \pm 0,09$	$+0,94 \pm 0,07$	$+0,96 \pm 0,08$	$+0,88 \pm 0,16$
2—3	$-1,29 \pm 0,06$	$-1,42 \pm 0,08$	$-1,12 \pm 0,07$	$-1,18 \pm 0,08$	$+0,92 \pm 0,15$
1—3	$-0,33 \pm 0,06$	$-0,43 \pm 0,09$	$-0,18 \pm 0,07$	$-0,22 \pm 0,08$	$-0,04 \pm 0,15$

Tab. 20.

Differenz im Untergewicht zwischen den einzelnen Abteilungen während verschiedener Tage in % des Geburtsgewichts (ohne Extra-Abt. II 0 Ringer).

Tag	Differenzen							
	Abt. I—Abt. II Ringer + 0 Ringer		Abt. I—Abt. II Ringer		Abt. I—Abt. II 0 Ringer		Abt. II Ringer—Abt. II 0 Ringer	
1	−0,15 ± 0,09	* = 0,27	−0,10 ± 0,09	* = 0,27	−0,31 ± 0,13	* = 0,39	−0,21 ± 0,13	* = 0,39
2	−0,25 ± 0,11	* = 0,33	−0,17 ± 0,12	* = 0,36	−0,51 ± 0,18	* = 0,54	−0,34 ± 0,17	* = 0,51
3	−0,65 ± 0,13	* = 0,39	−0,48 ± 0,14	* = 0,42	−1,21 ± 0,21	* = 0,63	−0,73 ± 0,21	* = 0,63

* Dreif. mittl. Abw.

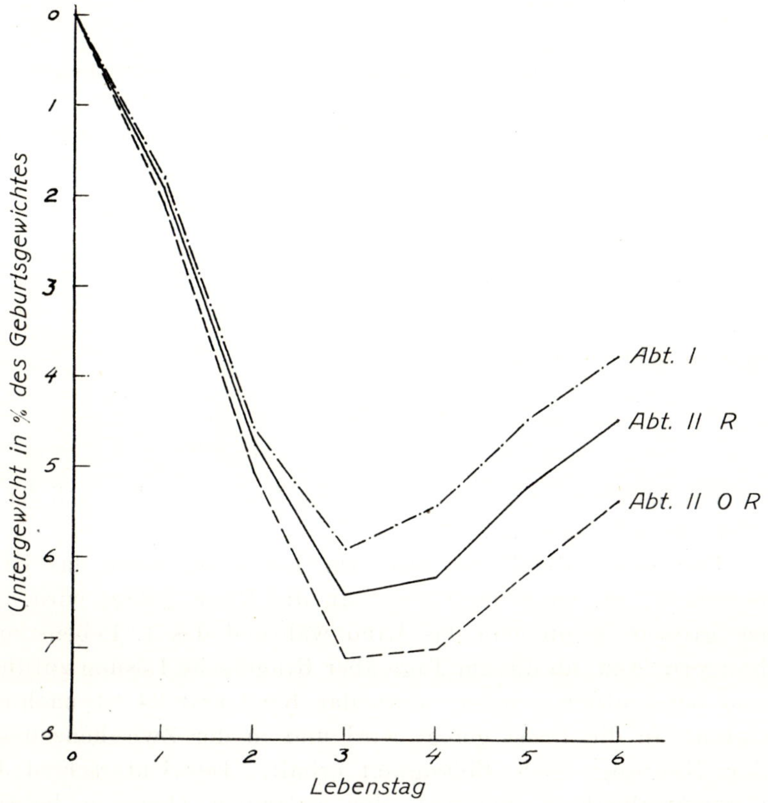

Abb. 3 b. Untergewicht in % des Geburtsgewichts (Gewichtsfall und Gewichtszunahme) während der ersten 6 Lebenstage bei verschiedener Nahrungs- und Flüssigkeitszufuhr.

in allen Abteilungen die gleiche. Das Untergewicht wird daher in allen dasselbe.

Auch während des 2. Tages liegt kein sicherer Unterschied zwischen den Abteilungen hinsichtlich des Untergewichts vor. Dagegen tritt ein sicherer solcher am 3. Tage in Erscheinung.

Die gesamte Gewichtsabnahme während des 1.—3. Tages beträgt für das ganze Material zusammen in % des Geburtsgewichts

$$6{,}21 \pm 0{,}07\ \%;$$

in Abt. I macht die zusammengerechnete Gewichtsabnahme

$$5{,}90 \pm 0{,}10\ \%,$$

in Abt. II (Ringer + 0 Ringer zusammengelegt)

$$6{,}55 \pm 0{,}09\ \%,$$

in Abt. II Ringer

$$6{,}38 \pm 0{,}10\ \%,$$

und in Abt. II 0 Ringer

$$7{,}11 \pm 0{,}18\ \%,$$

aus.

Die Differenzen in bezug auf das Untergewicht am 3. Tage sind überall gesichert.

Der Gewichtsfall ist also am kleinsten, wenn das Kind bereits 12 St. nach der Geburt an die Brust gelegt wird. Er ist grösser, wenn man das Kind während des 1. Lebenstages hungern lässt, an diesem Tage aber Ringersche Lösung zuführt, und beträchtlich grösser, wenn das Kind erst 24 St. nach der Geburt an die Brust gelegt wird und in der Zwischenzeit weder Nahrung noch Flüssigkeit erhält. Der Unterschied der Gewichtsabnahme zwischen den extremen Gruppen beträgt 20 % der Abnahme in derjenigen Abteilung, welche den geringsten Gewichtsfall aufweist. Das durchschnittliche Geburtsgewicht ist für Knaben und Mädchen zusammen $3\,458 \pm 9$ ($\sigma = 448$) g. Der Unterschied in der Gewichtsabnahme zwischen Abt. II Ringer und 0 Ringer wird, absolut betrachtet, $\frac{0{,}73}{100} \cdot 3\,458 = 25{,}2$ g. Der Unterschied in der Gewichtsabnahme entspricht also nur ungefähr der Hälfte der Menge zugeführte Ringersche Lösung (ca. 50 g).

Der Wiedergewinn des Gewichts zeigt denselben Unterschied zwischen den Abteilungen wie die Gewichtsabnahme. Am 6. Tage betragen Untergewicht und Wiedergewinn in % des Geburtsgewichts:

in Abt. I	Untergewicht	3,73 %,	Wiedergewinn	2,17 %
» » II (Ringer + 0 Ringer)	»	4,68 »	»	1,87 »
» » II Ringer	»	4,47 »	»	1,91 »
» » II 0 Ringer	»	5,35 »	»	1,76 »

Der Wiedergewinn erfolgt auch, prozentual betrachtet, in derjenigen Gruppe erheblich rascher, in welcher die Kinder schon während des 1. Tages an die Brust gelegt wurden, als in den Gruppen, wo Nahrung erst vom 2. Tage an zugeführt worden war (Abt. II). Das zusammengelegte Material nimmt daher eine Mittelstellung zwischen Abt. I und Abt. II ein.

Die Kinder in Abt. II Ringer gewinnen ihr Gewicht rascher wieder als die Kinder in Abt. II 0 Ringer (siehe Abb. 3 b).

Die Gewichtszunahme weist also in den verschiedenen Abteilungen einen der Abnahme entsprechenden, wenn auch umgekehrten, Verlauf auf. Je früher Nahrung und Flüssigkeit zugeführt werden, desto rascher steigt das Gewicht.

Gewichtsveränderungen des Kindes während verschiedener Jahreszeiten.

Die Gewichtsveränderungen während verschiedener Jahreszeiten lassen denselben prinzipiellen Verlauf erkennen wie bei Zusammenlegung des Materials für das ganze Jahr (Tab. 21).

Das Gewicht sinkt während aller Vierteljahre Tag für Tag während der 3 ersten Tage. Die Abnahme ist am grössten während des 2. Tages, dann folgt der 1. Tag und zuletzt der 3. Eine einzige Ausnahme könnte möglicherweise bestehen, nämlich das Vierteljahr Dezember—Februar, wo der 1. Tag eine geringere Gewichtsabnahme aufweist als der 3. Die Differenz ist indessen kleiner als die doppelte mittlere Abweichung ($0{,}18 \pm 0{,}099$). Der Unterschied ist also zufallsbetont.

Das grösste zusammengelegte Untergewicht tritt am 3. Tage auf. Während des 4.—6. Tages steigt das Gewicht überall. Die Zunahme ist am grössten während des 5. Tages, dann kommt der 6. und zuletzt der 4. Tag.

T

Gewichtsveränderungen des Kindes während verschiede

Jahreszeit	Leben											
	1				2				3			
	n	$M \pm \varepsilon(M)$	σ	Untergewicht	n	$M \pm \varepsilon(M)$	σ	Untergewicht	n	$M \pm \varepsilon(M)$	σ	Un gew
												Gesamtmaterial
März–Mai	405	−2,02 ± 0,08	± 1,62	2,02	404	−2,68 ± 0,07	± 1,48	4,70	582	−1,84 ± 0,07	± 1,58	6
Juni–Aug.	326	−2,29 ± 0,09	± 1,62	2,29	328	−2,71 ± 0,07	± 1,33	5,00	453	−1,25 ± 0,08	± 1,60	6
Sept.–Nov.	462	−1,68 ± 0,08	± 1,79	1,68	461	−3,04 ± 0,08	± 1,78	4,72	509	−1,62 ± 0,07	± 1,69	6
Dez.–Febr.	543	−1,65 ± 0,07	± 1,71	1,65	544	−2,82 ± 0,07	± 1,67	4,47	629	−1,83 ± 0,07	± 1,65	6
März–Mai	112	−2,70 ± 0,17	± 1,84	2,70	110	−2,50 ± 0,15	± 1,59	5,20	288	−1,04 ± 0,09	± 1,58	6
Juni–Aug.	101	−3,26 ± 0,15	± 1,53	3,26	101	−2,25 ± 0,14	± 1,40	5,51	225	−0,81 ± 0,10	± 1,44	6
Sept.–Nov.	227	−1,31 ± 0,12	± 1,87	1,31	227	−3,01 ± 0,12	± 1,87	4,88	274	−1,50 ± 0,10	± 1,73	6
Dez.–Febr.	336	−1,35 ± 0,09	± 1,69	1,35	337	−2,86 ± 0,10	± 1,84	4,21	421	−1,76 ± 0,08	± 1,71	5
												Ab
März–Mai	293	−1,76 ± 0,08	± 1,44	1,76	294	−2,74 ± 0,08	± 1,44	4,50	294	−1,64 ± 0,09	± 1,52	6
Juni–Aug.	225	−1,85 ± 0,10	± 1,46	1,85	227	−2,92 ± 0,08	± 1,24	4,77	228	−1,69 ± 0,11	± 1,63	6
Sept.–Nov.	235	−2,03 ± 0,11	± 1,62	2,03	234	−3,07 ± 0,11	± 1,68	5,10	235	−1,77 ± 0,11	± 1,63	6
Dez.–Febr.	207	−2,13 ± 0,11	± 1,64	2,13	207	−2,76 ± 0,09	± 1,34	4,89	208	−1,97 ± 0,10	± 1,49	6
												Ab
März–Mai	293	−1,76 ± 0,08	± 1,44	1,76	294	−2,74 ± 0,08	± 1,44	4,50	294	−1,64 ± 0,09	± 1.52	
Juni–Aug.	225	−1,85 ± 0,10	± 1,46	1,85	227	−2,92 ± 0,08	± 1,24	4,77	228	−1,69 ± 0,11	± 1,63	
Sept.–Nov.	122	−2,12 ± 0,15	± 1,67	2,12	121	−3,02 ± 0,14	± 1,58	5,14	122	−1,47 ± 0,15	± 1,62	
Dez.–Febr.	101	−1,99 ± 0,16	± 1,59	1,99	101	−2,70 ± 0,14	± 1,39	4,69	101	−1,91 ± 0,15	± 1,47	
											Abt. II 0	*R*
März–Mai	132	−2,26 ± 0,13	± 1,51	2,26	132	−3,15 ± 0,11	± 1,23	5,41	132	−1,79 ± 0,12	± 1,32	
Juni–Aug.	106	−2,55 ± 0,16	± 1,60	2,55	108	−3,01 ± 0,15	± 1,60	5,56	115	−1,27 ± 0,15	± 1,62	
Sept.–Nov.	113	−1,92 ± 0,15	± 1,56	1,92	113	−3,12 ± 0,17	± 1,78	5,04	113	−2,08 ± 0,15	± 1,59	
Dez.–Febr.	106	−2,27 ± 0,16	± 1,68	2,27	106	−2,82 ± 0,12	± 1,28	5.09	107	−2,02 ± 0,15	± 1,51	

ıreszeiten Tag für Tag in % des Geburtsgewichts.

g											
4				5				6			
ı	$M \pm \varepsilon(M)$	σ	Unter-gewicht	n	$M \pm \varepsilon(M)$	σ	Unter-gewicht	n	$M \pm \varepsilon(M)$	σ	Unter-gewicht
ra-Abt. II 0 Ringer											
0	+0,52 ± 0,08	± 1,91	5,52	587	+0,98 ± 0,06	± 1,32	4,54	575	+0,64 ± 0,05	± 1,30	3,90
8	+0,34 ± 0,07	± 1,47	5,91	470	+0,84 ± 0,06	± 1,26	5,07	468	+0,75 ± 0,06	± 1,21	4,32
1	+0,46 ± 0,08	± 1,75	5,88	511	+0,96 ± 0,07	± 1,57	4,92	508	+0,92 ± 0,06	± 1,38	4,00
2	+0,10 ± 0,07	± 1,64	6,20	627	+0,97 ± 0,06	± 1,39	5,23	619	+0,72 ± 0,06	± 1,39	4,51
6	+0,67 ± 0,08	± 1,39	5,57	293	+0,91 ± 0,08	± 1,39	4,66	285	+0,56 ± 0,06	± 1,33	4,10
0	+0,55 ± 0,09	± 1,38	5,77	242	+0,84 ± 0,08	± 1,29	4,93	242	+0,78 ± 0,09	± 1,34	4,15
6	+0,68 ± 0,11	± 1,88	5,70	276	+0,90 ± 0,10	± 1,70	4,80	276	+0,96 ± 0,09	± 1,49	3,84
4	+0,18 ± 0,08	± 1,64	5,79	421	+1,07 ± 0,07	± 1,38	4,72	419	+0,71 ± 0,07	± 1,39	4,01
ıger + 0 Ringer)											
4	+0,36 ± 0,14	± 2,32	5,78	294	+1,05 ± 0,06	± 0,95	4,73	290	+0,93 ± 0,03	± 0,47	4,00
8	+0,12 ± 0,10	± 1,53	6,34	228	+0,84 ± 0,08	± 1,23	5,50	226	+0,72 ± 0,07	± 1,05	4,78
5	+0,19 ± 0,10	± 1,56	6,68	235	+1,04 ± 0,09	± 1,36	5,64	232	+0,87 ± 0,08	± 1,23	4,77
8	−0,06 ± 0,11	± 1,63	6,92	206	+0,77 ± 0,10	± 1,40	6,15	200	+0,74 ± 0,11	± 1,53	5,41
ger.											
4	+0,36 ± 0,14	± 2,32	5,78	294	+1,05 ± 0,06	± 0,95	4,73	290	+0,93 ± 0,03	± 0,47	3,80
3	+0,12 ± 0,10	± 1,53	6,34	228	+0,84 ± 0,08	± 1,23	5,50	226	+0,72 ± 0,07	± 1,05	4,78
2	+0,15 ± 0,15	± 1,61	6,46	122	+1,12 ± 0,12	± 1,36	5,34	119	+0,90 ± 0,11	± 1,24	4,44
1	−0,13 ± 0,18	± 1,80	6,73	101	+0,82 ± 0,12	± 1,22	5,91	97	+0,74 ± 0,13	± 1,31	5,17
rz–Mai und Juni–August »Extramaterial» 1937).											
)	+0,15 ± 0,11	± 1,29	7,05	130	+1,15 ± 0,11	± 1,25	5,90	130	+0,46 ± 0,12	± 1,32	5,44
5	+0,24 ± 0,15	± 1,59	6,94	117	+0,97 ± 0,12	± 1,27	5,97	117	+0,77 ± 0,12	± 1,28	5,20
3	+0,24 ± 0,14	± 1,51	6,88	113	+0,95 ± 0,13	± 1,35	5,93	113	+0,84 ± 0,12	± 1,27	5,09
'	± 0,00 ± 0,14	± 1,40	7,11	105	+0,72 ± 0,15	± 1,52	6,39	103	+0,74 + 0,15	± 1,50	5,65

T

Gewichtsveränderung des Kindes in Gruppen mit verschiedenem Gebu
Abt.

	Gewichtsgruppe	Leben								
		1			2			3		
		n	$M \pm \varepsilon(M)$	σ	n	$M \pm \varepsilon(M)$	σ	n	$M \pm \varepsilon(M)$	σ
Gesamtmaterial mit Extra-Abt. II 0 Ringer	2 200–3 099	467	$-1{,}75 \pm 0{,}08$	$\pm 1{,}62$	470	$-2{,}55 \pm 0{,}07$	$\pm 1{,}54$	556	$-1{,}40 \pm 0{,}07$	±[illegible]
	3 100–3 699	935	$-1{,}88 \pm 0{,}06$	$\pm 1{,}71$	935	$-2{,}93 \pm 0{,}05$	$\pm 1{,}58$	1 158	$-1{,}54 \pm 0{,}05$	±[illegible]
	3 700–>	572	$-2{,}14 \pm 0{,}08$	$\pm 1{,}83$	571	$-3{,}04 \pm 0{,}07$	$\pm 1{,}57$	706	$-1{,}62 \pm 0{,}06$	±[illegible]
Gesamtmaterial ohne Abt. II 0 Ringer	2 200–3 099	406	$-1{,}66 \pm 0{,}08$	$\pm 1{,}60$	407	$-2{,}51 \pm 0{,}08$	$\pm 1{,}55$	492	$-1{,}40 \pm 0{,}07$	±[illegible]
	3 100–3 699	826	$-1{,}78 \pm 0{,}06$	$\pm 1{,}67$	826	$-2{,}92 \pm 0{,}06$	$\pm 1{,}62$	1 045	$-1{,}57 \pm 0{,}05$	±[illegible]
	3 700–>	504	$-2{,}16 \pm 0{,}08$	$\pm 1{,}80$	503	$-3{,}02 \pm 0{,}07$	$\pm 1{,}57$	636	$-1{,}57 \pm 0{,}07$	±[illegible]
Abt. I	2 200–3 099	194	$-1{,}45 \pm 0{,}12$	$\pm 1{,}65$	195	$-2{,}55 \pm 0{,}12$	$\pm 1{,}68$	277	$-1{,}26 \pm 0{,}10$	±[illegible]
	3 100–3 699	326	$-1{,}62 \pm 0{,}12$	$\pm 1{,}95$	325	$-2{,}83 \pm 0{,}10$	$\pm 1{,}79$	543	$-1{,}41 \pm 0{,}07$	±[illegible]
	3 700–>	256	$-2{,}25 \pm 0{,}12$	$\pm 1{,}95$	255	$-3{,}06 \pm 0{,}12$	$\pm 1{,}78$	388	$-1{,}35 \pm 0{,}09$	±[illegible]

Das grösste Untergewicht trifft während des Vierteljahrs September—November ein, das nächstkleinere während Dezember—Februar. Dann folgt das Vierteljahr Juni—August und zuletzt März—Mai. Die Gewichtsabnahme scheint also während des Herbstes und Winters am grössten und im Frühjahr und Sommer kleiner zu sein, wie es auch bei der Temperatursteigerung der Fall war.

Der Unterschied zwischen den Gewichtsabnahmen während September—November und Juni—August ist an allen drei Tagen gesichert.

Die Differenzen betragen:

am 1. Tage $0{,}61 \pm 0{,}12$, dreifache mittl. Abw. $= 0{,}36$
» 2. » $0{,}33 \pm 0{,}11$, » » » $= 0{,}33$
» 3. » $0{,}37 \pm 0{,}11$, » » » $= 0{,}33$.

vicht. Gesamtmaterial mit und ohne Extra-Abt. II 0 Ringer sowie
sich.

g											
4			5			6			Summa	
	$M \pm \varepsilon (M)$	σ	n	$M \pm \varepsilon (M)$	σ	n	$M \pm \varepsilon (M)$	σ	1—3	4—6
…8	+0,38 ± 0,07	± 1,63	556	+0,90 ± 0,06	± 1,52	555	+0,90 ± 0,06	± 1,38	−5,70	+2,18
…1	+0,27 ± 0,05	± 1,55	1 172	+0,99 ± 0,04	± 1,32	1 156	+0,72 ± 0,04	± 1,29	−6,35	+1,98
…7	+0,39 ± 0,06	± 1,56	714	+0,94 ± 0,05	± 1,35	706	+0,65 ± 0,05	± 1,29	−6,80	+1,98
…6	+0,39 ± 0,07	± 1,59	494	+0,90 ± 0,07	± 1,51	492	+0,90 ± 0,06	± 1,38	−5,57	+2,19
…8	+0,28 ± 0,05	± 1,62	1 059	+0,91 ± 0,05	± 1,53	1 043	+0,73 ± 0,04	± 1,31	−6,27	+1,92
…7	+0,42 ± 0,06	± 1,53	642	+0,90 ± 0,05	± 1,36	634	+0,68 ± 0,05	± 1,30	−6,75	+2,00
…1	+0,54 ± 0,10	± 1,65	281	+0,88 ± 0,10	± 1,60	281	+0,86 ± 0,08	± 1,40		
…5	+0,38 ± 0,07	± 1,64	556	+0,98 ± 0,06	± 1,39	546	+0,71 ± 0,06	± 1,41		
…0	+0,58 ± 0,08	± 1,52	395	+0,94 ± 0,07	± 1,42	395	+0,71 ± 0,07	± 1,34		

Die Gewichtsabnahme am 1. Tage ist während Juni—August am grössten. An den folgenden Tagen ist sie während September—November am grössten. Die Temperatur verhält sich ebenso: am 1. Tage ist sie während Juni—August am höchsten, an den folgenden Tagen während September—November. Die Gewichtsabnahme ist also am grössten, wenn die Temperatur am höchsten ist.

In den verschiedenen Abteilungen liegen kleinere Schwankungen vor, was nicht zu verwundern ist, wenn die Unterschiede im zusammengelegten Material so relativ klein sind. Es lässt sich jedoch durchweg konstatieren, dass die grösste Gewichtsabnahme während eines Tages und das grösste zusammengelegte Untergewicht in jeder Abteilung entweder in einem Herbst- oder Wintervierteljahr, gewöhnlich im Herbst

Tab.

Differenz in der Gewichtsveränderung zwischen verschiede-

	Gewichtsgruppe	Lebens- 1 Differenz	1 Dreif. mittl. Abw.	2 Differenz	2 Dreif. mittl. Abw.	3 Differenz	3 Dreif. mittl. Abw.
Gesamtmaterial mit Extra-Abt. II 0 Ringer	2 200–3 099= =3 100–3 699	+0,13±0,100	0,300	+0,38±0,086	0,258	+0,14±0,086	0,258
	3 100–3 699= =3 700–>	+0,26±0,100	0,300	+0,11±0,086	0,258	+0,08±0,078	0,234
	2 200–3 099= =3 700–>	+0,39±0,113	0,339	+0,49±0,099	0,297	+0,22±0,092	0,276
Gesamtmaterial ohne Extra-Abt. II 0 Ringer	2 200–3 099= =3 100–3 699	+0,12±0,100	0,300	+0,41±0,100	0,300	+0,17±0,086	0,258
	3 100–3 699= =3 700–>	+0,38±0,100	0,300	+0,10±0,092	0,276	±0 ±0,086	0,258
	2 200–3 099= =3 700–>	+0,50±0,113	0,339	+0,51±0,092	0,276	+0,17±0,099	0,297
Abt. I	2 200–3 099= =3 100–3 699	+0,17±0,17	0,51	+0,28±0,16	0,48	+0,15±0,12	0,36
	3 100–3 699= =3 700–>	+0,63±0,17	0,51	+0,23±0,16	0,48	−0,06±0,11	0,33
	2 200–3 099= =3 700–>	+0,80±0,17	0,51	+0,51±0,17	0,51	+0,09±0,13	0,39

23.

nen Abteilungen während verschiedener Beobachtungstage.

t a g							
4		5		6		Summa	
Differenz	Dreif. mittl. Abw.	Differenz	Dreif. mittl. Abw.	Differenz	Dreif. mittl. Abw.	1—3	4—6
−0,11 ± 0,086	0,258	+0,09 ± 0,072	0,216	−0,18 ± 0,072	0,216	+0,65	−0,20
+0,12 ± 0,078	0,234	−0,05 ± 0,064	0,192	−0,07 ± 0,064	0,192	+0,45	±0
+0,01 ± 0,092	0,276	+0,04 ± 0,078	0,234	−0,25 ± 0,078	0,234	+1,10	−0,20
−0,11 ± 0,086	0,258	+0,01 ± 0,086	0,258	−0,17 ± 0,072	0,216	+0,70	−0,27
+0,14 ± 0,078	0,234	−0,01 ± 0,071	0,213	−0,05 ± 0,064	0,192	+0,48	−0,08
+0,03 ± 0,092	0,276	±0 ± 0,086	0,258	−0,22 ± 0,078	0,234	+1,18	−0,19
−0,16 ± 0,12	0,36	−0,10 ± 0,12	0,36	−0,15 ± 0,10	0,30	+0,60	−0,41
+0,20 ± 0,11	0,33	−0,04 ± 0,09	0,27	±0 ± 0,09	0,27	+0,80	+0,16
+0,04 ± 0,13	0,39	+0,06 ± 0,12	0,36	−0,15 ± 0,11	0,33	+1,40	−0,05

Tab.

Temperatur der Mutter. Gesamt-

Tag	n	Gesamtmaterial	σ	n	Abt. I	σ
1	2 055	37,30 ± 0,01	± 0,39	1 097	37,28 ± 0,01	± 0,38
2	2 205	37,09 ± 0,01	± 0,39	1 244	37,10 ± 0,01	± 0,41
3	2 205	37,18 ± 0,01	± 0,42	1 243	37,19 ± 0,01	± 0,43
4	2 202	37,24 ± 0,01	± 0,44	1 240	37,23 ± 0,01	± 0,45
5	2 196	37,19 ± 0,01	± 0,39	1 236	37,19 ± 0,01	± 0,38
6	2 173	37,19 ± 0,01	± 0,38	1 229	37,20 ± 0,01	± 0,39

vierteljahr, und niemals im Sommer. Das Material in Abt. II 0 Ringer aus einem späteren Jahre (März—August) macht in dieser Beziehung keine Ausnahme. Das Untergewicht ist während des Vierteljahrs März—Mai sogar am grössten, dann kommt das Vierteljahr Juni—August. Während des 1. Tages finden wir im Vierteljahr Juni—August eine grössere Gewichtsabnahme als während eines der übrigen Vierteljahre, dann nimmt das Vierteljahr September—November diesen Platz ein. Wie in bezug auf die Temperatursteigerung rückt auch betreffs der Gewichtsabnahme das Extramaterial Abt. II 0 Ringer an diejenige Stelle im Verhältnis zum Hauptmaterial, welche es mit Rücksicht auf Nahrungs- und Flüssigkeitszufuhr einnehmen müsste. Dasselbe weist mit denen der Abt. II 0 Ringer im Hauptmaterial gut übereinstimmende Werte auf und eine Gewichtsabnahme, welche grösser ist als in irgendeiner anderen Abteilung im letzteren.

Gewichtsveränderung des Kindes im Verhältnis zum Geburtsgewicht.

Wie die Temperatur desto höher ist, je grösser das Geburtsgewicht war, so steht auch der Gewichtsverlust in derselben Beziehung zu letzterem. Je grösser das Geburtsgewicht ist,

24.

material ohne Abt. II 0 Ringer.

n	Abt. II Ringer + 0 Ringer	σ	n	Abt. II Ringer	σ	n	Abt. II 0 Ringer	σ
958	37,33 ± 0,01	± 0,39	738	37,32 ± 0,01	± 0,39	220	37,35 ± 0,03	± 0,38
961	37,08 ± 0,01	± 0,36	741	37,06 ± 0,01	± 0,35	220	37,16 ± 0,02	± 0,36
962	37,16 ± 0,01	± 0,41	742	37,13 ± 0,01	± 0,40	220	37,25 ± 0,03	± 0,41
962	37,24 ± 0,01	± 0,44	742	37,22 ± 0,02	± 0,44	220	37,32 ± 0,03	± 0,42
960	37,20 ± 0,01	± 0,40	742	37,17 ± 0,02	± 0,42	218	37,27 ± 0,02	± 0,36
944	37,17 ± 0,01	± 0,37	728	37,14 ± 0,01	± 0,38	216	37,25 ± 0,02	± 0,36

desto grösser wird der prozentuale Gewichtsfall. Die Verhältnisse während des 4.—6. Lebenstages, wo die Kinder zunehmen, sind nicht ebenso klar. Ob hier irgendeine Tendenz vorliegt, lässt sich nicht entscheiden. Existiert eine solche, so geht sie scheinbar in die entgegengesetzte, in Wirklichkeit aber in dieselbe Richtung wie die Gewichtsabnahme. Je geringer das Geburtsgewicht des Kindes ist, desto mehr nimmt dasselbe prozentual zu. Im Verhältnis zum Geburtsgewicht wird also die Gewichtsabnahme kleiner und die Gewichtszunahme grösser, je kleiner das Geburtsgewicht des Kindes gewesen war.

Temperatur der Mutter.

Da die Berechnungen für Mütter von Morgenkindern auf Grund der Morgentemperatur, für Mütter von Abendkindern auf Grund der Abendtemperatur vorgenommen worden sind, wird die Temperatur der Mütter eine mittlere Temperatur aus Morgen- und Abendtemperatur.

Die Temperatur der Mütter während der 6 ersten Tage nach der Entbindung weist erheblich kleinere Differenzen zwischen den einzelnen Tagen auf als die Temperatur der Kinder (Tab. 24).

Der Verlauf der Temperaturkurve ist ausserdem ein anderer.

So finden wir die höchste Temperatur, 37,3°, am 1. Tage, die niedrigste, 37,09°, am 2. Dann steigt die Temperatur wieder am 3. Tage auf 37,18° und am 4. auf 37,24°. Am 5. und 6. Tage schliesslich stabilisiert sich die Temperatur auf 37,19°. Die Mütter haben also die höchste Temperatur an dem Tage, wo die der Kinder am niedrigsten ist.

Die Differenzen in der Temperatur während der 5 ersten Tage sind gesichert (Tab. 25).

Eine Einteilung in die betreffenden Abteilungen ergibt denselben Verlauf in allen. Der Unterschied hinsichtlich der Temperaturentwicklung, welchen die Kinder in den verschiedenen Abteilungen untereinander im Rahmen eines prinzipiell gleichen Verlaufs aufgewiesen haben, hat also bei den Müttern kein Gegenstück.

Interessant ist indessen, dass die Mütter in Abt. II 0 Ringer durchweg und schon vom 1. Tage an während der ganzen Beobachtungszeit eine etwas höhere Temperatur aufweisen als die Mütter in den übrigen Abteilungen, ganz wie es sich mit den Kindern in dieser Abteilung verhielt.

Temperatur der Mutter während verschiedener Jahreszeiten.

Während der 2 ersten Tage nach der Entbindung ist die Temperatur der Mütter während aller Jahreszeiten dieselbe (Tab. 26).

Nach diesen Tagen macht sich ein gewisser numerischer Unterschied geltend. Dieser ist indessen nicht der Ausdruck einer statistischen Differenz. Interessant ist aber einmal, dass der besagte Unterschied erst im späteren Teil des Wochenbetts auftritt, und sodann, dass die Tendenz davon abgesehen in dieselbe Richtung geht wie die Temperatur bei den Kindern. Herbst—Winter weisen höhere Temperatur auf als Frühjahr—Sommer. Dies könnte dafür sprechen, dass doch ein wirklicher Unterschied vorliegt, wenn auch ein so unerheblicher, dass er sich an Hand eines Materials vom Umfang des hier vorliegenden nicht statistisch sichern lässt.

Tab. 25.

Differenz in der Temperatur der Mütter von Tag zu Tag innerhalb verschiedener Abteilungen ohne Extra-Abt. II 0 Ringer.

Tag	Gesamtmaterial		Abt. I		Abt. II Ringer + 0 Ringer		Abt. II Ringer		Abt. II 0 Ringer	
	Differenz	Dreif. mittl. Abw.	Differenz	Dreif. mittl. Abw.	Differenz	Dreif. mittl. Abw.	Differenz	Dreif. mittl. Abw.	Differenz	Dreif. mittl. Abw.
1—2	−0,21 ± 0,014	0,042	−0,18 ± 0,014	0,042	−0,25 ± 0,014	0,042	−0,26 ± 0,014	0,042	−0,19 ± 0,036	0,108
2—3	+0,09 ± 0,014	0,042	+0,09 ± 0,014	0,042	+0,08 ± 0,014	0,042	+0,07 ± 0,014	0,042	+0,09 ± 0,036	0,108
3—4	+0,06 ± 0,014	0,042	+0,04 ± 0,014	0,042	+0,08 ± 0,014	0,042	+0,09 ± 0,022	0,066	+0,07 ± 0,042	0,126
4—5	−0,05 ± 0,014	0,042	−0,04 ± 0,014	0,042	−0,04 ± 0,014	0,042	−0,05 ± 0,028	0,084	−0,05 ± 0,036	0,108
5—6	±0 ± 0,014	0,042	+0,01 ± 0,014	0,042	−0,03 ± 0,014	0,042	−0,03 ± 0,022	0,066	−0,02 ± 0,028	0,084

Tab.

Temperatur der Mutter während verschiedener Jahres-

Jahreszeit	Lebens- 1			2			3		
	n	$M \pm \varepsilon(M)$	σ	n	$M \pm \varepsilon(M)$	σ	n	$M \pm \varepsilon(M)$	σ
März–Mai	550	37,31 ± 0,02	± 0,40	590	37,09 ± 0,02	± 0,39	589	37,13 ± 0,02	± 0,39
Juni–Aug.	401	37,28 ± 0,02	± 0,43	468	37,09 ± 0,02	± 0,44	471	37,18 ± 0,02	± 0,47
Sept.–Nov.	491	37,31 ± 0,02	± 0,36	513	37,07 ± 0,02	± 0,37	512	37,18 ± 0,02	± 0,44
Dez.–Febr.	613	37,30 ± 0,01	± 0,37	634	37,11 ± 0,01	± 0,35	633	37,21 ± 0,02	± 0,39

Tab

Temperatur der Mutter bei verschiedenem Geburtsgewicht

Geburts-gewicht des Kindes	Lebens- 1		2		3	
	$M \pm m(\varepsilon)$	σ	$M \pm m(\varepsilon)$	σ	$M \pm m(\varepsilon)$	σ
2 200—3 099	37,27 ± 0,02	± 0,41	36,93 ± 0,02	± 0,35	37,05 ± 0,02	± 0,46
3 100—3 699	37,32 ± 0,01	± 0,37	37,09 ± 0,01	± 0,38	37,18 ± 0,01	± 0,42
3 700—>	37,29 ± 0,02	± 0,39	37,09 ± 0,01	± 0,38	37,16 ± 0,02	± 0,41

Temperatur der Mutter und verschiedenes Geburtsgewicht des Kindes.

Es wäre denkbar, dass die Entbindung im allgemeinen länger dauerte und dass die Temperatur der Mutter infolgedessen wenigstens während des ersten Tages nach der Entbindung eine höhere wäre, wenn das Kind ein hohes Geburtsgewicht hat. Dies ist indessen nicht der Fall.

Die Temperatur der Mutter ist weder erhöht oder gesenkt, wenn das Geburtsgewicht hoch oder niedrig ist.

26.

zeiten. Gesamtmaterial ohne Extra-Abt. II 0 Ringer.

t a g								
4			5			6		
n	$M \pm \varepsilon(M)$	σ	n	$M \pm \varepsilon(M)$	σ	n	$M \pm \varepsilon(M)$	σ
588	37,21 ± 0,02	± 0,42	585	37,16 ± 0,02	± 0,41	573	37,18 ± 0,01	± 0,35
469	37,21 ± 0,02	± 0,47	471	37,16 ± 0,02	± 0,38	469	37,16 ± 0,02	± 0,41
512	37,24 ± 0,02	± 0,46	512	37,20 ± 0,02	± 0,39	509	37,20 ± 0,02	± 0,37
633	37,28 ± 0,02	± 0,44	628	37,25 ± 0,01	± 0,37	622	37,24 ± 0,02	± 0,40

27.

des Kindes. Gesamtmaterial ohne Extra-Abt. II 0 Ringer.

t a g					
4		5		6	
$M \pm m(\varepsilon)$	σ	$M \pm m(\varepsilon)$	σ	$M \pm m(\varepsilon)$	σ
37,26 ± 0,02	± 0,43	37,20 ± 0,02	± 0,35	37,24 ± 0,02	± 0,34
37,24 ± 0,01	± 0,44	37,20 ± 0,01	± 0,42	37,20 ± 0,01	± 0,38
37,22 ± 0,02	± 0,46	37,18 ± 0,01	± 0,37	37,18 ± 0,02	± 0,40

Wechselbeziehungen.

Die drei Beobachtungen, deren Wechselbeziehungen im Hinblick auf die im Schrifttum wiedergegebenen Anschauungen besonderes Interesse beanspruchen dürften, sind:

Temperatur des Kindes und Gewichtsabnahme,
Temperatur des Kindes und Temperatur der Mutter und im Anschluss hieran möglicherweise Temperatur der Mutter und Gewichtsabnahme des Kindes.

Tab. 28.

Wechselbeziehung.
Gesamtmaterial ohne Extra-Abt. II 0 Ringer.

Abteilung	Lebens-tag	n	Temperatur und Gewichtsabnahme des Kindes $r \pm \varepsilon(r)$	n	Temperatur des Kindes und Temperatur der Mutter $r \pm \varepsilon(r)$	n	Temperatur der Mutter und Gewichtsabnahme des Kindes $r \pm \varepsilon(r)$
Abt. I	1	776	$+0{,}23 \pm 0{,}03$	1097	$+0{,}02 \pm 0{,}03$	770	$-0{,}11 \pm 0{,}04$
	2	775	$+0{,}06 \pm 0{,}04$	1244	$+0{,}05 \pm 0{,}03$	773	$-0{,}02 \pm 0{,}04$
	3	1208	$+0{,}19 \pm 0{,}03$	1243	$+0{,}04 \pm 0{,}03$	1218	$+0{,}02 \pm 0{,}03$
Abt. II Ringer	1	741	$+0{,}33 \pm 0{,}03$	738	$-0{,}15 \pm 0{,}04$	738	$-0{,}16 \pm 0{,}04$
	2	743	$+0{,}06 \pm 0{,}04$	741	$+0{,}02 \pm 0{,}04$	741	$-0{,}01 \pm 0{,}04$
	3	745	$+0{,}09 \pm 0{,}04$	742	$+0{,}01 \pm 0{,}04$	742	$-0{,}01 \pm 0{,}04$
Abt. II 0 Ringer	1	219	$+0{,}28 \pm 0{,}06$	220	$-0{,}14 \pm 0{,}07$	219	$-0{,}20 \pm 0{,}06$
	2	219	$+0{,}11 \pm 0{,}07$	220	$-0{,}05 \pm 0{,}07$	219	$+0{,}06 \pm 0{,}07$
	3	220	$+0{,}15 \pm 0{,}07$	220	$+0{,}03 \pm 0{,}07$	220	$-0{,}03 \pm 0{,}07$
Gesamt-material	1	1736	$+0{,}28 \pm 0{,}02$	2055	$-0{,}06 \pm 0{,}02$	1727	$-0{,}14 \pm 0{,}02$
	2	1737	$+0{,}07 \pm 0{,}02$	2205	$+0{,}03 \pm 0{,}02$	1733	$-0{,}01 \pm 0{,}02$
	3	2173	$+0{,}15 \pm 0{,}02$	2205	$+0{,}03 \pm 0{,}02$	2180	$+0{,}01 \pm 0{,}02$

Diesbezügliche Berechnungen für die 3 Tage, während welcher das Kind an Gewicht abnimmt, sind in Tab. 28 zusammengestellt. Die Wechselbeziehung wird sowohl für das ganze Material wie für jede Abteilung für sich wiedergegeben.

Temperatur und Gewichtsabnahme des Kindes lassen eine positive Beziehung an allen drei Tagen erkennen. Die Beziehung muss indessen als schwach bezeichnet werden. Am 1. Tage, wo sie am stärksten ist, beträgt dieselbe 0,28. Während des 2. Tages ist sie am geringsten, 0,07, und am 3. Tage 0,15.

Die Beziehung ist demnach am stärksten, bevor irgendein Unterschied in der Nahrungs- und Flüssigkeitszufuhr Platz greift (am 1. Tage). Während des Tages, wo ein Unterschied in der Nahrungs- und Flüssigkeitszufuhr vorliegt, und wo

Temperatursteigerung und Gewichtsabnahme am grössten sind (am 2. Tage), ist sie sehr schwach. Sie ist immer noch sehr schwach, wenn auch etwas stärker, an dem Tage (am 3.), wo sowohl Temperatur wie Untergewicht ihren schliesslichen, höchsten Wert erreichen.

In den verschiedenen Abteilungen spiegelt sich dasselbe Verhalten wider. Irgendein Unterschied zwischen denselben in der Stärke der Wechselbeziehung liegt nicht vor.

Temperatursteigerung und Gewichtsabnahme weisen also nur einen sehr schwachen Zusammenhang miteinander auf, und die Möglichkeit, diese Faktoren durch Änderung der Flüssigkeits- und Nahrungszufuhr zu beeinflussen, ist sehr begrenzt.

Temperatur des Kindes und Temperatur der Mutter weisen eine sehr schwache Wechselbeziehung auf, und zwar nur während des 1. Tages. Die Beziehung ist reziprok. Soweit ein Zusammenhang besteht, würde einer höheren Temperatur der Mutter während dieses Tages also eine niedrigere Temperatur des Kindes entsprechen.

Temperatur der Mutter und Gewichtsabnahme des Kindes lassen ebenfalls eine sehr schwache reziproke Wechselbeziehung während des ersten Lebenstages, nicht später, erkennen. Die Beziehung geht in die Richtung, dass das Kind um so weniger abnimmt, je höher die Temperatur der Mutter ist. Das Verhältnis stimmt gut damit überein, dass bei höherer Temperatur der Mutter die des Kindes desto niedriger ist, und dass Kinder mit niedriger Temperatur weniger abnehmen als solche mit höherer Temperatur.

Es ist bereits darauf hingewiesen worden, dass ein gewisser Zusammenhang zwischen der *Temperatur des Kindes und dem Geburtsgewicht desselben* besteht. Je höher das Geburtsgewicht des Kindes ist, desto grösser wird die Temperatursteigerung, welche es bekommt. Der Zusammenhang ist indessen, wenn auch sicher, so doch im Verhältnis zum Grade der Temperatursteigerung überhaupt nicht besonders augenfällig. Die Wechselbeziehung kann also als ziemlich schwach bezeichnet werden.

Tab. 29 A.

Temperatur des Kindes und Länge der Wehenzeit.

Abt. I.

Länge der Wehenzeit in St.	Temperatur des Kindes am 1. Tage.																
	35,0–35,1	35,2–35,3	35,4–35,5	35,6–35,7	35,8–35,9	36,0–36,1	36,2–36,3	36,4–36,5	36,6–36,7	36,8–36,9	37,0–37,1	37,2–37,3	37,4–37,5	37,6–37,7	37,8–37,9	38,2–	> 38,7
0—6	1		1	3	6	17	31	38	31	23	18	19	13	6	1		
6,5—12	3	2	4	3	12	25	66	40	31	36	23	14	8	3	3		
12,5—18	1	2	2	2	1	16	9	22	22	29	18	14	11	1	2		
18,5—24		1	2	1	3	11	13	21	16	15	21	9	6	2	2		
24,5—30			2	1		8	6	9	11	8	4	2	2				
30,5—36		1	1	2	3	3	2	6	7	9	3	2					
36,5—42			1			1	1	4	6	3	1	1		1			
42,5—48				1		4		4	2	2	1	1		1		1	
48,5—54					1		3	2	4	2	1	1		1			
54,5—60						2	1	1	1	2	2						
60,5—66							1	2	2	1	2	1					
66,5—72						1	2		1								
72,5—78						2	1	1				1					
0—30	5	5	10	10	22	77	125	130	111	111	84	58	40	12	8		2
30,5—60		1	2	3	4	10	7	17	20	18	8	5		3		1	
60,5—90			1			3	5	4	4	1	2	2					
90,5—120	1				1			1	1		1						
120,5—150						2		1	1								
150,5—180						1											
180,5—210																	
210,5—240								1	1		2						
— 336											1		1				

Tab. 29 B.

Temperatur des Kindes und Länge der Wehenzeit.

Abt. I.

Länge der Wehenzeit in St.	Temperatur des Kindes am 2. Tage																
	< 35,8	35,8–35,9	36,0–36,1	36,2–36,3	36,4–36,5	36,6–36,7	36,8–36,9	37,0–37,1	37,2–37,3	37,4–37,5	37,6–37,7	37,8–37,9	38,0–38,1	38,2–38,3	38,4–38,5	38,6–38,7	> 38,7
0—6		2	8	21	23	38	51	45	29	18	3		1	3			1
6,5—12		2	14	15	41	39	47	37	32	23	12	4	5	3		1	2
12,5—18	1		13	13	20	27	36	25	20	7	9	5		2		1	1
18,5—24			2	12	20	20	25	18	15	12	5	6	1	2	1		
24,5—30		1	2	3	5	12	13	9	5	4		1	2		1		
30,5—36		1	1	4	3	10	11	6	4		2	1		1	1		1
36,5—42			1	2	3	3	3	4	3	2			1				
42,5—48			3	2	6	4	1	1	3	1	2		1				
48,5—54					3	2	2	6	1	4				1			
54,5—60			1	1	2		3	1	1	1					1		
60,5—66			1		1	3		1	1			1		1			
66,5—72					1	1	1			1							
72,5—78				1	1	1	1		1	1		1					
0—30	1	5	39	64	109	136	172	134	101	64	29	16	9	10	2	2	4
30,5—60		1	6	9	17	19	20	18	12	8	4	1	2	2	2		1
60,5—90			2	3	3	5	5	1	2	2		2		1			
90,5—120				1			2	1	1								
120,5—150				1		1		1	1								
150,5—180							1										
180,5—210					1												
210,5—240					1		1	1					1				
— 336							1		1								

Temperatur des Kindes und Dauer der Entbindung.

Aus einer Zusammenstellung der Temperatur des Kindes am 1. Tage und am Tage des Temperaturmaximums (2. Tag) und der Länge der Wehenzeit wird ersichtlich, dass der Grad der Temperatursteigerung *nicht* von der Dauer der Entbindung abhängig ist (Tab. 29).

Es gibt im Gegenteil eine schwache Tendenz zur reziproken Wechselbeziehung (die freilich nicht gesichert ist), also Untertemperatur wenn die Entbindung langwierig war. Auch Entbindungen, bei welchen sehr lange Wehenzeiten angegeben wurden, sind in die Tabelle aufgenommen worden, wenn die betreffende Angabe sehr bestimmt gemacht wurde. Die Angaben sind mit einer gewissen Zurückhaltung zu betrachten, aber die Anzahl derartigen Entbindungen ist, wie aus der Tabelle ersichtlich wird, so klein, dass die Resultate hierdurch nicht beeinflusst werden.

Nur die Mütter in Abt. I wurden bei der Zusammenstellung berücksichtigt. Eine Erweiterung des Materials durch die übrigen Abteilungen würde keine weiteren, der Mehrarbeit entsprechenden Aufschlüsse liefern. Die Entbindung erfolgte in der grossen Mehrzahl der Fälle nach einer Wehendauer von 6—18 St. Eine Wehendauer von mehr als 24 St. ist verhältnismässig selten, wenn sich auch die Entbindungen manchmal sehr lange hinziehen können.

Temperatur der Mutter und Dauer der Entbindung.

Wenn die zu Abt. I gehörenden Mütter nach der Temperatur während des ersten Tages (12 St.) nach der Entbindung und nach der Länge der Wehenzeit gruppiert werden, ergibt sich, dass die Temperatur der Mutter nicht in nachweisbarem Grade von der Dauer der Entbindung an und für sich beeinflusst wird, wenn, wie es hier der Fall ist, ansteckend kranke und damit im allgemeinen fiebernde Mütter ausgeschaltet werden (Tab. 30). Eine Ausdehnung der Untersuchung auf Abt II ist offenbar auch hier bedeutungslos.

Tab. 30.

Länge der Wehenzeit und Temperatur der Mutter am Tage nach der Entbindung.

Abt. I.

Länge der Wehenzeit in St.	Temperatur der Mutter am 1. Tage											
	36,2–36,3	36,4–36,5	36,6–36,7	36,8–36,9	37,0–37,1	37,2–37,3	37,4–37,5	37,6–37,7	37,8–37,9	38,0–38,1	38,2–38,3	> 38,3
0—6		6	11	25	40	47	50	23	11	6	2	1
6,5—12	1	2	16	26	56	53	47	28	18	5	2	
12,5—18		1	8	20	35	30	37	22	10	2		2
18,5—24		3	6	8	30	23	39	13	4	5	1	
24,5—30			2	5	13	15	12	5	1	1		1
30,5—36			4	2	11	9	4	6	3	1		
36,5—42			1	2	3	3	7	1		3		
42,5—48			2	5	1	9	3	1			1	
48,5—54			1	1	3	7	3	1	1			
54,5—60			1	1	1	2	1	2	1			
60,5—66			2	1	3		2	2				
66,5—72					1		2			1		
72,5—78			2	2		3						
0—30	1	12	43	84	174	168	185	91	44	19	5	4
30,5—60			9	11	19	30	18	11	5	4	1	
60,5—90			4	3	5	6	5	2		1		
90,5—120				2	2		1					
120,5—150				1			2					1
150,5—180									1			
180,5—210					1							
210,5—240			1				2	1				
—												
336			1			1						

Tab. 31.

Geburtsgewicht der Kinder und Länge der Wehenzeit.

Abt. I.

Länge der Wehenzeit in St.	Geburtsgewicht des Kindes													
	2200–2400	2410–2600	2610–2800	2810–3000	3010–3200	3210–3400	3410–3600	3610–3800	3810–4000	4010–4200	4210–4400	4410–4600	4610–4800	4810–5000
0—6	5	3	11	24	35	37	35	33	28	12	11		4	
6,5—12	3	6	15	18	37	43	38	53	26	22	19	3	1	3
12,5—18	2	4	11	22	20	34	28	20	22	9	4	3	1	
18,5—24	1		4	10	16	29	18	26	23	6	5	3	2	
24,5—30	1	1	6	3	8	9	12	9	4	3	3			
30,5—36	1	2	2	1	8	8	9	6	5	3	1			
36,5—42			2	2	4	2	1	5	4	1	1			1
42,5—48			2	3	6	5	2	1	3		3			
48,5—54			2		2	6	3	1		3		1		
54,5—60					2	4	1	1	2		1			
60,5—66		1	1		2	2	1		2		2			
66,5—72					1		1	1	1					
72,5—78				1	2				3	1				
0—30	12	14	47	77	116	152	131	141	103	52	42	9	8	3
30,5—60	1	2	8	6	22	25	16	14	14	7	6	1		1
60,5—90		4	1	2	5	2	2	1	6	2	3			
90,5—120		1			1	2	1							
120,5—150					1	1		1				1		
150,5—180								1						
180,5—210									1					
210,5—240				1						1	1	1		
—														
336									1		1			

Länge der Wehenzeit und Geburtsgewicht des Kindes.

Eine Gruppierung des Materials in Abt. I in bezug auf die Länge der Wehenzeit nach dem Geburtsgewicht der Kinder zeigt auch keinen merkbaren Zusammenhang zwischen diesen Faktoren. Die Einschränkung ihrer eigenen Kost während des letzten Teils der Schwangerschaft, welche werdende Mütter manchmal in der Meinung vornehmen, sie könnten dadurch eine kürzere Entbindung herbeiführen, ist also völlig sinnlos, auch wenn das Geburtsgewicht des Kindes hierdurch beeinflusst werden würde. Andere Faktoren als das Geburtsgewicht des Kindes spielen die entscheidende Rolle für die Dauer der Entbindung.

Zusammenfassung und Erörterung der Untersuchungsergebnisse.

Mit der Untersuchung wird bezweckt, an Hand eines grösseren, systematisch untersuchten Materials zu ergründen, ob ein im Schrifttum gewöhnlich als »Durstfieber» bezeichneter Fieberzustand während der ersten Lebenstage vorkommt, und, wenn dies der Fall sein sollte, die Ursachen desselben festzustellen. In erster Linie wurde beabsichtigt, den Einfluss der Zufuhr von Nahrung und Flüssigkeit bzw. von Nahrungs- und Flüssigkeitsabstinenz auf die Temperatur des Kindes während seiner 6 ersten Lebenstage sowie einen eventuellen Zusammenhang zwischen der Temperatur und der Gewichtsabnahme des Kindes zu studieren. Das Material besteht aus 2 481 Kindern von während einiger Jahre in den allgemeinen Abteilungen der Allgemeinen Entbindungsanstalt der Stadt Stockholm stationär behandelten Müttern. Auf diesen Abteilungen werden keine Kinder mit einem Geburtsgewicht unter 2 200 g und keine ansteckend kranken Mütter oder Kinder derselben behandelt. Die Kinder wurden in 3 Abteilungen eingeteilt. In einer Abteilung wurden die Kinder 12 St. nach der Geburt an die Brust gelegt, in einer zweiten 24 St. nach der Geburt, erhielten aber nach 12 St. Ringersche Lösung, und in einer dritten Abteilung wurde den Kindern während 24 St. weder Nahrung noch Flüssigkeit zugeführt.

Nach $^1/_2$ Lebenstag hat das Kind eine Durchschnittstemperatur von 36,54°. Während des 2. und wahrscheinlich auch während des 3. Tages steigt die Temperatur und erreicht einen höchsten Durchschnittswert von 36,90°. Die Steigerung beträgt 0,35°. Die Variationsbreite ist ±0,54°. Die Maximaltemperatur übersteigt also in $^2/_3$ der Fälle nicht 37,5° in $^1/_3$ kann sie 38,5° erreichen. Während des 4. Tages sinkt die Temperatur wieder, um am 5. Tage auf 36,65° herabgegangen zu sein, wo sie sich auch während des 6. Tages hält.

Die Temperatursteigerung, welche normalerweise am 2.—4. Lebenstage vorkommt, erreicht also nur seltener eine solche Höhe, dass man sie als Fieber bezeichnen kann.

Die Temperatursteigerung gelangt am raschesten auf ihren höchsten Wert, und dieser Wert selbst wird höher, wenn das Kind frühzeitig Nahrung (und Flüssigkeit, Muttermilch) erhält. Sie tritt langsamer ein, erreicht aber dieselbe Höhe, wenn dem Kinde nur Flüssigkeit (Ringersche Lösung) zugeführt wird, oder wenn es weder Nahrung noch Flüssigkeit bekommt.

Die Zufuhr von Nahrung (Muttermilch) fördert also die Temperatursteigerung. Die Zufuhr von lediglich Flüssigkeit (Ringerscher Lösung) beeinflusst die Temperaturerhöhung nicht, weder in bezug auf den Zeitpunkt ihres Einsetzens noch hinsichtlich ihrer maximalen Höhe. Umgekehrt ruft Mangel an Flüssigkeit auch keine Temperatursteigerung hervor.

Nahrungszufuhr beeinflusst indessen die Temperatursteigerung, wenn auch sicher, so doch in verhältnismässig geringem Grade. Der wesentlichste Teil der Steigerung kommt unabhängig davon zustande, ob das Kind Nahrung erhält, wenn ihm nur Flüssigkeit zugeführt wird, oder wenn es seine ersten 24 Lebensstunden bei Nahrungs- und Flüssigkeitsabstinenz zubringt.

Die maximale Temperatursteigerung des Kindes beruht nicht auf der Dauer der Entbindung, wenn infektiös-fiebernde Mütter nicht mitberücksichtigt werden.

Während des 1. Tages ist die Temperatur des Kindes am höchsten (die Untertemperatur niedriger) während des Sommers (Juni—August), an den übrigen Tagen ist sie während des

Herbstes und Winters am höchsten. Der Unterschied, welcher während des 2.—6. Tages vorliegt, ist jedoch nur ein Gradunterschied. Eine Temperatursteigerung tritt auch unabhängig von der Jahreszeit ein.

Am Morgen ist die Temperatur etwas höher als am Abend.

In einer ausführlichen Untersuchung hat JUNDELL (1904) die Temperaturen während der verschiedenen Lebensperioden und zu den verschiedenen Tagesstunden derselben Periode sowie die Faktoren, die auf dieselben einwirken, eingehend untersucht. Betreffs der Neugeborenenperiode umfasst die Untersuchung hauptsächlich den 5.—8. Lebenstag. Die Untersuchung JUNDELLS und die meinige beziehen sich also auf verschiedene Probleme und haben nur 2 Tage, die gemeinsam sind. Die Übereinstimmung ist indessen für diese sehr gut. Da die soeben genannten Fragen ausserhalb der Problemstellung der vorliegenden Untersuchung stehen, sei hier im übrigen auf JUNDELLS Arbeit für näheres Studium verwiesen.

Kinder mit grösserem Geburtsgewicht haben höhere Temperatur als Kinder mit niedrigerem Geburtsgewicht.

Knaben haben eine höhere Temperatur als Mädchen, aber deren Geburtsgewicht ist durchschnittlich etwas höher. Im Gesamtmaterial betrug das durchschnittliche Geburtsgewicht der Knaben 3 532 ± 14 g gegenüber 3 370 ± 14 g bei den Mädchen. Die Differenz war 162 ± 20 g. Ein geschlechtsbedingter Unterschied im Temperaturverlauf scheint nicht zu bestehen.

Irgendein sicherer Unterschied im Geburtsgewicht zwischen während verschiedener Jahreszeiten geborenen Kindern liegt im Material nicht vor.

Das Gewicht des Kindes sinkt während des 1.—3. Lebenstages, am meisten während des 2., weniger während des 1. und am wenigsten während des 3. Tages. Der 1. Tag enthält jedoch eine Beobachtungszeit von nur 12 St. Im ganzen sinkt das Gewicht um etwa 6 % des Geburtsgewichts. Das Gewicht sinkt am wenigsten, wenn dem Kinde frühzeitig Muttermilch zugeführt wird, etwas mehr, wenn das Kind lediglich Flüssigkeit erhält, und am meisten, wenn es weder Flüssigkeit noch Nahrung bekommt. Ein kleinerer Teil des Gewichtsverlusts lässt sich durch Zufuhr von Flüssigkeit vermeiden, ein etwas grösserer durch Zufuhr von Nahrung (und Flüssigkeit), aber der grösste Teil trifft unabhängig davon ein, ob das Kind während der ersten 24 Lebensstunden Nahrung oder Flüssigkeit erhält.

Während des 4.—6. Lebenstages tritt eine Gewichtszunahme ein. Diese ist jedoch verhältnismässig geringer als die Abnahme. Das Untergewicht beträgt noch am 6. Tage etwa 4 % des Geburtsgewichts. Nur $^1/_3$ des Gewichtsverlusts während der 3 ersten Lebenstage ist also in den 3 dann folgenden eingeholt worden. Der Gewichtsfall ist, ebenso wie die Temperatursteigerung, freilich in weniger ausgesprochenem Grade als diese, während des Herbstes und Winters am grössten, im Frühjahr und Sommer geringer. Je niedriger das Geburtsgewicht des Kindes war, desto weniger verliert es an Gewicht. Leichtere Kinder scheinen auch den Gewichtsverlust rascher einzuholen als schwerere, wenn auch die Tendenz hier nicht ebenso deutlich ist. Knaben nehmen durchschnittlich etwas mehr ab als Mädchen, aber dies lässt sich durch das durchschnittlich höhere Geburtsgewicht der ersteren erklären. In allen erwähnten Beziehungen stimmen die Verhältnisse mit den Bewegungen der Temperatur überein.

Die Temperatur der Mutter ist während des ersten Tages nach der Entbindung am höchsten, 37,30°. Dann sinkt sie während des 2. Tages auf 37,09°, um am 3. und 4. Tage wieder eine Erhöhung auf 37,18° bzw. 37,24° aufzuweisen. Am 5. und 6. Tage stabilisiert sich die Temperatur bei 37,19°. Während des Herbstes und Winters ist die Temperatur nach den ersten 2 Tagen möglicherweise etwas höher als während des Frühjahrs und Sommers.

Die Temperatur der Mutter ist von dem Geburtsgewicht des Kindes und von der Dauer der Entbindung unabhängig, wenn fiebernde Entbindungsfälle unberücksichtigt bleiben.

Die Dauer der Entbindung hängt nicht von dem Geburtsgewicht des Kindes ab.

Es scheint also ein gewisser Zusammenhang zwischen der Temperatur des Kindes und der Gewichtsabnahme desselben vorzuliegen.

Wenn das ganze Material zusammengelegt wird, fällt der Zeitpunkt des Temperaturmaximums des Kindes mit dem des grössten Untergewichts desselben zusammen. Ebenso fallen die Zeitpunkte der stärksten Temperatursteigerung und des grössten Gewichtsfalls zusammen.

Die Temperatursteigerung folgt aber der Gewichtsabnahme nicht wie ein Schatten.

Während des 1. Lebenstages liegt ein gewisser Grad von Untertemperatur vor, obwohl das Gewicht einen starken Fall aufweist. Umgekehrt erreicht die Temperatur ihr Maximum am 3. Tage, wo der Gewichtsfall am geringsten ist.

Die zahlenmässig bestimmte Wechselbeziehung zwischen der Temperatur des Kindes und der Gewichtsabnahme desselben ist schwach. Am stärksten ist sie am 1. Tage, wo die Temperatur am niedrigsten, der Gewichtsfall aber am nächstgrössten ist. Sie ist während des 2. Tages am allerschwächsten, wo die Temperatur am stärksten steigt und der grösste Gewichtsfall eintrifft. Am 3. Tage, wo Temperatur- und Untergewichtsmaximum zusammenfallen, ist die Wechselbeziehung etwas stärker als am 2. Tage, aber doch sehr schwach.

Im grossen ganzen handelt es sich also um zwei Erscheinungen, welche zwar in gewissem Grade parallel, aber im allgemeinen ziemlich unabhängig voneinander verlaufen.

Die Temperatursteigerung wird höher und tritt rascher ein, wenn Nahrung (und Flüssigkeit) eher nach der Entbindung zugeführt werden, als wenn dies später der Fall ist. Die Zufuhr von lediglich Flüssigkeit vermag weder die Temperatursteigerung zu hemmen noch die Temperatur zu senken, vermindert aber den Gewichtsfall etwas.

Sowohl Temperatursteigerung wie Gewichtssturz treffen indessen zum grössten Teil unabhängig von Zufuhr von Flüssigkeit oder Nahrung oder von voller Abstinenz während des 1. Lebenstages ein. Die Wechselbeziehung zwischen der Temperatur und der Gewichtsabnahme des Kindes ist am stärksten, bevor irgendein diesbezüglicher Unterschied Platz greift.

Weder Temperatursteigerung noch Gewichtsfall ist im Sommer am grössten.

Die Temperatursteigerung beruht also nicht auf Flüssigkeitsmangel und wird auch nicht durch Zufuhr von Flüssigkeit »geheilt».

Sie beruht ebensowenig auf dem Gewichtsfall als Ausdruck einer Austrocknung. Die Temperatursteigerung wird im Gegenteil am grössten und trifft am raschesten ein, wenn der Gewichtssturz am geringsten ist. Wenn der Gewichtsverlust die Temperatursteigerung verursachen würde, müsste jener zuerst und diese später auftreten. Im Falle einer frühzeitigen Nahrungszufuhr erreicht im Gegenteil die Temperatursteigerung ihren Höhepunkt, bevor das Maximum des Untergewichts eintrifft. Die Temperatursteigerung kommt also tatsächlich etwas vor dem Untergewichtsmaximum, nicht gleichzeitig mit oder nach demselben. Würde der Gewichtsfall die Temperaturveränderungen verursachen, so wäre ferner zu erwarten, dass die Veränderungen des Gewichts grösser und sicherer wären, als die Veränderungen der Temperatur. Es verhält sich aber gerade umgekehrt. Überhaupt treten die Veränderungen in der Temperatur des Kindes deutlicher hervor, als die hinsichtlich irgendwelcher anderer untersuchter Verhältnisse.

Die Temperatursteigerung, welche zweilfelsohne während des 2.—4. Lebenstages vorliegt, ist also weder dem Gewichtsfall noch einem Flüssigkeitsverlust zur Last zu legen. Dass die Temperatur bei einem Fieber während eines dieser Lebenstage nach Zufuhr von Flüssigkeit ein Sinken aufweist, kann durchaus nicht als Gegenbeweis angeführt werden. Einen solchen Verlauf zeigt die Temperaturkurve während dieser Tage normalerweise, ungeachtet, ob Extraflüssigkeit zugeführt wird oder nicht.

Es wäre vielleicht darauf hinzuweisen, dass stark ausgetrocknete Säuglinge mit Untergewicht eher Untertemperatur als Fieber zu haben pflegen. In dieselbe Richtung tendiert die Temperatur des Kindes nach langwieriger Entbindung. Die Erklärung der Temperatursteigerung muss in anderen Ursachen als Flüssigkeitsverlust und Gewichtsabnahme zu suchen sein.

Die Temperatursteigerung stellt sich am raschesten ein, wenn das Kind frühzeitig Muttermilch erhält. Der Gewichtssturz wird gleichzeitig geringer, die Temperatur stabilisiert sich, nachdem sie wieder gesunken ist, am schnellsten und gleichmässigsten und der Wiedergewinn des Gewichts wird grösser. Für Kinder, welche sowohl hungern wie dürsten mussten, ist es am schwersten, mit Temperatursteigerung zu reagieren und dann die Temperatur zu stabilisieren und den Gewichtsverlust einzuholen. Kinder mit höherem Geburtsgewicht reagieren mit stärkerer und rascherer Temperatursteigerung als Kinder mit niedrigerem Geburtsgewicht. Je kräftiger das Kind bei der Geburt entwickelt ist, und je »normaler» sich dann die Lebensumstände desselben gestalten, desto schneller stellt sich also die Temperaturerhöhung ein und desto grösser wird sie. Äussere Umstände haben jedoch verhältnismässig geringen Einfluss. Der Grad der Temperatursteigerung wie auch der des Gewichtsfalls kann zwar von Nahrungszufuhr beeinflusst werden, aber zum grösseren Teil kommen und verlaufen Temperaturerhöhung und Gewichtssturz unabhängig davon, ob das Kind bei der Geburt mehr oder weniger gewogen hat, ob es ein Knabe oder ein Mädchen ist, ob die Entbindung kurze oder längere Zeit gedauert hat, ob das Kind früher oder später an die Brust gelegt worden ist oder während des 1. Lebenstages überhaupt nichts erhalten hat, sowie schliesslich, ob es im Sommer oder Winter, im Frühjahr oder Herbst geboren wurde. All das zeigt, dass die Temperatursteigerung wie der Gewichtsfall ein normaler, kein pathologischer, Prozess ist. Die relativ rasche und vorübergehende Temperatursteigerung deutet auf einen kurzdauernden Vorgang hin. Das gesetzmässige Auftreten derselben, ihre nur graduelle, aber nicht prinzipielle, Abhängigkeit von äusseren Umständen, wie Geburtsgewicht des Kindes (innerhalb und sogar unter der Grenze des Ausgetragenseins), Jahreszeit, Geschlecht, Flüssigkeits- und Nahrungszufuhr, deuten auf einen endogenen Ursprung hin. Die Änderungen sind als eins von vielen Symptomen der gewaltigen Umwälzung auszulegen, welche bei der Umstellung des Organismus vom intra- zum extrauterinen Leben Platz greift.

Die Temperatursteigerung als einen Fieberzustand zu bezeichnen, ist unberechtigt. Durchschnittlich erreicht dieselbe kaum 37,0°. Ihre höchste Grenze liegt in 2/3 der Fälle bei 37,5°, wenn sie auch 38,5° betragen kann.

Alle Bezeichnungen, welche den Gedanken auf ein Fieber lenken, sollten daher vermieden werden. Dies gilt besonders für solche Namen wie Durstfieber, Inanitionsfieber, Salzfieber, mit welchen ein Kausalzusammenhang angedeutet oder behauptet wird, für den die jetzt vorliegenden Tatsachen keinerlei Beleg bieten.

Die Bezeichnung soll das wirkliche Verhalten zum Ausdruck bringen. In Analogie zur Bezeichnung physiologische Gewichtsabnahme bei Neugeborenen wird der Name *physiologische Temperaturerhöhung bei Neugeborenen* vorgeschlagen.

Irgendeine spezielle Behandlung erheischt der Zustand nicht. Vor kühlenden Packungen wird bestimmt gewarnt. Sie senken zwar die Temperatur, aber dem hier Nachgewiesenen zufolge muss man annehmen, dass dies auf Kosten der Reaktionsfähigkeit geschieht, und dass die Packungen demgemäss direkt schädlich wirken.

Die beste »Behandlung» besteht darin, dass das Stillen möglichst frühzeitig in Gang kommt. Je eher dies geschieht, je früher das Kind an die Brust gelegt wird, desto rascher stabilisiert sich die Temperatur, desto geringer wird der Gewichtsfall und desto schneller wird das Gewicht wiedergewonnen. Der Grad, in welchem Temperaturerhöhung und Gewichtsabnahme durch derartige Massnahmen beeinflusst werden, ist jedoch verhältnismässig gering. Im grossen ganzen kann man das Phänomen sich selbst überlassen. Die Richtung, in welcher die besagten Massnahmen wirken, gibt gleichwohl darüber klar Bescheid, dass das Kind möglichst bald nach der Geburt, jedenfalls eher 12 St. als 24 St. nach derselben, an die Brust gelegt werden soll. Eine Pause von 24 St. nach der Geburt gereicht dem Kinde keineswegs zum Vorteil.

Eine Temperatursteigerung über 37,5° hinaus am 3. Lebenstage muss den Verdacht auf eine andere Ursache als eine physiologische Temperaturerhöhung bei Neugeborenen wachrufen; steigt die Temperatur über 38,5°, so muss man eine andere Ursache annehmen und sich bei der Behandlung nach der Art der Krankheit richten. Zufuhr von Flüssigkeit, ganz besonders von Ringerscher Lösung subkutan, ist meinen Erfahrungen nach bei den meisten von Fieber begleiteten Krankheitszuständen in diesem Alter von grossem therapeutischem Wert.

Die höhere Temperatur der Kinder während des Herbstes und Winters dürfte sich mit Rücksicht auf den höheren Infektionsindex als während des Frühjahrs und namentlich während des Sommers durch einen Zusammenhang mit einem Infektionszustand leichter Art erklären lassen und deutet hierauf hin. Hierfür spricht auch die Tendenz in gleicher Richtung, welche die Temperatur der Mütter erkennen lässt. Sowohl Kinder wie Mütter würden eine leichte Infektion durchmachen. Die schwache Wechselbeziehung zwischen der Temperatur der Mütter und der Kinder gibt zu der Annahme Anlass, dass es nicht die Mütter sind, welche zuerst erkranken und dann ihre Kinder anstecken, sondern dass es sich für beide Teile um eine Nosokomialinfektion handelt. Das spätere Eintreten der Temperatursteigerung bei den Müttern als bei den Kindern würde eine bei den ersteren längere Inkubationszeit als bei den Neugeborenen andeuten, eine Annahme, welche sich mit der starken Empfänglichkeit der letzteren für Infektionen namentlich der oberen Luftwege, ihrer schwachen Widerstandsfähigkeit gegen dieselben und der sich daraus ergebenden hohen Mortalität an derartigen Infektionen recht wohl vereinbaren lässt.

Die etwas geringere Untertemperatur am 1. Tage während der Sommermonate im Vergleich zu den 3 kälteren Vierteljahren dürfte ebenso wie die etwas höhere Morgentemperatur im Verhältnis zur Abendtemperatur während der 5 ersten Lebenstage in der Empfindlichkeit besonders der neugeborenen Kinder für die Aussentemperatur ihre Erklärung finden. Die Morgentemperatur wird gemessen, bevor das Kind gepflegt wird oder Nahrung erhalten hat. Vor der Abendmessung ist es den Strapazen des Tages mit dem Risiko der Abkühlung ausgesetzt gewesen. Dieser Umstand bildet auch seinerseits einen Hinweis darauf, dass die Neugeborenen auf jede erdenkliche Weise geschützt werden müssen.

Von besonderem Interesse ist neben dem Umstand, dass ein äusserer Einfluss sich während des 1. Tages am meisten geltend macht, noch dass der Unterschied der Morgen- und Abendtemperatur am 6. Tage ausgeglichen zu sein scheint. Die unvergleichlich grösste Anzahl Todesfälle während des Säuglingsalters treffen in den 5 ersten Tagen nach der Geburt ein.

Da ein Zusammenhang zwischen der Dauer der Entbindung und der Temperatursteigerung des Kindes nicht besteht, wenn infektiös-fiebernde Mütter nicht mitberücksichtigt werden, kann ein Fieberzustand im Neugeborenenalter nach schwerer Entbindung nicht in Beziehung zur *physiologischen Temperaturerhöhung* bei Neugeborenen stehen.

Die Zustände, welche in der Literatur als Durstfieber, Inanitionsfieber etc. beschrieben worden sind, scheinen aus einer Verquickung zweier Erscheinungen mit ganz verschiedener Ätiologie zu bestehen, nämlich einmal einer normalen, physiologischen Temperaturerhöhung, die in der Mehrzahl der Fälle 37,5° nicht übersteigt und praktisch niemals 38,5° erreicht, und ferner wirklicher Fieberzustände mit pathologischer Genese.

Schrifttum.

ABT, Handbuch II, 374. — ADAIR u. STEWART, Amer. J. Dis. Ch. *31,* 846, 1926. — ERÖSS, Jb. Kinderheilk. *24,* 189, 1886. — HELLER, Z. Kinderheilk. *4,* 55, 1912. — HOLT, Arch. of Pediatrics, *12,* 560, 1895. — —, Lehrbuch, 1909. — JUNDELL, Jb. Kinderheilk. *59,* 521, 1904. — LINDERS, Om sambandet mellan nyfödda barns längd och vikt och moderns havandeskapstid, Stockholm 1930. — VON REUSS, Z. Kinderheilk. *4,* 32, 1912. RIETSCHEL, Ergebn. d. Inn. Med. u. Kinderheilk. *47,* 220, 1934. — SALMI, Acta Pædiatrica, *17,* 469, 1934. — WOLLSTEIN, Die Erhöhung der Körperwärme in den ersten Lebenstagen. Inaug.-Diss. Berlin 1934. — Stockholms stads hälsovård, Service sanitaire de la ville de Stockholm, *63,* 1940, Stockholm 1941. — Ausführliche Literaturangaben findet man, ausser in den Handbüchern, u. a. bei RIETSCHEL, SALMI und WOLLSTEIN.

Renal rickets and cystinuria.

By

Prof. Dr. S. van CREVELD and Dr. A. GRUNBAUM, Amsterdam.

In 1924 the pathologist LIGNAC (1) was the first to draw the attention to a syndrome which principally was characterized by renal affections, stunted growth, rickets and a disturbance in the cystine metabolism. The existence of the last mentioned disturbance was derived from the presence of cystine deposits found post mortem in different organs, especially in the spleen. In one of the cases of LIGNAC moreover cystine stones were found in the urinary tract. These cystine deposits in the tissues had been found already formerly in a case, communicated by KAUFMANN (2) in 1902. No deviations in the skeletal development nor the existence of a nephritis were, however, mentioned here. In this case of KAUFMANN the heredity of the disturbance in the cystine metabolism was placed in the foreground, because ABDERHALDEN (3) diagnozed cystinuria in two other children of the family and in the father and grand-father of the patient.

The cases described by LIGNAC in 1924 and later on have generally been regarded as being rare ones. In discussions on renal rickets the disturbance in the cystine metabolism was scarcely mentioned in the beginning, depending for the greater part on the fact that this disturbance had not been established during life. Of late this has altered for several reasons. Firstly cases of renal rickets have been described in which definite clinical and biochemical symptoms were failing, which till yet had been considered as being characteristic for renal rickets. Furthermore some cases have been described corresponding to those of LIGNAC, in which cystinuria or other signs of a disturbance in the cystine metabolism have been established during life. To this small group of cases also our case belongs, which we communicated in 1939 for the first time (4). — Besides from physiological side many researches have been performed in recent years on the metabolism of cystine and allied substances, which gave rise to new aspects of the problem. From these facts firstly the question arises whether in the etiology of many cases of renal rickets dietetic factors must be put in the foreground and secondly whether, with regard to the same etiology, a disturbance in the cystine metabolism should not be stressed more than thus far. In recent studies on cystine-disease by different authors from Basel (5 a—e) this second question, on other grounds, was answered by HOTTINGER in the affirmative for the cases of so-called renal rickets with renal glycosuria and for the cases of resistant rickets with glycosuria, described by different authors. — Before going into a more detailed discussion of some of the problems here concerned we report upon the above mentioned observation of our own.

The boy X. was admitted on 11.9.1939 to the Children's Department of the Binnengasthuis at the age of 2 1/2 years. Admittance had been demanded by the house-physician on account of severe rickets and glycosuria. The principal complaints were: vomiting, abnormal thirst and great retardation of growth. The boy was the 7th child of healthy parents. During her last three pregnancies the mother was put on diet on account of albuminuria. No relationship between the parents. Next to our patient only two boys of the seven children were still alive and healthy; two had been still born, two had died resp. when 10 years (sepsis?) and one year old (whooping cough followed by pneumonia). The 8th child had been still born one month too early. The patient had been born spontaneously in due time in the surroundings of Amsterdam; birth weight about 2500 Gm. Condition at birth normal. The boy was breast fed only for a few weeks, then he got for a long time goat's milk with floor, first diluted milk, then undiluted (compare later on). When he was 6 months old, fruit juice was added. During the first year no cod-liver oil, but the child was very often in the open air. Teeth appeared in due time. Mental development normal. Sitting was retarded; he could not walk until the age of 2 years. Till X-mas 1937 the growth should have been normal; much vomiting. After that retardation in growth. In Febr. 1938 abscess in front of the left ear, which showed a bad healing. On account of this abscess the boy came medio April 1938 in the Emma-Children's Clinic in Amsterdam (HOORNSTRA (6)). The weight of the boy, then 14 months old, was only 6400 Gm, his length 69.5 cM; he had rickets and albuminuria with in the beginning many granulated casts in the urine. Treatment of the rickets with Vitamin D (Davitamon AD) and calcium, later on with ultraviolet irradiation. The abscess healed promptly. During the stay in the Clinic once suddenly symptoms of strong exsiccation appeared, which apparently could not be explained by severe vomiting, severe diarrhea or marked decrease of water intake. With subcutaneous administration of physiological salt solution these symptoms soon disappeared. Some weeks later a glycosuria was present (the glucose being identified as such), which just as the albuminuria, was persistent. No acetonuria with exception on the day of entrance into the Emma Children's Clinic. (No glycosuria in the history of the family.) Urea-content of the blood 500 mGm pro liter; concentration power of the kidneys slightly diminished. No increase of the blood pressure, no edema. The glycosuria appeared to be a renal one. The concentration of serum calcium and of inorganic phosphorus of the serum were resp. 8.6 and 4.6 mGm. pCt. After the child had been discharged (at the end of June 1938) the parents withdrew from control.

Further anamnesis showed that the child from then on always was very thirsty, also during the night. Stools mostly came with difficulty, were very firm. During the last weeks before the entrance into the Pediatric Clinic of the Binnengasthuis (Sept. 1939) the child complained of pains in the legs, especially in the knees; going was impeded. — In the Pediatric Clinic the child did not make the impression of being ill. Feeding condition very moderate with a thin subcutaneous layer of fat. Bad turgor. Weight 7 KG, length 71 cM, sitting height 42 cM; so the boy according to age was greatly retarded in weight and length. No anemia. Intellect normal; the boy has a grave face. He can stand without help. Caput quadratum, the fontanel is about 2 cM wide. Teeth are complete but worn off and covered with a brown layer. The tongue is humid, rather glib. Thorax shows a strong rhachitic deformation. Heart is not enlarged, the first sound is impure. No deviations of the lungs. The liver is palpable one fingerbreadth below the costal margin, has a sharp edge.

Table I. Values for different constituents of the blood, determined on different dates.

Date	Calcium Mg. per 100 cc.	Inorganic phosphorus Mg. per 100 cc.	Serum phosphatase (Bodansky-units).	Sodium Mg. per 100 cc.	Chloride Mg. per 100 cc.	Carbon dioxyde, volumes per cent.	Cholesterol Mg. per 100 cc.	Urea Mg. per 1000 cc.
12.9.'39	—	1.9	17.9	—	—	34	—	250
18.9	10.8	—	—	—	—	—	—	—
4.10	11	2	23.8	—	385	—	263	—
300.000 Units of vitamin D_3								
16.10	12.8	2.7	29.7	—	—	34	183	—
23.10	—	2.6	34.3	—	—	—	259	—
30.10	11.3	2.8	—	292	—	—	—	—
6.11	—	2.6	27.2	—	—	42.5	—	29.3[1]
30.11	—	2.6	14.9	—	—	—	174	260
11.12	11.6	2.4	12.5	—	—	—	—	—
12.1.'40	—	2.5	7.9	—	—	—	—	280
2.2	—	2.3	—	—	—	—	—	—
29.2	—	2.0	12.0	—	—	—	—	—
2.4	11.0	2.2	—	—	—	—	—	28[1]
16.10	—	1.9	—	—	—	—	—	170

The spleen can be palpated one fingerbreadth below the costal margin. Slight kyphosis of the vertebral column. Testes can be palpated in the groin canal. Epiphyses are thickened, the fingers rather long. Tibiae are somewhat crooked. Bilateral pes planus. Normal reflexes. So in this extremely emaciated and small child, in poor condition, distinct rachitic symptoms were present. Fundus oculi normal. The appetite was good but in the beginning the child often vomited, also after the food had been changed. The child showed polydipsia and polyuria. The specific gravity of the urine was usually very low. The fresh urine was neutral to alcaline, clear, had a strikingly light colour (like grape fruit juice) and very soon became badly smelling (presence of ptomaines); it contained albumin (the quantity was never more than 0.1 per cent) and often a small amount of aceton; no sugar,

[1] non-protein Nitrogen, in Mg. per 100 cc.

diacetic acid or urobilin. The sediment usually contained some erythrocytes and no or a few casts. The concentration test showed a highly diminished power of concentration. After intramuscular injection of phenolsulfonpthalein there was an excretion of 45.5 per cent in the urine in two hours. Urea clearance normal. — The morphological bloodpicture at repeated examination showed no particularities. The inorganic phosphorus content of the blood was very low, the amount of serum alcaline phosphatase was increased. The cholesterol content of the blood was normal. The calcium content of the serum and the residual nitrogen or urea content of the blood were not increased. (A number of determinations in blood and serum have been repeated on different dates and the results are summarised in table I). — The v. Pirquet test with human and bovine tuberculin was negative, as also the v. Wassermann and Kahn tests.

In performing the tolerance tests with glucose (in relation to the finding of a glycosuria of the renal type in an earlier stade of the disease) the first time a diabetic curve with glycosuria and acetonuria was obtained, a second and third time a normal curve without glycosuria and without distinct acetonuria. With a view to the persistant glycosuria formerly found, and to the glycosuria present this time at admittance to the hospital, these curves are of importance. The diabetic curve was obtained in the test performed shortly after the entrance into the hospital, when on the preceeding day the child had vomited a great deal; this had given rise to a certain degree of exsiccation. It is known that under such circumstances diabetic curves in childhood may occur (7). The two normal curves with a normal fasting blood sugar and with absence both of glycosuria and distinct acetonuria are in striking contrast with the first curve and with the glycosuria of a renal type, found in an earlier stade of the disease. We can add here that also outside the days of these experiments an often repeated examination of the urine nevermore showed any glycosuria. The fact that the boy was put on a diet rather poor in fat, probably plays a role here.

With a view to the fact that the boy had vomited a good deal we composed his diet during the examination of the calcium- and phosphorus-balance as follows: 900 Gm. »concentrated» buttermilk (2 pCt floor and 12 pCt dextri-maltose) and 50 cc fruit juice. This diet was given for 5 days before the Ca- and inorganic P-balance with the same diet was examined during 3 days. During the 3 weeks preceeding these test-days the child daily got 2×5 to 2×10 drops of a vitamin D preparation (1500—3000 I.U.). Before the feces were collected and at the beginning

Table II.

Calcium balance: 4 Oct.—7 Oct. 1939.

Ca in »concentrated» buttermilk:	Ca in urine:	Ca in faeces:
3 × 1.28 = 3.84 gram	0.0158 gram	
	0.0112 »	
	0.0084 »	
	0.0354 »	3.10 gram
	= 0.92 per cent	= 80.73 per cent

Phosphor balance; 4 Oct.—7. Oct. 1939.

P in »concentrated» buttermilk:	P in urine:	P in faeces:
3 × 0.989 = 2.97 gram	0.1325 gram	
	0.1341 »	
	0.0802 »	
	0.3468 »	1.63 gram
	= 11.68 per cent	= 54.88 per cent

Excretion of	Ca	P
in urine	0.0354 gram	0.3468 gram
in faeces	3.10 »	1.63 »
In total	3.1354 »	1.9768 »
Added in diet	3.84 »	2.97 »
Balance	+ 0.7046 »	+ 0.9932 »
Daily retention:	$\frac{0.7046}{3} = 0.2349$ gram.	$\frac{0.9932}{3} = 0.3311$ gram.

and end of the 3 days' period orally carmine was given. The results of this balance experiment are given in table II. So a small retention of Ca and inorganic P was found, with a relation Ca : P in favour of P. The excretion of Ca and especially that of the inorganic P with the urine was small.

The X-ray examination of the skeleton showed typical rachitic changements: general osteoporosis, fraying, broadening and cupping of the epiphyseal ends of the shaft, coarse and irregular trabeculation especially of the metaphyses.

In order to examine the function of the liver the following tests were performed. A galactose test gave negative results. — The blood sugar curve after 16 Gm. of fructose gave the following values: in fasting condition 1.03 pro mille, after $^1/_2$ hour 1.85, after 1 hour 1.69, after 1 $^1/_2$ hour 1.63, after 2 $^1/_2$ hour 1.30;

so the rise was *abnormally high.* The voided urine gave no reduction and no positive Seliwanoff-test however, and did not contain aceton. — The fibrinogen content of the blood plasma was normal (0.38 Gm. per 100 cc; e.g. upper limit of normal) as well as the prothrombin time of the blood (after Quick). — The Takata-Ara test in the serum was negative. The sedimentation rate of the erythrocytes was normal.

The vitamin A content of the blood was very low (1.3 I.U. per 10 cc.); with a daily extra-dose of a concentrated vitamin A preparation this content soon became normal.

The stools contained temporarily a rather large quantity of soaps; no worns or worm-eggs.

With a view to the rather discouraging results of oral ingestion of vitamin D to patients as ours we gave the boy on Oct. 10, 1939, parenterally one single massive dose of 300.000 units of vitamin D_3. (The preceeding oral application of vitamin D had not resulted in any effect on the inorganic P content or on the alcaline phosphatase.) This healing shock-therapy was followed by a roentgenological cure of the rachitic process at the epiphyseal ends of the shaft, combined with a moderate local deposit of calcium; the structure of the shaft, however, was only slightly influenced (compare fig. 1—4). Further only a small transitory rise of the inorganic P content of the blood took place, whereas the increased value of the number of units of alcaline phosphatase after several weeks decreased to normal values. A transitory slight rise of the Ca content of the serum also appeared, but without any disagreeable symptom. — The improved roentgenological picture of the skeleton was still unchanged seven months after the massiv dose of vitamin D was given. Local sclerosis of the skeleton as observed with this treatment in an analogous case recently published by HOTTINGER (5) was not noticed in our case.

The consideration that the urine of the boy always contained an increased content of organic acids (determined after PALMER and VAN SLYKE) caused us to establish a nearer examination into the nature of these acids. These acids amounted in the 24 hours'urine on different dates to values of 3.9, 2.3, 2.9 and 4.1 cc of normal acid pro KG of body weight (normal values according to HOTTINGER and FANCONI 1.25 cc normal HCl pro KG). The ammonia-coefficient of the 24 hours' urine was in this boy 3.8 pCt (normal value 2.5 pCt). — The nearer examination of the nature of these organic acids learned in the first place that the urine contained much lactic acid (once even 28 mGm. pCt). Secondly the presence of cystinuria could be established several

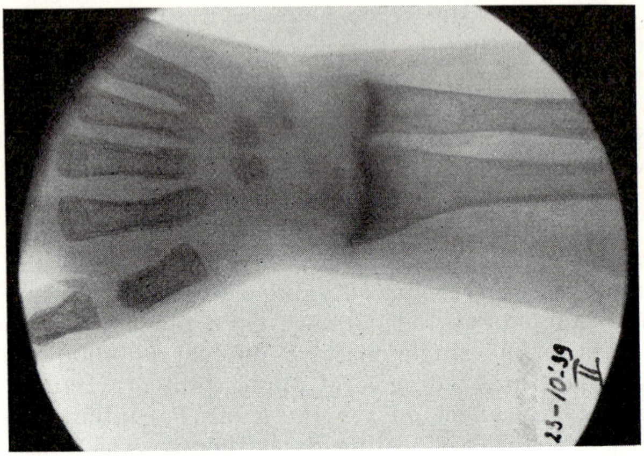

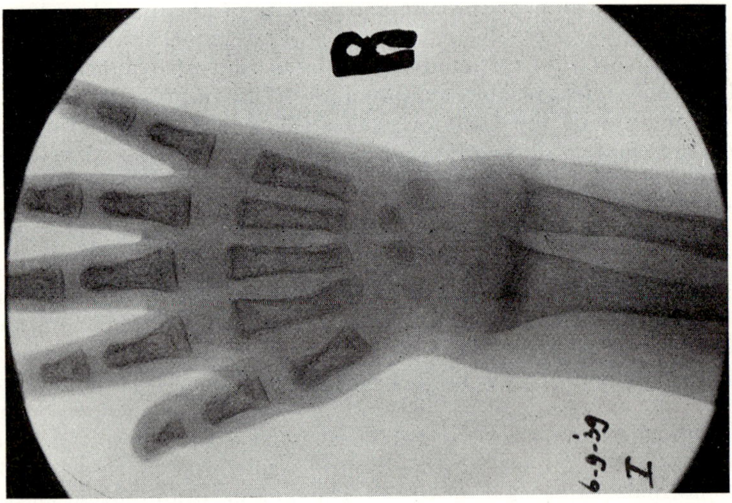
R

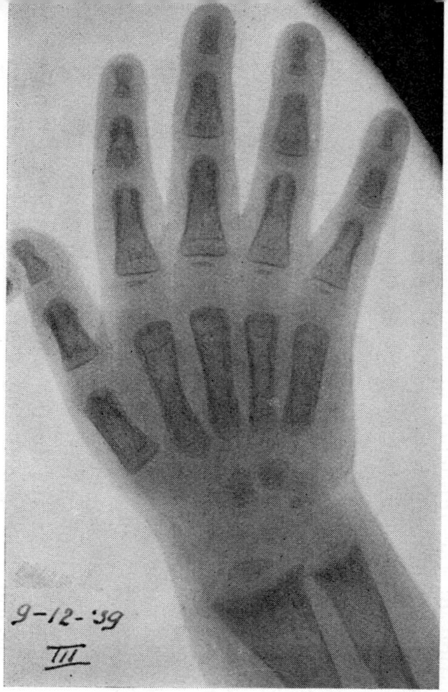

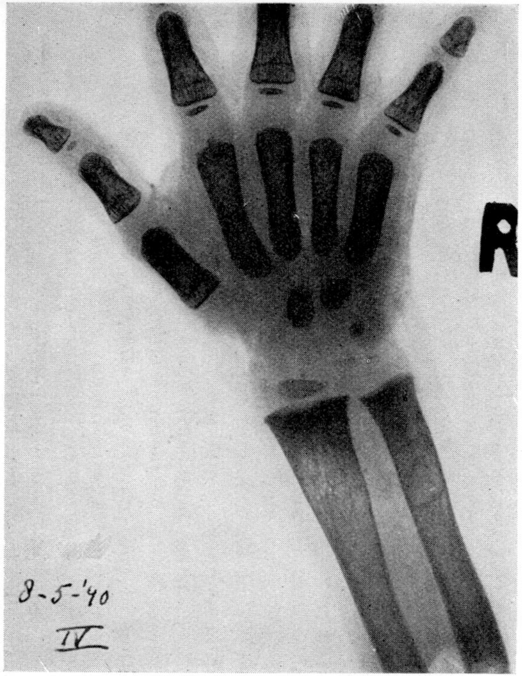

Roentgenograms of the wrist taken before and at different dates after the injection of one massive dose of vitamin D_3.

I. Taken 6.9.1939. Marked cupping of the epiphyses of radius and ulna; widening and irregular calcification of the metaphyses. Periostal reaction at radius and ulna. Centers of ossification small and indistinct.

II. Taken 23.10.1939. Improvement of the rachitic process at the distal ends of radius and ulna. Centers of ossification more distinct.

III. Taken 9.12.1939. Process at the distal ends of radius and ulna still more improved. Widening and irregular calcification of the metaphyses still clearly visible.

IV. Taken 8.5.1940. Distal ends of radius and ulna have maintained a normal aspect during several months. Findings in metaphyses analogous to those in the previous roentgenograms.

times: The sediment of the acidified urine after standing for several weeks contained typical cystine crystals which were identified as such. — Further from the urine benzoylcystine was isolated according to GOLDMANN und BAUMANN, und V. UDRANSZKY and BAUMANN (8). After recrystallisation the melting point of the obtained crystals was determined in a micro-melting point apparatus. This melting point corresponded to the date (180—181° C). The crystals in solution gave a black precipitate with lead-acetate and potassium hydroxyde. — Further the freshly passed urine often gave a more or less positive qualitative reaction for cystine (nitroprussid test after reduction with sodium cyanide). Later we succeeded in demonstrating cystine-crystals also in the fresh urine after having precipitated the cystine present as a cysteine-copper compound (method of ROSSOUW and WILKEN-JORDEN, compare later on). — Finally now and then also tyrosine-crystals could be isolated from the urine.

At examination of the relatives of the boy, also in the urine of his father once cystinuria was found.

The possibility of a pituitary dysfunction as a cause of the disease had to be considered in this patient. CHOWN (9) especially has defended this conception for analogous cases. Röntgenologically the turcic sella of our patient did not show deviations. In order to examine whether the polydipsia was primary in our boy we followed different ways, though a priori the disturbed renal function made an exact judgment not well possible.

A. Examination of the influence of restriction of the intake of fluid on diuresis, sodiumchloride content of the blood, hemoglobin content and on the specific gravity of the voided portions of urine.

1. For this purpose the patient from March 11 at 6 p.m. till March 12 at 10 a.m. remained in fasting condition; at 8.50 and 9.50 a.m. blood examination was performed. From 7 a.m. on the specific gravity was determined in each hour's portion of urine. Slight increase of the number of erythrocytes, relative volume and hemoglobin content was noticed. The specific gravity of the urine remained the same during the period of the withdrawal of fluid. — On March 14, in the middle of the day, the NaCl content of the serum was however about the same as that found at the end of the period of thirst (at 10 a.m. on March 12).

2. After a period of 3 days during which the patient got only small quantities of fluid, he got no fluid at all on the fourth day till 12 o'clock; at breakfast he got 2 gram of NaCl. The specific gravity of each hour's portion of urine remained the same from 6 a.m. till 12 o'clock; during the same time there was no in-

crease of Sahli, nor of the number of erythrocytes (rather a slight decrease). The NaCl content of the serum showed during that time a slight increase, as a consequence of the insufficient excretion of the extra NaCl at breakfast. The patient greatly objected to the restriction of fluid.

B. 1. The influence of injection of pituitrin on the quantity and specific gravity of the urine, while the use of fluid was unlimited.

	27/3, from	12 a.m.	—28/3, 8 a.m.	he drank	675 cc
1/2 cc pituitr. →	28/3, »	8 »	—29/3, 8 »	» »	1425 »
1 » » →	29/3, »	8 »	—30/3, 8 »	» »	1300 »
	30/3, »	8 »	—31/3, 8 »	» »	1400 »

Urine:	27/3—28/3	(from 8 a.m.—8 a.m.)	710 cc;	spec.gr.	1006
»	28/3—29/3	» 8 » —8 »	715 »	»	1006
»	29/3—30/3	» 8 » —8 »	485 »	»	1004
»	30/3—31/3	» 8 » —8 »	575 »	»	1004
»	31/3—1/4	» 8 » —8 »	920 »	»	1007.

So the influence of the pituitrin was clearly demonstrated, though the specific gravity of the urine did not increase. Thus it is highly improbable that we have to do with a pituitary influence in our boy.

2. Finally we examined the influence of injection of pituitrin on a day when the patient got no fluid till 12 o'clock:

4/4 after 8 a.m. no fluid
» 9 o'clock: 1 cc of pituitrin.

The specific gravity of each hour's portion of urine from 8—12 showed nearly no difference, rather a small decrease than an increase.

These experiments generally did not point to a pituitary origin of the polydipsia.

We have to deal here with a patient showing a remarkable type of rickets, where it is questionable whether we may speak of primary renal rickets. It is not a case of renal rickets in the former sense of the word. There is o. a. no hyperphosphatemia, on the contrary hypophosphatemia permanently was found by us. The residual nitrogen (urea) content of the blood always is normal. At least temporarily glycosuria and ketonuria were present and there were signs of chronic acidosis; several times cystinuria could be demonstrated. The result of the fructose-test and the occasional finding of tyrosine crystals in the urine also pointed to a disturbed liver function and perhaps also the very low vitamin A-content of the blood and the effect of the parenteral administration of vitamin D could be regarded as such. The disease began at an earlier age than the renal rickets usually start. The true nature of the renal deviations in this patient cannot be ascertained at present. Clinically and clinical-chemically — with exception of the cystinuria — there is a great resemblance to the cases described for the first time by DEBRÉ (10), DE TONI (11) and FANCONI (12), and further on by several authors (13—21); and moreover, as regards the cystinuria, to a small group of cases described for the first time by LIGNAC (1). We do not intend to enter into details of the manyfold questions to which the study of our case gives rise, especially not after the different extensive allied publications from other sides (compare especially the recent publication of GITTLEMAN and PINCUS (20)). We only want to make a remark on the permanent low concentration of inorganic phosphorus in the blood of our patient, which was not or only slightly influenced by the administration of vitamin D, even when given in one very large amount. There is a tendency to ascribe the chronic hypophosphatemia as well as the rachitic changes in such cases to the acidosis. However, there is no agreement as to the way in which the chronic acidosis gives rise to the rachitic changes and the hypophosphatemia. The most recent theory in this question is that of HARRISON and HARRISON (22). According to these authors vitamin D should influence the reabsorption of phosphates in the renal tubules. In the group of cases of rickets in which the existing low concentration of phosphate in the serum is not increased by the administration of vitamin D (DEBRÉ—DE TONI—FANCONI and others), there should exist a marked loss of phosphate in the urine. HARRISON and HARRISON assume, that the development of low phosphorus rickets in such cases is due to a failure of the renal tubular mechanism concerned with the reabsorption of phosphate[1] and that this tubular dysfunction is not corrected by the administration of vitamin D. The renal tubular reabsorption of phosphates should be greatly diminished by severe acidosis. However attractive the theory may be, we find it difficult to accept it in the explanation of our case, as the phosphate excretion with the urine at repeated examination was found to be small.

In the further discussion of this case we will restrict ourselves to the communication of some experiments and a discussion of one essential problem in our case: the combination of renal lesions with cystinuria.

The combination of a disturbance in the cystine metabolism, symptoms of a chronic renal affection and of (renal) rickets, and sometimes a disturbance in the carbohydrate metabolism, described for the first time by Lignac, has a special significance from the pediatric point of view. The disturbance in the cystine metabolism in these cases provisionally has to be separated from the well known familial cystinuria (belonging to the »inborn errors of metabolism» as Garrod (23) called them), from cystinuria occurring sometimes in severe parenchymal liver affections and from the formation of cystine stones as a separate affection.

Here follows first a short review of the cases which are reckoned to belong to the Lignac's syndrome.

The first case which is usually mentioned in speaking of this syndrome dates from 1902; then Kaufmann (2) found peculiar deposits in kidneys, intestinal wall, mesenterial glands, liver and spleen of a boy, 21 months old, who had died of inanition. In this case nothing was reported on the existence of nephritis or of skeletal lesions. Abderhalden (3) examined the chalky deposits in this case; they consisted in angular or more rounded crystals, which were identified as cystine crystals. Further he could demonstrate that in the family of the child cystinuria occurred in three generations, namely in two other children of the same family, in the father and in the grandfather.

The first description of cystine deposits in organs in children

[1] Compare in this regard the case of Goldmann and Ekstein (18), described under the title: »Renal dwarfism due to tubular dysfunction».

who during life showed a. o. disturbances in growth and symptoms of a severe renal affection, has been given by LIGNAC (1). In 1924 and 1925 he could observe 3 cases in non allied families; from this fact could already be deduced that this morbid condition perhaps is not so very rare. His patients were two boys of 3 and 2 years old, and a girl of 14 months. The children showed great developmental retardation and rachitic symptoms of different degrees. It is of importance that the first patient showed in the beginning pentosuria, always albuminuria and ketonuria and later on slight glycosuria without increase of bloodsugar. The anatomical and histological findings in the kidneys were greatly varying. In the first case there was a severe albuminuric degeneration (nephrosis). In the second case an acute non-purulent pyelonephritis was present. In the third patient in the left pelvis and in the right ureter cystine stones were found; the left kidney showed a cloudy swelling, the right one a non-purulent pyelonephritis. In two of the cases there existed an internal hydrocephalus. In none of the families of all three children cystinuria could be found; however, the fact that in the third child cystine stones were present in the urinary tract undoubtedly proves that at least temporarily cystinuria has been present in this case.

In 1936 RUSSELL and BARRIE (24) could augment the number of cases with three more. In only two of them deposits of cystine were found in the tissues after death. The first case of RUSSELL was that of a girl, aged 12 years; she died with symptoms of uremia. During life there was great retardation of growth and severe rickets; occasionally also glycosuria was present. At the autopsy greatly reduced kidneys were found; microscopically there was a diffuse fibrosis of the kidneys. Many glomeruli were completely destroyed and the tubuli were atrophied to a large extent. — The second case was that of a boy of 16 years old with a rather unknown history; *severe deformities of the skeleton and dwarfism were absent.* The kidneys showed the same picture as those of the former patient and the deposits of cystine in different organs corresponded to those found in the first case. In both cases no cystinuria had been found during life and also no cases of cystinuria could be found in the families of both children. — The third patient of RUSSELL and BARRIE was a boy, 13 years old; he is the first patient of the group of morbid cases in question where, at least during an early stade of the disease, cystinuria had been found during life, and also the presence of cystine stones. When the chronic nephritis had developed in this boy, the cystinuria disappeared, and after death no accumulations of cystine were found in the organs. The boy died with symptoms of uremia. The anatomical and histological picture of the kidneys of this case was quite in agreement with that found in the first two patients. This boy was not underdeveloped and showed no bony deformities.

BEUMER and WEPLER (25) in 1937 could describe a case in a boy who died at the age of 17 months. The clinical diagnosis was: renal diabetes and renal dwarfism, perhaps based on deformities of the kidneys. In spleen, liver, kidneys and thymus grey-white deposits were found which proved to consist in cystine crystals. The kidneys also here showed the picture of an interstitial nephritis. Next to this a retardation in development of the kidneys was derived especially from the aspect of many glomeruli. No cystinuria in the family of the patient.

In 1939 we communicated for the first time (4) our case, where during life the cystinuria was recognized and which was extensively described above. The boy is still alive.

In 1940 some cases have been published where the cystinuria also has been established during life. VAN DER ZYL and HESLINGA (26) reported on a case of renal dwarfism combined with cystinuria and *pyramidal and extra-pyramidal symptoms.* It concerned a boy of 12 years old, oldest of 6 children. The birth weight had been 3 KG; since birth the child always had been remarkably thirsty, and the urine always had a very light colour; it greatly resembled grape fruit juice. When the boy was 12 years old, the cystinuria had been established; the morning urine contained the greater part of the excreted cystine. When the renal symptoms became worse, more cystine was excreted. The residual N content of the blood was increased as well as the content of inorganic phosphorus. The urine of the patient's parents did not contain cystine. The authors do not mention whether the cystinuria in their patient regularly could be found.

In the same year PACHE (27) gave a description of two children where also during life the cystinuria has been recognized. The first child, a girl, when 11 months old had shown a transitory strong hypoglycemia and acetonuria. After the 8th month of life the growth of the child had been greatly retarded; there was anorexia, inclination to severe vomiting, further deviations in the urine and in the skeleton (renal rickets). Inorganic phosphorus of the serum 2,97 mgr. pCt. In 1937, when the child was 2 years old, FREUDENBERG in this case established cystinuria; at that time the child also showed strong polydipsia. Two years later the child had but little gained in weight, but its length had increased by $8 \frac{1}{2}$ cM in $2 \frac{3}{4}$ years. Intellect normal. Urine:

slight albuminuria, in sediment erythrocytes, hyaline casts and leucocytes. Specific gravity of the urine ranges within normal limits. Residual nitrogen normal. — During treatment with $^1/_2$ teaspoon of yeast daily the weight of the child temporarily increased in a striking way, and then no cystine could be demonstrated anymore in the urine in using the same method as formerly. — We must remark here that no mention is made by PACHE whether directly before the yeast-treatment was started cystine still could be demonstrated in the urine with the method he used. Further the method which could have proved that the cystinuria was favorably influenced by the yeast therapy, namely the performance of a tolerance test with cysteine or with methionine (compare later on) has not been applied in this patient.

The second patient of PACHE was a boy of the same family; by means of a sensitive method the cystine could be found in the urine when this child was two years old. After giving orally 0,5 gm of cysteine the excretion of cystine increased moderately. Severe rickets; slight albuminuria. In the sediment many casts. Hypertension. Residual nitrogen normal. Specific gravity of the urine normal.

Finally very recently (1941) a group of doctors from Basel (5 a—e) (HOTTINGER, FREUDENBERG, ROULET, BÜRKI, ESSER) in a series of articles communicated a case in a boy who at the age of 7 $^1/_2$ years died and where, as expected by FREUDENBERG before death, post mortem extensive deposits of cystine were found. In 1937 HOTTINGER (28) had described this boy as a case of dwarfism with renal rickets. Cystinuria has not been found during life. The post mortem examination has been very extensive and in different directions. From the diagnostical point of view of great interest are the cystine deposits found shortly before death in corneae and in conjunctivae, and the finding of cystine crystals in the slides of the bone marrow punctate. — In a newly born brother of this patient *cysteinuria* was established by HOTTINGER (5 a).

Summarising: the total number of cases in which the syndrome was present in a more or less complete form (especially dwarfism, renal lesions and disturbance in the cystine metabolism) amount to 14 (included the second case of HOTTINGER); of these 14 cases 10 have been published after 1936. — In the cases which came to autopsy and in which accumulations of cystine have been found in the tissues, cystinuria has not been established during life. In the third patient of RUSSELL and BARRIE, a boy aged 13, described in 1936, two small cystine stones have been removed at the age of 4 years (in 1921), and the *urine contained some cystine crystals.* One year later at operation a cystine stone was removed from the right ureter and about six small stones from the kidney substance. No cystinuria was found at the next admittance at the age of 13 years, and at the autopsy no cystine crystals were found in kidneys and other organs.[1] — So with the exception of this case the disturbance in the cystine metabolism and by this fact the true nature of the complex of symptoms during life has been established only a few times (two cases of PACHE, described in 1940, in one of which FREUDENBERG could demonstrate the cystinuria in 1937, our case, and the case of VAN DER ZYL and HESLINGA).

Considering the fact that stunted growth and renal rickets were no constant phenomena in all the above mentioned cases, one has to include also those cases in which cystinuria in childhood was combined with signs of disturbed kidney function only. As such may be considered the two cases, two sisters respectively aged 12 and 10 years, discribed by HICKMANS and SMALLWOOD (29). The albuminuria present in these cases was not associated with other evidence of kidney damage, but »it increased and decreased with increased or decreased output of urinary cystine».

In the studies — explanation of the cause and therapeutic attempts — of morbid cases, accompanied by cystinuria, one has to pay special attention to some results of recent experimental researches on the metabolism of the sulfur containing amino acids. Next to the

cystine $COOH \cdot CHNH_2 \cdot CH_2 \cdot S{-}S \cdot CH_2(NH_2)CH \cdot COOH$ are belonging to these sulfur containing amino acids:

methionine $CH_3{-}S{-}CH_2 \cdot CH_2 \cdot CHNH_2 \cdot COOH$, isolated in 1923 by MÜLLER, which is present especially in casein; BARGER has determined its composition and name;

[1] In his recent anatomical study of the case of Basel ROULET (5 b) emphasises the fact how easily the presence of cystine can be overlooked in the tissues.

cysteine, a reduction product of cystine: $SHCH_2 \cdot CHNH_2 \cdot COOH$;

homocystine: $COOH \cdot CHNH_2 \cdot CH_2 \cdot CH_2S—SCH_2 \cdot CH_2 \cdot CHNH_2 \cdot COOH$;

and *homocysteine* (methionine freed from cystine): $SHCH_2 \cdot CH_2 \cdot CHNH_2 \cdot COOH$.

Concerning the metabolism of a patient suffering from cystinuria it was known already for a long time, that administration of cystine did not give rise to an increase of the degree of cystinuria. BRAND and coworkers (30) were able to demonstrate, however, that cysteine and methionine, administered to a patient with cystinuria, are excreted for an important part as cystine.[1] »The fundamental difficulty in the cystinuric individual arises not from an inability to handle the cystine but rather the methionine in the food and also the cysteine which can be formed during protein digestion» (BRAND, CAHILL and HARRIS). The authors concluded from these facts that the oxydation of S—S- and of S—H-compounds probably is brought about by separate mechanisms.

Of the facts resulting from recent studies on the metabolism of sulfur containing amino acids (34), we must mention here the following:

1. The conception that cystine can be built up by the living organism out of methionine, and that, contrary to the current conception, cystine is no indispensable amino acid, has got new support.

---

[1] Already in 1908, as BRAND c. s. remember, GROSS (31) determined in a case of cystinuria the amount of cystine excreted in daily morning specimens in using the GASKELL method (acetone-acetic acid precipitation). He administered cystine and cysteine to the patient and found that the cystine precipitate in the morning specimen was increased after ingestion of cysteine only. An analogous experiment of WOLF and SHAFFER (32) gives no conclusive evidence in the opinion of BRAND c. s. — Sometimes the degree of cystinuria was also increased by giving amino acids which did not contain sulfur. So HESS and SULLIVAN (33) in a case of cystinuria found an increase of the cystinuria after giving alanine. In this case increased excretion was also noted after giving methionine, which increase had not been found in an earlier case.

2. In young animals methionine can be replaced, as regards its influence on growth, by homocystine and homocysteine. However, this growth promoting influence is dependent on certain dietetic factors, to which a. o. choline belongs.

3. If choline is absent from the food of young animals, an insufficient growth is the consequence, with fatty degeneration of the liver (no cirrhosis) and renal hemorrhages.

4. Addition of cystine to a choline-poor diet increases the frequency and intensity of the renal lesions and of other morbid symptoms in the young animals. When choline-chloride is added to the choline-poor diet, the renal lesions disappear and also (though more slowly) the fatty degeneration of the liver.

5. The presence of methionine or of proteins relatively high in methionine in the choline-poor diet has a retarding influence on the occurrence of renal lesions, or it prevents them totally. So methionine and cystine in this regard are exerting an antagonistic influence.

6. The old conception that cystine and methionine are able to increase the glycogen content of the liver, has not been confirmed by newer researches. So the explanation of the disturbances in the carbohydrate metabolism and of the ketonuria in patients with cystinuria must be sought in another direction.

In the light of these new facts, which a. o. stress the relation of choline to the metabolism of sulfur containing amino acids, we have to consider once again the experiments performed by many workers on mice, rats and rabbits on the effect of oral or intramuscular application of cystine on the kidneys. The first experiments of this kind have been done by LEWIS (35) (1925) and by LIGNAC (36) (1926). LEWIS gave large doses of cystine orally to rabbits. Usually one week later the animals died after having developed albuminuria with casts and nitrogen retention. At autopsy the kidneys showed cloudy swelling, casts and once inflammatory foci. LIGNAC injected cystine intramuscularly into mice and at the autopsy the kidneys showed a severe cloudy swelling of tubuli contorti and even necrosis of tubuli recti of the medulla, whereas cystine deposits were found in spleen, liver and kidneys. — This nephrotoxic action of cystine has been studied with analogous results by CURTIS and NEWBURGH and coworkers (37), by COX, SMYTHE and FISHBACK (38), BRAND, BEUMER and HÜCKEL (39) and by DORNUF (40). The general conclusion of these experiments was that young animals react on extra administration of cystine with severe renal lesions.

The same renal lesions occurred when certain proteins were present in the food of laboratory animals, whereas other proteins had no nephrotoxic effect. So for instance NEWBURGH and CURTIS (37), in studying the nephropathogenic effect of diets very rich in casein, beef protein or lactalbumin, were able to keep the animals over long periods on either of the first two proteins. In the case of lactalbumin they reported that many young rats died, without exception in 7 days or less. COX, SMYTHE and FISHBACK were of opinion that the toxicity of the lactalbumin might be due to its high content of cystine (more than 4 percent). Further HARTWELL (41) observed renal injuries and death in young rats when they were fed rations low in vitamin B and containing 20 percent of edestin as the sole protein. The kidney injuries found were similar to those observed by others in young rats after adding free cystine to the diet. Casein fed at the same level as edestin was harmless. An important increase of the vitamin B content of the diet protected the rats entirely from the kidney damage. The protecting factor present in the vitamin B preparation used (marmite) which was responsible for this protective activity, was not indicated, but aneurin could be excluded as such. In HARTWELL's opinion it was possible that some specific amino acids, present in edestin to a greater extent than in other proteins used, was responsible for the amount of marmite required. Cystine was accepted as such a specific amino acid (COX c. s.).

The factor in the vitamin B complex which prevented the nephrotoxic effect of cystine was further studied. GRIFFITH and WADE (42) arrived at the conclusion that this factor was choline and that methionine in this regard had a cholin-like action. These authors fed young white rats on diets low in choline content. Hemorrhagic lesions of the kidneys soon developed. Presence of cystine in the diet increased this nephrotoxic effect, while methionine delayed the effect. The same difference existed between proteins in the rations containing much cystine as fibrine, and proteins containing more methionine as caseine. GRIFFITH and WADE are of opinion that choline plays an important role in the maintenance of normal kidney structure in young rats. The choline requirement is principally dependent on certain other factors among which the methionine-cystine ratio, and the total amount of either, present in the protein may be particularly important. — The injurious effect of cystine on the kidneys of the rat could be prevented by choline and by methionine.

Analogous results were obtained by DU VIGNEAUD and coworkers (43). DU VIGNEAUD, ROSE and RICE (44) had found that the ability of the young white rat to utilize dietary homocystine (or homocysteine) instead of methionine, was dependent on secondary dietary factors other than the amino acids. Completion of the ration with the various components of the vitamin B complex available in pure form had no effect on the utilization of homocystine. However when the B-complex was furnished by milk concentrate and tiki-tiki (rice-bran concentrate) positive results were obtained. As unknown factors in these vitamin concentrates DU VIGNEAUD c. s. (45) could indicate choline, which was isolated in relatively large amounts from these vitamin concentrates.[1] When choline was fed with homocystine, the rat was able to utilize homocystine for purposes of growth instead of methionine.

These investigations stress a relation between the metabolism of choline and that of the sulfur containing amino acids, and in this way also to the kidney function, analogous

[1] We must remark, however here, that there remains the possibility that next to choline also another unknown factor with biochemical activity and different from the known members of the vitamin B complex plays a role here (compare the recent observations of STOKSTAD c. s. and of JUKES (47)).

to the relation demonstrated between choline and the production of fatty livers (Best c. s.).

The demonstration of the significance of certain dietetic factors to the nephrotoxic effect of cystine can further explain the fact, at least partly, that the number of cases of cystinuria combined with renal lesions, till yet is relatively small and that the intensity of an existing renal lesion is often greatly varying.

The fact that our patient got goat's milk from shortly after birth during a long time perhaps has had some aetiologic influence in so far as goat's milk has a larger content of lactalbumin than cow's milk and this lactalbumin has a high cystine content (4.3 per cent).

We have put ourselves the question in how far the application of these experimental findings, next to possessing a more general significance, may be of benefit in cases of cystinuria, and especially in the cases showing Lignac's syndrome. When in such cases the renal lesions are severe and exist already for a long time — as probably in our case — it hardly can be expected that these lesions can be cured totally. However, an eventual improvement of the »error of metabolism» (Garrod (8)) by dietetic measures (administration of vitamin B complex rich in choline, proteins rich in methionine and poor in cystine) can only have a favourable influence on the general condition of the young patient.

Hartwell's findings have been clinically applied in one of the two cases showing Lignac's syndrome, described by Pache (27). In this case, as already remarked, the impression was obtained that the general condition was favourably influenced by giving half a teaspoon of yeast daily.

With a view to study the influence of dietetic factors upon the cystinuria we performed some tolerance tests in our patient. First we performed two tests in our patient. Each time we gave him with an interval of 24 hours, 0.5 gram of cysteine hydrochloride. A great increase in the excretion of cystine with the urine followed, as could be judged from the very strong qualitative reaction for cystine given in the urine of these test days. At that time circumstances did not enable us to do quantitative determinations of cystine in the urine. However, we have estimated this cystine content by performing the qualitative test (nitroprusside test after reduction with sodium cyanide) also with urine of the patient collected outside the test days to which different quantities of cystine were added. In this way we arrived at the conclusion that in this series of two tests, considering the cystine already present in the urine, more than 40 percent of the ingested cysteine was excreted with the urine in the form of cystine. No cysteine was found in the urine as could be derived from the negative result of the nitroprusside test before reduction with sodium cyanide.

After these tests had been performed the patient got daily 3 grams of a dried brewers' yeast preparation containing choline and deprived from its bitter taste. One month later the tolerance test with cysteine was repeated in this way that the patient on one day twice (in the morning and at night) got 0.5 gram of cysteine hydrochloride. This time the qualitative reactions for cystine in the urine of the test day and in that of the two succeeding days were only weakly positive; they were not stronger than those often found on days when no cysteine hydrochloride was given to the patient. — The yeast treatment was continued, and 5 weeks later a third series of tests was performed. This time the patient on two successive days got each morning 1 gram of cysteine hydrochloride. The qualitative reactions for cystine of the urine of the two test days and one succeeding day were again only weakly positive. Also this time no cysteine was found in the urine. The quantitative determination of cystine in the urine of this last experiment was done by the method of Rossouw and Wilken-Jorden (48) as indicated by Brand and coworkers (49). The result is given in table I.

We must remark that with the method used in the urine of our patient on days when no cysteine was given, for the

Table III.

Day	Amount of cysteine HCl given	Quantity of urine in 24 hours	Amount of cystine in urine	Percentage of cystine in urine
1	1 gram	1790 cc	170.68 mg.	9.53 mg. pCt
2	1 »	1820 »	122.6 »	6.73 » »
3	—	1910 »	124.15 »	6.5 » »

percentage of cystine in the urine were found values, ranging between 4 and 8.5 mg. pCt., whereas the amount of urine in 24 hours was always about equally large. The oscillations in the cystine output on days when no cysteine was given are due to the fact, that it was practically impossible to keep the boy on a constant diet. — Accepting that during the days preceeding these tests the urine contained only 4 mg. pCt. of cystine, we arrive at the conclusion that of the administered 2000 mg. of cysteine hydrochloride about 7.5 pCt. is excreted as extra cystine; this is in contrast to the extra excretion of more than 40 pCt. of cystine in the tolerance test at the time when no yeast was yet given. (The patient of Brand c. s. excreted out of 8.8 gm. of cysteine HCl 2.13 gm. as extra cystine, e. g. more than 24 pCt.).

Instead of the yeast preparation we now gave our patient a combination of rice-bran and choline, especially in connection with the findings of Du Vigneau and coworkers, cited above. We added choline, in order to be sure that the rice-bran contained a sufficient amount of choline, as a rice-bran concentrate was not available.[1] We gave our patient thrice daily one teaspoon of rice-bran and 200 mg. of choline pro day. After the patient had used these two preparations for 18 days and while he continued to take them a fourth series

[1] We are indebted to Hoffmann-La Roche & Co at Basel for procuring us the cysteine hydrochloride and the choline hydrochloride, to the N. V. Beiersch Bierbrouwery »De Amstel» at Amsterdam for giving us the unbittered brewers' yeast, and to the N. V. Koninklyke Pellery »Mercurius» at Wormerveer for the rice-bran.

Table IV.

Day	Amount of cysteine HCl given	Quantity of urine in 24 hours	Amount of cystine in urine	Percentage of cystine in urine
1	—	1840 cc	154.56 mg.	8.4 mg. pCt.
2	0.5 gram	1910 »	177.63 »	9.3 » »
3	0.5 »	1920 »	131.33 »	6.84 » »
4	—	1920 »	84.48 »	4.4 » »

of tests was done. In this series the cystine excretion was determined during four successive days, whereas on the morning of the 2nd and 3rd day each time 0.5 gram of cysteine hydrochloride was given. The results are given in table II.

Thus also in this series of tests the extra cystine excretion is very small.

During the many weeks that the boy regularly made use of the yeast preparation or of rice-bran and choline, the deviations in the urine (large amount, low specific gravity, very light colour, quick putrification of the urine on standing when no preservative was added, in the sediment constantly one or some erythrocytes) remained the same. The general condition apparently slightly improved, and some increase in length and weight was noticed.

In the treatment of different forms and stades of renal rickets now and then a diet was indicated as logical which combatted the losses of calcium and phosphates with urine and stools, established by the study of the metabolism, and which also counteracted the chronic acidosis. Only occasionally temporary improvement was noted after the application of such and other therapeutic endeavours. Do the above mentioned considerations and experiments give reason to support these therapeutic endeavours also into other directions? In this regard we want to conclude with the following.

Cystinuria as occurring in certain patients with renal rickets is usually regarded as a constitutional (sometimes hereditary) anomaly of metabolism. The above cited animal experiments and in childhood a. o. our own experiments make it probable that the condition may also be caused by dietetic factors. One has to consider the possibility that the use of a diet of low choline content or of a diet which contains too much protein of a high cystine content by the pregnant mother or by the new born (perhaps the use of undiluted goat's milk by the new born may be regarded as such a diet) may give rise during the later stade of fetal life or in the young infant to lesions of the liver. These liver lesions may cause an abnormal metabolism of the sulfur containing amino-acids which in its turn in the young individual may give rise to severe kidney lesions. If this conception is right — and the results of our experiments speak in favour of it — perhaps it also contains some consequences of therapeutic value. Patients with renal rickets showing cystinuria, or in whom a disturbance of the cystine metabolism may be suspected, should get a diet which does not contain proteins with a high cystine content, and next to this should receive a total vitamin B complex which must contain sufficient choline.

Summary.

Report of a case of renal rickets with absence of azotemia and presence of hypophosphatemia in which cystinuria was demonstrated several times. Temporarily glycosuria existed. The metabolism was studied into different directions. No evidence of pituitary dysfunction was found, but there were some indications of a disturbed liver function.

A survey is given of the results of some recent experimental studies on the metabolism of sulfur containing amino acids. These studies stress the relation existing between certain dietetic factors, particularly choline, and the metabolism of sulfur containing amino acids, especially in young animals. The possible etiologic significance of such dietetic factors for the arise of hepatic and renal lesions in infancy is pointed out. The influence of dietetic factors upon the cystinuria was studied in our patient by performing some tolerance tests with cysteine hydrochloride. It appeared that the important extra excretion of cystine occurring after ingestion of cysteine hydrochloride was greatly reduced by the regular use of a yeast preparation or of a combination of rice-bran and choline.

In the treatment of patients with renal rickets and particularly of those patients in which cystinuria is demonstrated, the probability that dietetic factors have an etiologic significance should be taken in greater consideration. In this regard it is recommendable to give to such patients only proteins poor in cystine and a total vitamin B complex which must contain enough choline.

References.

1. LIGNAC, G. O. E., a. o. D. Arch. Klin. Med. *145,* 1924, 139; Münch. Med. W. *71,* 1924, 1016; Ned. Tydschr. v. Geneesk. *68,* 1924, 2987 and *69,* 1925, 819; Amer. J. Med. Sc. *196,* 1938, 542. — 2. KAUFMANN, E., Lehrb. d. spez. path. Anatomie, 7th and 8th Ed. II, 1922, 1107. — 3. ABDERHALDEN, E., Zeitschr. physiol. Chem. *38,* 1903, 557. — 4. CREVELD, S. VAN, Clinical demonstration Med. Society Amsterdam Nov. 28, 1939; Ned. Tydschr. v. Geneesk. *84,* 1940, 2373. — 5 a. HOTTINGER, A., Ann. Paediatrici *156,* 1941, 257. — 5 b. ROULET, F., Ann. Paediatrici *156,* 1941, 284. — 5 c. BÜRKI, E., Ann. Paediatrici *156,* 1941, 324. — 5 d. FREUDENBERG, E. Ann., Paediatrici *156,* 1941, 335. — 5 e. ESSER, M.. Ann. Paediatrici *156,* 1941, 344. — 6. HOORNSTRA, CHR. S., Maandschr. v. Kindergeneesk. *7,* 1938, 440. — 7. JOHN, H. J., J. Paediatr. *14,* 1939, 737. — 8. See C. NEUBERG: »Der Harn», I, 1911, 627 (Berlin). — 9. See a. o. CHOWN, B. and LEE, M., Am. J. Dis. Childr. *53,* 1937, 117. — 10. DEBRÉ, R., MARIE, J., CLÉRET, F. and MESSIMY, R., Bull. Soc. Péd. Paris 1934, 305. — 11. TONI, G. de, Acta Pædiatr. *16,* 1933, 479. — 12. FANCONI, G., Jahrb. f. Kinderh. *133,* 1931, 257 and *147,* 1936, 299; see also STURZENEGGER, H., Ann. Paediatr. *153,* 1939, 1. — 13. FORNARA, P., Il Lattante *8,* 1937, 437. — 14. GUILD, H. G., PIERCE, J. A. and LILIENTHAL, J. L.: Am. J. Dis. Child. 54, 1937, 1186; see also ELIOT, M. and PARK, E. A., Brennemann Pediatrics I, 36, p. 76. — 15. DEBRÉ, R. and MARIE, J., Bull. et Mém. Soc. méd. Hôp. Paris, July 22, 1938, nr. 26. — 16. NOBÉCOURT, P., CATHALA, J., BRISKAS, S. and MOREL, Arch. Méd. Enfants *41,* 1938, 204. — 17. LELONG, M., Bull. et Mém. Soc. méd. Hôp. Paris, 1938, nr. 25 (séance 8 July). — 18. GOLDMANN, F. and EKSTEIN, G., Journ. Pediatr. *15,* 1939, 53. — 19. MCCUNE, D. J., MASON, H. H. and

CLARKE, H. F., Am. J. Dis. Child. *58*, 1939, 673. — 20. GITTLEMAN, I. F. and PINCUS, J. B., Am. J. Dis. Child. *60*, 1940, 1351. — 21. ALBRIGHT, F. C. S. Johns Hopkins Hosp. *66*, 1941, 7. — 22. HARRISON, H. E. and HARRISON H. C., J. Clin. Investig. *20*, 1941, 47. — 23. GARROD, A. »Inborn errors of metabolism». Oxford Medical Public. 1923. — 24. RUSSELL, D. S. and BARRIE, H. J., Lancet 1936 (Oct. 17), 899. — 25. BEUMER, H. and WEPLER, W., Klin. Wochenschr. *16*, 1937, 8. — 26. ZYL, M. O. v. D. and HESLINGA, E. M., Nederl. Tydschr. v. Geneesk. *84*, 1940, 2120. — 27. PACHE, H. D., Zeitschr. Kinderh. *62*, 1940, 1. — 28. HOTTINGER, A., Schweiz. med. W. 1937, p. 977. — 29. HICKMANS, E. M. and SMALLWOOD, W. C., Biochem. J. *29*, 1935, 357. — 30. BRAND, E., CAHILL, G. F., and HARRISS, M. M., J. Biol. Chem. *109*, 1935, 69. — 31. GROSS, W. Sitzungsber. Ges. Morphol. u. Physiol. *24*, 1908, 97. — 32. WOLF, C. G. L. and SHAFFER, P. A., J. Biol. Chem. *4*, 1908, 439. — 33. HESS, W. C. and SULLIVAN, M. X., J. Biol. Chem. 133, XLIII, 1940 (Scientif. Proc.), and ibid. 123, LV, 1938 (Scientif. Proc.). — 34. For literature see Ann. Review of Biochem. IX, 1940, p. 220 and 293, and GUGGENHEIM, M.: »Die biogenen Amine», 3rd ed. Basel 1940. — 35. LEWIS, H. B., J. Biol. Chem. *65*, 1925, 187. — 36. LIGNAC, G. O. E., Krankheitsf. *2*, 1925, 43. — 37. See a. o. CURTIS, A. C. and NEWBURGH, L. H., Arch. Int. Med. *39*, 1927, 817, and NEWBURGH, L. H. and CURTIS, A. C., Proc. Soc. Exp. Biol. a. Med. *24*, 1927, 963. — 38. COX, G. J., SMYTHE, C. N. and FISHBACK, C. F., J. Biol. Chem. *82*, 1929, 95. — 39. BEUMER, H. and HÜCKEL, R., Klin. Wochenschr. *16*, 1937, 78. — 40. DORNUF, G., Mon. Kinderh. *82*, 1940, 120. — 41. HARTWELL, G. A., Biochem. J. *22*, 1928, 1212. — 42. See a. o. GRIFFITH, W. H. and WADE, N. J., Proc. Soc. Exp.. Biol. a. Med. *41*, 1939, 333 and J. Biol. Chem. *132*, 1940, 627. — 43. Vigneaud, V. DU, DYER, H. M. and KIES, M. W., J. Biol. Chem. *130*, 1939, 325. — 44. ROSE, W. C. and RICE, E. S., J. Biol. Chem. *130*, 1939, 305. — 45. VIGNEAUD, V. DU, CHANDLER, J. P., MOYER, A. W. and KEPPEL, D. M., J. Biol. Chem. *131*, 1939, 57. — 46. See a. o. BEST, C. H. and MACLEAN, D. L., Brit. Journ. of Exp. Path. *15*, 1934, 193. — 47. STOKSTAD, E. L. R., MANNING, P. D. V. and ROGERS, R. E., J. Biol. Chem. *132*, 1940, 463, and JUKES, TH. H., J. Biol. Chem. *133*, 1940, 631. — 48. ROSSOUW, S. D. and WILKEN-JORDEN, T. J., Biochem. J. *29*, 1935, 219. — 49. BRAND, E., CAHILL, G. F. and KASSELL, B., J. Biol. Chem. *133*, 1940, 431.

AUS DER KINDERKLINIK DES UNIVERSITÄTSKRANKENHAUSES IN UPPSALA. CHEF: PROF. DR. IVAR THORLING.

Zur Kenntnis der anämischen und polyzytämischen Zustände bei Neugeborenen sowie des Icterus gravis neonatorum.

(With an english summary.)

Von

GILLIS HERLITZ, Dozent.

Neben einer Anzahl anämischer Zustände in der Neugeborenenperiode, welche durch bekannte äussere oder innere schädigende Faktoren hervorgerufen werden, wie Blutungen, Lues, Sepsis, Malaria, Röntgenbehandlung, Bleivergiftung der Mutter usw., oder Begleiterscheinungen anderer, stärker dominierender Krankheitsbilder sind, wie Hydrops foetalis und Icterus gravis, findet sich in diesem Lebensabschnitt eine Gruppe von Blutmangelzuständen, deren klinische und pathologisch-anatomische Eigentümlichkeiten Anlass gegeben haben, sie von den übrigen, ihrer Natur nach mehr oder weniger symptomatischen Anämien abzusondern. Dieselben werden in der Literatur mit verschiedenen Namen bezeichnet: primäre, idiopathische oder essentielle Anämie des Neugeborenen, hämolytische Anämie des Neugeborenen, kongenitale Anämie, Anämie von Ecklin-Typus usw. In neuerer Zeit scheint indes der Name Anaemia neonatorum (Neugeborenenanämie, anemia of the new-born, anémie du nouveau-né) immer allgemeiner angewandt zu werden, um die hierhergehörigen Krankheitszustände zusammenzufassen.

Die Krankheitsfälle sind selten und in ihren Äusserungen durchaus nicht immer gleichartig. Ein Teil der Fälle zeigt weitgehende Übereinstimmungen mit den untereinander verwandten, familiären Krankheitszuständen Hydrops foetalis und

Icterus gravis, so dass man bisweilen geradezu von fliessenden Übergängen wenigstens zwischen der letzteren Krankheit und diesen Fällen sprechen kann. Mehrere Forscher fassen auch alle drei — Hydrops foetalis, Icterus gravis und Anaemia neonatorum — unter der gemeinsamen Bezeichnung Erythroblastosis foetalis zusammen, nach dem Teilsymptom, das, wie man im allgemeinen gefunden hat, allen dreien gemeinsam ist, und in dem manche das Essentielle der Krankheit erblicken, nämlich das reichliche Vorkommen von Erythroblasten im Blut. Andere Fälle von Anaemia neonatorum dagegen bieten ein klinisches Bild, welches in so wichtigen Beziehungen von dem eines Icterus gravis abweicht, dass man die Frage aufgeworfen hat, ob man nicht mit mindestens zwei wesensverschiedenen Formen der Krankheit zu rechnen hat, von denen die eine nahe mit Icterus gravis und deshalb auch mit Hydrops foetalis verwandt ist, während die andere diesen beiden völlig selbständig gegenübersteht.

Kennzeichnend für die erste Form soll sein: ein schwereres Krankheitsbild mit früh einsetzender und oft starker Anämie, charakterisiert durch kräftige Regenerationserscheinungen, z. B. Reichtum des Blutes an Erythroblasten und unreifen weissen Zellen, mit einer meist erheblichen Leukozytose, einem ausgesprocheneren Icterus, Milz- und Lebervergrösserung sowie einer schlechten Prognose. Post mortem haben bei dieser Form der Krankheit vor allem die ausgebreiteten extramedullären Blutbildungsherde die Aufmerksamkeit auf sich gezogen. Diese klinischen und pathologisch-anatomischen Züge lassen die Krankheit nahe verwandt mit Icterus gravis erscheinen, zu dem sie also, wie man sagen kann, einen Übergang bildet. — Für die zweite, selbständige Form dagegen, welche die gewöhnlichere von beiden ist, soll im Gegensatz zur ersten charakteristisch sein: eine später eintretende Anämie von mehr »torpider» Art ohne regeneratorische Zeichen in Form unreifer roter oder weisser Blutkörperchen im Blut und ohne Leukozytose, kein oder nur unbedeutender Icterus, keine oder bloss geringe Leber- und Milzvergrösserung sowie eine gute Prognose. Pathologisch-anatomisch findet man praktisch nichts ausser der Anämie. Man hat auch hervorgehoben, dass man häufiger die schwerere Form in familiärer Anhäufung zusammen mit Icterus gravis und Hydrops foetalis sieht als die leichtere, welche also mehr sporadisch auftreten würde.

Es will indes scheinen, als ob keiner der Faktoren, die man als geeignet zur Unterscheidung der beiden Formen angeführt hat, ein wirkliches Trennungsmerkmal von grundsätzlicher oder definitiver Bedeutung ist. Vielmehr handelt es sich nur um Gradunterschiede desselben Symptoms. Dies gilt auch für die Erythroblastämie, die ja schon normalerweise in den ersten Lebenstagen mit ungefähr 500 kernhaltigen roten Blutkörperchen auf 1 mm^3 oder gegen 0,01 % der roten Blutkörperchen vorkommt und keineswegs eine Reaktionsart zu sein scheint, die nur für die hierhergehörigen Krankheiten spezifisch ist. Es liegt auf der Hand, dass der Forschung, solange Unklarheit über die Ätiologie einer Krankheit herrscht, nur an Versuchen gelegen sein kann, verschiedene Typen derselben zu unterscheiden, aber je mehr Fälle man später findet, welche Übergangsformen zwischen diesen Krankheitstypen darstellen, um so mehr verliert die Typeneinteilung an Interesse.

Nachstehend will ich über zwei Fälle von Anämie bei Neugeborenen berichten, die ich beobachtet habe, und die in grossem Umfang gleichzeitig Züge von beiden oben genannten Formen der Krankheit aufweisen. Es handelt sich nämlich in beiden Fällen um eine früh eintretende Anämie mit ausgesprochener — in dem einen Fall sogar exzessiver — Erythroblastämie, aber ohne Icterus, ohne Leber- und Milzvergrösserung und mit einer guten Prognose. Die Fälle sind unter anderem auch deshalb interessant, weil sie beide je einen Zwilling eines eineiigen Zwillingspaares betreffen, während der andere Zwilling jedes Paares gesund war, aber in beiden Fällen ein Blutbild aufwies, dass in gewissen Beziehungen dem der kranken Kinder gerade entgegengesetzt war, nämlich das Bild einer Polyzytämie. Ausserdem zeigten die Thrombozytenzahlen bei den beiden kranken Kindern Veränderungen, die ich bei diesen Krankheitszuständen bisher nicht beschrieben gefunden habe. In einem der Fälle war auch ein Umstand hinsichtlich der Blutverteilung in der Plazenta zu konstatieren, der in diesem Zusammenhang bemerkenswert ist. (Über die Fälle ist im Verein der schwedischen Kinderärzte am 29.5.1935 berichtet worden.)

Fall 1. Eltern gesund, nicht verwandt. Mutter 1905 geboren, der Vater 1910, Landarbeiter. In den Familien sind keine Fälle von Wasserfötus, schwerer Gelbsucht oder früher, auffallender Blässe der Neugeborenen bekannt, ebensowenig wiederholte Fehlgeburten. Keine Venerien bei den Eltern. Wassermanns Reaktion bei der Mutter negativ. Erster Partus der Mutter 1932; hatte während der Schwangerschaft Cystopyelitis und Hyperemesis gravidarum. Der Partus war unkompliziert; das Kind, ein Mädchen, gesund. Zweiter Partus 1933; hatte Albuminuria sub et post partum. Im übrigen unkomplizierte Schwangerschaft und Entbindung; das Kind, ein Mädchen, gesund. Keine Fehlgeburten.

Die dritte Schwangerschaft resultierte in dem Zwillingspaar, welches hier beschrieben werden soll. Die letzte Menstruation begann am 31.7.1934. Fötusbewegungen Anfang Dezember. Während der ganzen Schwangerschaft ziemlich viel Erbrechen, am wenigsten im 5. und 6. Monat. Am 20.3.1935 Leibschmerz und Schüttelfröste, Temp. 39.6°: Cystopyelitis ac., die sich bald besserte. Am 27.3. unkomplizierter Partus 5 Minuten nach Sprengung der Eihäute mit Abgang von Fruchtwasser, dessen Menge und Aussehen normal war. Die Zwillinge wurden mit 15 Minuten Zwischenraum geboren, und die Plazenta ging nach weiteren 20 Minuten spontan ab. Abnabelung erfolgte nach 1—2 Minuten. Blutung vor Abgang der Plazenta 300 g, nach demselben 200 g (normal). Die Plazenta war zusammenhängend und rundlich elliptisch, ihr Gewicht betrug 1050 g (normal). Zwei Blätter in der Scheidewand zwischen den Eihautsäcken. Die beiden Nabelstränge waren symmetrisch in der Längsachse der Plazenta befestigt, jeder ungefähr im Zentrum seiner Plazentahälfte. Die Hälfte, die zu dem blassen Kind gehörte (siehe unten), war auffallend blass im Vergleich mit der andern, welche normale Farbe hatte; die Grenzlinie war ziemlich scharf und verlief längs der Querachse der Ellipse. Sonst keine auffallenden Veränderungen der Plazenta, die leider nicht näher untersucht wurde. Die Mutter wies zwei Tage nach dem Partus einen Hämoglobingehalt von 65 % auf (Sahli).

Zwilling Nr. I. Johan W., Knabe, Gewicht 1 580 g. Wurde unmittelbar nach der Geburt auf die Pädiatrische Abteilung gebracht. Sehr blasse Hautfarbe bei der Geburt, aber kräftiges Schreien und verhältnismässig guter Zustand im übrigen. Kein Icterus. Leber und Milz nicht tastbar. Im übrigen zeigte der Status nichts Bemerkenswertes. Die erste Blutprobe wurde etwa 3 Stunden nach der Geburt entnommen. Sie zeigte einen Hämoglobingehalt (Sahli) von 50 %, 1 940 000 rote Blutkörperchen und 10 600 kernhaltige Blutzellen je mm^3. Im Ausstrichpräparat 4 % unreife weisse Blutkörperchen sowie 50 Erythroblasten auf 100 weisse Blutkörperchen, entsprechend einem Wert von 3 500 Erythroblasten je mm^3 oder 0,18 % der roten Blutkörperchen (Näheres siehe Tab. 1).

Ohne therapeutische Massnahmen (abgesehen von einer kleinen Dosis Ferrum reductum, die erstmalig am 21.4. gegeben wurde) besserte sich die Anämie allmählich (siehe die Tabelle). Der Allgemeinzustand des Kindes war die ganze Zeit über erstaunlich gut. Es wurde mit der Milch der Mutter genährt. Die Gewichtszunahme war im ganzen eine gute, und am 21.9.1935 wurde Pat. in gutem Zustand entlassen. Die Leber war zeitweise eben noch tastbar, die Milz war niemals palpabel und auch nicht röntgenologisch vergrössert. Blutungen wurden nicht beobachtet, ebensowenig Icterus. Keine Zyanose. Die osmotische Resistenz der roten Blutkörperchen war normal. Am 20.4. wurden die Thrombozyten zum erstenmal gezählt, wobei der abnorme Wert von 1 915 000 je mm^3 festgestellt wurde. Umrechnungen ergaben dieselben hohen Werte. Hierauf sank die Thrombozytenzahl, lag aber auch in der Folge an der oberen Grenze des Normalen (siehe die Tabelle). Knochenmarkspunktion[1] (in der Tibiaepiphyse) am 26.5. zeigte ein Mark, dessen Reichtum an Zellen auf Hyperplasie deutete. Leichte Erhöhung der Prozentzahl Myeloblasten mit auffallend vielen Mikromyeloblasten. Im übrigen lagen die Prozentzahlen für die verschiedenen Zellarten innerhalb der Grenzen der normalen Variabilität. Keine pathologischen Zellformen.

Am 24.1.1936 kam Pat., der bis dahin gesund gewesen war und sich zu Hause normal entwickelt hatte, mit akuten Bauchersch einungen und einer Blutung per rectum ins Krankenhaus. Man konstatierte Invagination, deren Ursache, wie sich bei der Operation herausstellte, ein Meckelsches Divertikel war. Die Blutung rührte von dem etwa 2 Tage alten Invaginat her. Der Nachverlauf war komplikationsfrei, und Pat. wurde gesund entlassen. Das Blutbild zeigte eine Linksverschiebung (siehe die Tabelle), die wohl mit der akuten Baucherkrankung in Zusam-

[1] Für Gutachten über die Knochenmarkpunktate in Fall 1 und 2 spreche ich der Dozentin ELSA SEGERDAHL, Uppsala, meinen verbindlichsten Dank aus.

Tab. 1. Fall 1.

Tag	Hämoglobin in %	Erythrozyten in Millionen	Leukozyten in Tausenden	Thrombozyten in Tausenden	Weisses Blutbild: My + Jug	Neutro	Eo	Bas	Lympho	Mono	Erythroblasten in Tausenden	Bemerkungen
Zwilling Nr. I. Knabe, geb. 27.3.1935.												
27/3 1935	50	1,94	7,1		4	43	7	0	35	11	3,5 (= 1,8 ‰)	Polychromasie.
10/4	40—45	2,58										
20/4	45	2,06	13,7	1 915,0	1,5	51	11,5	0,5	26	9,5	0	Retikulozyten 3 %.
7/5	50	2,62	18,7	430,0	1	41	3,5	0	49	5,5	0	do.
18/5	65	3,32	9,9	438,0	1	20	9	0	64	6	0,1	Geringe Aniso- und Poikilozytose.
22/6	60	3,38	23,7	857,0	0	50	1	0	48	1	0	do.
26/7	65—70	3,69	10,7	591,0	0	16	11	0	67	6	0	do.
21/9	70	4,04	4,8	385,0	0	20	9	0	65	6		Retikulozyten 2,5 %.
24/1 1936	80	5,33	10,5		7	40	0	0	36	17		Invaginatio ileocolica.
6/12 1941	90	5,28	9,7	312,0	0	33	10,5	0,5	52	4		Nachuntersuchung.
Zwilling Nr. II. Knabe, geb. 27.3.1935.												
27/3 1935	160	7,02	10,7		0,5	53,5	2	0	34	10	0,6 (= 0,1 ‰)	Polychromasie.
12/4	140—150	6,27										
20/4	120	5,5	7,8	254,0	0	29,5	7	0	46	17,5	0	
19/9	80	4,05	8,2	399,0	0	17,5	13,5	0,5	64	4,5	0	
6/12 1941	83	4,35	7,5	341,0	0	31,5	5	0	59,5	4		Nachuntersuchung.

menhang gebracht werden kann, obgleich keine ausgesprochenen Peritonitiszeichen bei der Operation bestanden. Das Gewicht des Kindes bei der Operation betrug 5 490 g.

Eine Nachuntersuchung am 6.12.1941 ergab, dass sich der Knabe in allen Beziehungen gut entwickelt hatte, wenn er auch physisch noch etwas hinter dem Zwillingsbruder zurückgeblieben war (Länge 109 cm, Gewicht 17,3 kg). Seitens der inneren Organe nichts Pathologisches. Das Blutbild zeigte nichts Abnormes (siehe die Tabelle). Die Mutter hat keine Kinder mehr bekommen und keine Fehlgeburten gehabt.

Zwilling Nr. II. Evert W., Knabe, Gewicht 2 580 g. Normale, rosa Hautfarbe bei der Geburt. Guter Allgemeinzustand, aber in den ersten Tagen ziemlich anhaltende Zyanose von Gesicht und Extremitäten, die dann verschwand, ohne wiederzukehren. Bei der Geburt ein mässiges Ödem im Scrotum. Die Leber war eben noch tastbar. Die Milz war nicht palpabel. Im übrigen zeigte der Status nichts Bemerkenswertes. Die erste Blutprobe wurde 15 Stunden nach dem Partus entnommen. Sie ergab einen Hämoglobinwert (Sahli) von 160 %, 7 020 000 rote Blutkörperchen und 11 300 kernhaltige Blutzellen je mm^3. Im Ausstrich 0,5 % unreife weisse Blutkörperchen sowie 12 Erythroblasten auf 200 weisse, entsprechend einem Wert von 640 Erythroblasten je mm^3 oder 0,01 % der roten Blutkörperchen (Näheres siehe Tab. 1).

Das Kind, welches am Tage der Geburt in die Päd. Abt. gebracht wurde, entwickelte sich in allen Beziehungen normal. Die Leber war nach den ersten Tagen nicht mehr tastbar, die Milz niemals. Icterus trat nicht auf. Keine Blutungen. Die Thrombozytenzahl war normal (vgl. die Tabelle). Wurde am 30.4.1935 in gutem Zustand entlassen.

Bei Nachuntersuchung am 6.12.1941 wurde festgestellt, dass das Kind normal entwickelt war (Länge 110 cm, Gewicht 18,7 kg). Seitens der inneren Organe nichts Pathologisches. Das Blutbild zeigte nichts Abnormes (siehe die Tabelle).

Fall 2. Mutter 1915 geboren, unverheiratet. Über den Vater ist nichts Näheres bekannt. In der Familie der Mutter sind keine Fälle von Wasserfötus, schwerer Gelbsucht oder frühzeitiger auffallender Blässe der Neugeborenen bekannt. Mutter gesund, keine Venerien, Wassermann neg. Ihre erste Schwangerschaft resultierte in den unten beschriebenen Zwillingen.

Die letzte Menstruation begann Mitte August 1934. Die Schwangerschaft hatte normalen Verlauf. Partus am 3.5.1935. Die Zwillinge wurden mit 15 Minuten Zwischenraum geboren, nachdem Eihautsprengung für den zweiten Zwilling vorgenommen worden war. Das abgegangene Fruchtwasser war in bezug auf Farbe und Menge normal. Abnabelung erfolgte nach 1—2 Minuten. Die Plazenta ging ein paar Minuten nach dem zweiten Zwilling spontan ab. Blutung vor und während des Abgangs der Plazenta 630 g, nach demselben 870 g, also mehr als normal. Die Plazenta wog 1 050 g und zeigte nichts Bemerkenswertes. Zwei Blätter in der Scheidewand zwischen den Eihautsäcken. Blutwerte der Mutter drei Tage nach dem Partus: Sahli 65, rote Blutkörperchen 3 250 000; Differentialzählung der weissen Blutkörperchen ergab nichts Pathologisches.

Zwilling Nr. I. Maj Britt J., Mädchen, Gewicht 3 030 g. Schon bei der Geburt auffallend stark dunkelrote allgemeine Hautfarbe. Ziemlich kräftige zyanotische Färbung von Händen, Füssen und Gesicht. Kräftiges Schreien und guter Allgemeinzustand im übrigen. Kein Icterus. Leber und Milz eben noch tastbar. Im übrigen zeigte der Status nichts Bemerkenswertes. Die erste Blutprobe wurde etwa 30 Stunden nach dem Partus entnommen. Der Hämoglobingehalt betrug ungefähr 200 % (das Sahli-Röhrchen reichte nicht aus) und die Anzahl der roten Blutkörperchen 6 520 000 je mm^3. Acht Stunden später betrug der Wert 7 200 000 und nach weiteren 15 Stunden 8 030 000 je mm^3. Die Zahl der kernhaltigen Blutzellen betrug in dem letzteren Zeitpunkt 4 800 je mm^3, und das Ausstrichpräparat zeigte 4 Erythroblasten auf 200 weisse, d. h. 96 je mm^3 (Näheres siehe Tab. 2).

Das Kind, das am Tage nach der Geburt in die Päd.Abt. gebracht wurde, entwickelte sich dann im ganzen normal. Die hohen Werte von Hämoglobin und roten Blutkörperchen blieben jedoch lange bestehen (siehe die Tabelle), und die dunkelrote Hautfarbe war noch 14 Tage nach der Geburt in die Augen fallend; danach wurde sie allmählich weniger ausgesprochen. Die Neigung zu Zyanose an Händen, Füssen und im Gesicht blieb gleichfalls während der ersten zwei Wochen bestehen, verschwand dann aber. Die bei Polyglobulie verschiedener Art sowohl bei Erwachsenen als bei Kindern (vgl. OPITZ) charakteristische Verfärbung der Schleimhäute lag nicht vor. Blutdruck 70—80, systolisch. Die Koagulationszeit des Blutes war normal. Icterus lag nicht vor, ebensowenig Ödeme. Urobilin und Urobilinogen waren nur bei einer Gelegenheit im Harn vorhanden (spurenweise). Leber und Milz waren nach 1—2 Wochen nicht mehr tastbar, auch röntgenologisch zeigte die Milz normale Grösse. Einen Beleg für kongenitales Vitium konnte man nicht erhalten. Das Herz zeigte sowohl bei physikalischer als bei röntgenologischer Untersuchung

Tab. 2. Fall 2.

Tag	Hämoglobin in %	Erythrozyten in Millionen	Leukozyten in Tausenden	Thrombozyten in Tausenden	Weisses Blutbild						Erythroblasten in Tausenden	Bemerkungen
					My+Jug	Neutro	Eo	Bas	Lympho	Mono		
					Zwilling Nr. I. Mädchen, geb. 3.5.1935.							
4/5 1935	200	6,52—7,20										
5/5	180	8,03	4,7		0	44	3,5	0,5	22	30	0,1	
8/5	160	7,24	7,1	170,0	0	45	2	0	26	27	0	
13/5	150	7,10	8,0	276,0	0	38	1	0	43	18	0	
21/5	150	7,16	8,8	264,0	1	20	4	1	68	6	0	
28/5	135	6,61	11,8	296,0	0	16	2	0	59	23	0	
6/12 1941	86	4,84	3,5	192,0	0	25	8,5	0,5	44,5	21,5		Nachuntersuchung.
					Zwilling Nr. II. Mädchen, geb. 3.5.1935, gest. 22.7.1935.							
4/5 1935	65	2,27	6,0	272,0	0	62,5	2,5	0	24,5	10,5	21,0 (= 9,2 ‰)	
9/5	65—70	3,13	4,7		0	25	5	0	57	13	4,8	Polychromasie. Aniso- und Poikilozytose. Mikrozytose. Retikulozyten 5 %.
13/5	75	3,50	12,2	1 250,0	3,5	42,5	4	0,5	31	18,5	0,4	
16/5	60—65	2,96	44,5	1 200,0	1	76	0	0	16	7	0,4	Retikulozyten 2 %.
20/5	65	2,82	11,6	1 070,0	4	31	1	1	46	17	0	Keine Retikulozyten.
27/5	60	2,86	17,0	1 610,0	4	33	0	0	56	7	0,2	do.
5/6	55	2,49	12,2	760,0	1	26	3	0	58	12	0	Retikulozyten 1 %.
19/6	45—50	2,43	8,9	506,0	0	24	4	0	65	7	0	» 4—5 %.
2/7	55—60	2,96	18,6	686,0	0	22	0	0	72	6	0	» 4 %.
16/7	55—60	3,10	12,8	586,0	1	40,5	1	0	54,5	3	0,1	» 4—5 %.

normale Verhältnisse. Keine Blutungen. Die Thrombozytenzahl war normal (siehe die Tabelle), ebenso die osmotische Resistenz der roten Blutkörperchen. Knochenmarkspunktion (in der Tibiaepiphyse) am 26.5.: sehr zellreiches Mark. Die Prozentzahl der Myeloblasten war erhöht. Im übrigen lagen die Werte innerhalb der Grenzen des Normalen. Keine pathologischen Zellformen. Die roten Zellelemente auffallend hämoglobinreich. — Entlassung am 1.6. in gutem Zustand.

Nachuntersuchung am 6. 12. 1941 ergab, dass sich das Mädchen in allen Beziehungen gut entwickelt hatte (Länge 122 cm, Gewicht 23,6 kg). Die Milz war indes durch die dünne Bauchwand fühlbar, sie schien unbedeutend vergrössert und weich zu sein. Sonst nichts Pathologisches seitens der inneren Organe. Das Blutbild wies nichts Abnormes auf (siehe die Tabelle). Die Mutter hat keine Kinder mehr bekommen und keine Fehlgeburten gehabt.

Zwilling Nr. II. Eva J., Mädchen. Gewicht 2 220 g. Schon bei der Geburt auffallende allgemeine Blässe, die stark gegen die dunkelrote Hautfarbe des andern Zwillings abstach. Im übrigen verhältnismässig guter Allgemeinzustand. 12 Stunden nach der Geburt war die Blässe noch ausgesprochener. Icterus war nicht vorhanden. Leber und Milz waren nicht tastbar, und der Status zeigte auch sonst nichts Bemerkenswertes. Die erste Blutprobe wurde etwa 30 Stunden nach der Geburt entnommen. Der Hämoglobinwert (Sahli) betrug damals 65 %, die Anzahl der roten Blutkörperchen 2 270 000 und die der kernhaltigen Blutzellen 27 000 je mm^3 (im übrigen siehe Tab. 2). Auf 200 weisse Blutkörperchen wurden im Ausstrichpräparat keine unreifen weissen festgestellt, aber nicht weniger als 700 kernhaltige rote, entsprechend einem Wert von 21 000 Erythroblasten je mm^3 oder nahezu 1 % der roten Blutkörperchen. Von den Erythroblasten hatten 6—7 % mehr als einen Kern.

Das Kind wurde am Tage nach der Geburt in die Päd. Abt. gebracht. Dort wurde es die ganze Zeit über mit Ammenmilch ernährt. Die Milch der Mutter reichte von Anfang an nicht aus und versiegte nach drei Wochen ganz. Anfangs wurde die Anämie überhaupt nicht behandelt. Am 31. 5. wurde mit Verabreichung einer täglichen kleinen Dosis Ferrum reductum begonnen, und am 12. 6. erhielt das Kind eine intramuskuläre Blutinjektion von 3 ccm, die dann in den nächsten drei Wochen wöchentlich einmal wiederholt wurde. Der Allgemeinzustand war die ganze Zeit über gut, und die Gewichtszunahme war nach den ersten 14 Tagen gleichmässig und gut. Die Erythroblastämie verschwand bald, und nach der allmählichen Vermehrung der Retikulozyten zu urteilen, ging der Zustand der Besserung entgegen, obgleich die Anämie hartnäckig war. Am zweiten Tage wurden die Thrombozyten zum erstenmal gezählt und hatten damals normale Werte. Wegen der Erfahrungen im vorhergehenden Fall (Fall 1, Zwilling Nr. I) wurde die Thrombozytenzahl indes auch weiterhin verfolgt und zeigte bald dieselben hohen Sprünge nach oben wie im vorhergehenden Fall (siehe die Tabelle). Die osmotische Resistenz der roten Blutkörperchen war normal. Leber und Milz waren nicht tastbar, die letztere zeigte auch bei röntgenologischer Untersuchung keine sichere Vergrösserung. Während der letzten Woche, als eine Kapillarbronchitis das Bild komplizierte, konnte die Milz jedoch unmittelbar unter dem Arcus gefühlt werden. Am vierten Tage trat leichter Icterus auf, der nach einigen Tagen verschwand. Keine Zyanose. Keine Blutungstendenz. Die Koagulationszeit des Blutes war auch normal. Knochenmarkspunktion (in der Tibiaepiphyse) am 26. 5. ergab zellreiches Mark. Prozentzahl der Myeloblasten erhöht. Im übrigen lagen die Prozentzahlen für die verschiedenen Zellarten innerhalb der Grenzen des Normalen. Keine pathologischen Formen.

Am 12. 7. traten Zeichen von Kapillarbronchitis auf, die nicht gehemmt werden konnte, sondern am 22. 7. zum Tode führte. Bei der Obduktion war ausser der allgemeinen Anämie und der Kapillarbronchitis nichts Pathologisches feststellbar. Jedoch lag Foramen ovale apertum vor, und die Milz wog 19 g. Keine Blutbildungsherde in Leber, Milz und Nieren.

In den beiden oben beschriebenen Fällen handelt es sich also um eine Anämie in der Neugeborenenperiode. Eine Blutung konnte bei den Kindern nicht konstatiert werden. Lues dürfte wegen der negativen Wassermannreaktion der Mütter und des gänzlichen Fehlens anderer für diese Krankheit charakteristischer Zeichen ausgeschlossen sein. Mit einer intrauterin entstandenen Sepsis braucht man wohl in den vorliegenden Fällen auch kaum zu rechnen. Eine kongenitale Leukämie , die in einigen Fällen beschrieben worden ist (LOMMEL, POLLMAN u. a.), kann bei diesem Blutbild und diesem Verlauf sowie wegen des Nichtvorhandenseins von Leber- und Milzvergrösserung nicht vorgelegen haben. Hämolytischer Icterus, der ja auch kongenital sein kann, verläuft nicht ohne herabgesetzte osmotische Resistenz der roten Blutkörperchen, ohne Icterus und ohne Leber- und Milzvergrösserung wie in diesen Fällen. Von Icterus gravis oder Hydrops foetalis kann man ja beim Fehlen von Icterus bzw. Ödem nicht sprechen. Vergiftung irgendwelcher Art hat, soweit bekannt, bei den Müttern nicht vorgelegen, ebensowenig eine Röntgen- oder Radiumschädigung. — Man hat also bloss das Fehlen aller anämisierenden Faktoren festzustellen. Es scheint also offen zutage zu liegen, dass die Fälle den Charakter einer »primären», »idiopathischen» oder »essentiellen» Anämie bei Neugeborenen hatten.

In beiden Fällen war die Anämie angeboren. Indes wird als charakteristisch für Anaemia neonatorum angegeben, dass die Blutmangelerscheinungen erst etwa eine Woche nach der Geburt auftreten, während das Kind vorher alle Zeichen völliger Gesundheit aufgewiesen hat. Dies scheint jedoch keine durchgehende Regel zu sein. Unter den bisher veröffentlichten einwandfreien Fällen, deren Zahl nicht mehr als 100 betragen dürfte, und für die der Zeitpunkt des ersten Auftretens der Anämie keineswegs immer mitgeteilt ist, findet man mehrere, wo die Anämie angeboren war oder schon am ersten Lebenstage beobachtet wurde [SANFORD, SCHLEUSSING, GELSTON-SAPPINGTON, STRANSKY 2 Fälle, DIAMOND-BLACKFAN-BATY 2 Fälle, VELDHUYSEN, YAGUDA, PASACHOW-WILSON (2), MANNHEIMER, GYLLENSWÄRD, CALDER, APPELBERG-ULFSPARRE, VAHLQUIST u. a.]. Anaemia neonatorum ist also nicht selten kongenital, was übrigens auch eine gewisse Verworrenheit der Nomenklatur zur Folge gehabt hat.

In einem der oben beschriebenen Fälle repräsentierte die Patientin mit ihrer Zwillingsschwester das »erste Kind». Man hat oft darauf hingewiesen, dass das erste Kind stets von Anaemia neonatorum ebenso wie von Hydrops foetalis und Icterus gravis verschont bleibt, auch wenn mehrere andere Geschwister von der Krankheit betroffen werden (LEHNDORFF in seiner Monographie 1937). Ausnahmen scheinen jedoch vorzukommen (SEGAR-STOEFFLER, ÅKERRÉN 2 Fälle, WYATT-COOPER-GROAT), und zu diesen ist also auch der oben beschriebene Fall zu zählen.

Das Geburtsgewicht war in unsern beiden Fällen geringer, als es im allgemeinen bei Anaemia neonatorum zu sein pflegt. Man gibt nämlich als charakteristisch an, dass die erkrankten Kinder bei der Geburt ausgetragen sind und keine Debilitätszeichen aufweisen. Diese Regel scheint auch für die Fälle zu gelten, wo die Erkrankung angeboren war. Indes finden sich in der Literatur auch mehrfach Angaben über Geburtsgewichte unter 3 000 g, und es sind sogar Fälle mit Geburtsgewichten von 2 000 g und weniger bekannt. [Pasachow-Wilson (2), Stalling-Schwab]. Ein niedrigeres Geburtsgewicht als das von 1 580 g in unserm ersten Fall scheint bisher kaum mehr als einmal festgestellt worden zu sein; auch in diesem Fall handelte es sich um einen Zwilling, welcher gesund wurde (Stalling-Schwab).

Das Blutbild war in unsern Fällen im grossen und ganzen dasselbe, wie es bisher überall in der Literatur bei dieser Krankheit beschrieben worden ist, abgesehen von den Thrombozytenzahlen. Als ein sehr charakteristischer Zug des Blutbildes wird ein Farbenindex bezeichnet, der »im Beginne und bis zur Höhe der Anämie sehr hoch, meist über 1», ist [Lehndorff (1)]. Indes muss man hier bedenken, dass ein hoher Farbenindex eine physiologische Erscheinung bei Neugeborenen ist. In der Mehrzahl der veröffentlichten Fälle liegt der Farbenindex kaum oberhalb der Grenze der normalen Variation. Die Bedeutung des hohen Farbenindex ist also in etlichen Fällen dieser Krankheit ein wenig überschätzt worden. Indes findet man in einigen Fällen von Anaemia neonatorum Indexwerte, die sicher vom Normalen abweichen, und zwar in der angegebenen Richtung (seltener dagegen in der Richtung nach unten). Dies gilt im Beginn der Krankheit und auf der Höhe der Anämie. Während der Rekonvaleszenz schlägt der Index dann um, und die Anämie wird hypochrom [Lehndorff (1)]. In unsern beiden Fällen erreichte der Index in den ersten Tagen sehr hohe Werte — 1,30 bzw. 1,44 —, um dann allmählich unter 1 zu sinken. Vergleicht man diese Werte mit den Normalwerten, so findet man indes, dass der Unterschied wenigstens im ersten Fall nicht allzu gross ist.

Der Indexwert 1,30 entspricht einem mittleren Hämoglobingehalt der roten Blutkörperchen von $40{,}7 \cdot 10^{-12}$ g; die Normalwerte liegen bei entsprechender Probeentnahmemethodik bei $39{,}3 \cdot 10^{-12}$ g (berechnet nach MERRITT-DAVIDSONS Tabellen) mit einer Streuung, welche angibt, dass die Abweichung in unserm Fall 1 auf einem blossen Zufall beruhen kann. In Fall 2 dagegen, mit einem mittleren Erythrozyten-Hb-Gehalt von $45 \cdot 10^{-12}$ g, liegt der Wert oberhalb der Variationsgrenze, die als vom Zufall bedingt angesehen werden kann. Hinzuzufügen ist, dass ein Farbenindex über 1 auch bei Neugeborenen mit niedrigem Geburtsgewicht eine physiologische Erscheinung ist (LICHTENSTEIN, MERRITT-DAVIDSON, MAGNUSSON u. a.), aber wenigstens die zweite der beiden oben angegebenen Indexzahlen übersteigt doch die Normalwerte weit.

Das Blutbild war in unsern beiden Fällen durch eine ziemlich ausgesprochene Polychromasie der roten Blutkörperchen während der ersten Tage gekennzeichnet. Dies hat man auch früher bisweilen bei Anaemia neonatorum beobachtet, aber dann in der Regel im Heilungsstadium. In unsern Fällen kann die Polychromasie möglicherweise mit den verhältnismässig niedrigen Geburtsgewichten (1 580 bzw. 2 200 g) zusammenhängen. LICHTENSTEIN hat darauf hingewiesen, dass man bei neugeborenen nichtausgetragenen Kindern konstant eine mehr oder weniger ausgeprägte, bisweilen recht starke Polychromasie findet, und dass diese besonders in den Fällen mit hoher Erythroblastenzahl hervortritt. Er sagt auch, dass bei ausgetragenen Zwillingen (in unserm Fall 2 betrug die Dauer der Schwangerschaft wahrscheinlich 8 $^1/_2$—9 Monate) in hämatologischer Beziehung oft Übereinstimmungen mit den nichtausgetragenen Kindern bestehen. Die Polychromasie würde bei unsern Fällen also eher als Ausdruck einer relativen Nichtausgetragenheit der Kinder als der Krankheit Anaemia neonatorum als solcher aufzufassen sein.

Bei den nichtausgetragenen Neugeborenen ist auch die bei allen Neugeborenen vorkommende Anisozytose besonders stark ausgesprochen, während Poikilozytose bei ihnen häufiger zu fehlen scheint. Beide Formen sind in unsern Fällen vorgekommen, wenn auch die Veränderungen in diesen Beziehungen nur mässig waren. Als besonders bemerkenswert bei Anaemia neonatorum wird hervorgehoben, dass bei dieser Krankheit niemals eine auffallende Aniso- und Poikilozytose auftritt, auch wenn die Anämie erhebliche Intensität erreicht. Das Fehlen dieser Strukturveränderungen der roten Blutkörperchen bei gleichzeitiger ausgeprägter Anämie wird als eines des charakteristischsten Merkmale der Krankheit bezeichnet, wodurch sie sich unter anderm bestimmt von COOLEYS Erythroblastenanämie unterscheiden soll [LEHNDORFF (1)]. Mässige Grade wenigstens von Anisozytose sind jedoch auch bei Anaemia neonatorum nichts Ungewöhnliches, ja sogar höhere Grade scheinen in manchen Fällen vorgelegen zu haben (ÅKERRÉN: »considerable», VELDHUYSEN: »+ + +», MANNHEIMER: »strong», ABBOTT-ABBOTT: »+ + +», KALBAK-WITH: »pronounced»). In unsern Fällen war der Grad von Aniso- und Poikilozytose nur mässig, und das Blutbild unterscheidet sich also in dieser Hinsicht nicht von den Verhältnissen, die von anderen Forschern bei Anaemia neonatorum beschrieben worden sind.

Fall 2 wies in den ersten Tagen eine der Anisozytose nahestehende Veränderung der roten Blutkörperchen auf, die seltener bei Anaemia neonatorum beobachtet worden ist, nämlich eine auffallende Mikrozytose. In der Regel hat ja die Krankheit eher makrozytären Charakter [LEHNDORFF (1)] mit hämoglobinreichen Zellen. Die in unseren Präparaten vorkommenden kleinen Zellen waren auch gut mit Hämoglobin gesättigt, was übrigens aus den Indexwerten hervorgeht. Es ist möglich, ja recht wahrscheinlich, dass auch diese Erscheinung ihre Erklärung in der relativen Unausgetragenheit des Kindes findet. So hat schon LICHTENSTEIN 1917 darauf hingewiesen, dass das Blut nichtausgetragener Neugeborener regelmässig eine auffallend grosse Anzahl intensiv gefärbter kleiner Erythrozytenformen enthält. Messungen der Erythrozytengrösse wurden in unseren Fällen leider nicht vorgenommen.

Eine Erythroblastämie von 21 000 je mm^3 oder nahezu 1 % der roten Blutkörperchen, wie sie in Fall 2 vorlag, hat man bei dieser Krankheit nur äusserst selten beobachtet. Auch ein Wert von 3 500 Erythroblasten je mm^3 (Fall 1) gehört zu den Ausnahmen. Bei Berechnung dieser Ziffern wurde gebührend berücksichtigt, dass bei Zählung der weissen Blutkörperchen auf gewöhnliche Weise in der Zählkammer nicht bloss die Leukozyten, auf deren Anzahl die Erythroblastenzahl bezogen werden muss, sondern sämtliche kernhaltige Elemente des Blutes mitgezählt werden. In ein paar Veröffentlichungen ist dies möglicherweise nicht beachtet worden, was, speziell wenn die Erythroblasten zahlreich waren, zur Folge gehabt haben muss, dass die Anzahl sowohl der Leukozyten als der Erythroblasten je mm^3 zu hoch angegeben ist. In Fall 2 waren bemerkenswert viele (6 %) Erythroblasten zweikernig, auch einige dreikernige und sogar ein vierkerniger wurden festgestellt. Buchan und Comrie haben solche Mehrkernigkeit auch bei Icterus gravis beobachtet (Kind A 4).

Eine Ursache der exzessiven Erythroblastenwerte in unsern Fällen kann, entsprechend dem früher Gesagten, darin zu suchen sein, dass nichtausgetragene Neugeborene überhaupt eine grössere Anzahl kernhaltige rote Blutkörperchen im Blut haben als ausgetragene; die Anzahl scheint auch mit dem Grad der Nichtausgetragenheit zu wachsen. Lichtenstein zählte sogar bei einem 3 Monate zu früh geborenen Kinde mit einem Geburtsgewicht von 1 040 g am ersten Tage 22 950 Erythroblasten je mm^3. Dass auch ausgetragene Neugeborene, ohne Anämie und sonstige Krankheitszeichen und mit einem Icterus, der die Grenzen des gewöhnlichen Icterus neonatorum nicht überschreitet, eine temporäre Erythroblastämie aufweisen können, die einen ausserordentlich hohen Grad erreicht, ist von Salomonsen nachgewiesen worden.

In unsern beiden Fällen nahm die Erythroblastämie rasch ab und verschwand, bevor die Anämie ihren Höhepunkt erreicht hatte. Es ist in früher veröffentlichten Fällen auch vorgekommen, dass sie, nachdem sie erst stark ausgesprochen war, verschwand, ehe die Anämie aufgetreten war. Hierin hat man einen Beweis dafür erblickt, dass keine ursächlichen Beziehungen zwischen Erythroblastose und Anämie bestehen [Lehndorff (1)]. Ein sicherer Zusammenhang zwischen der

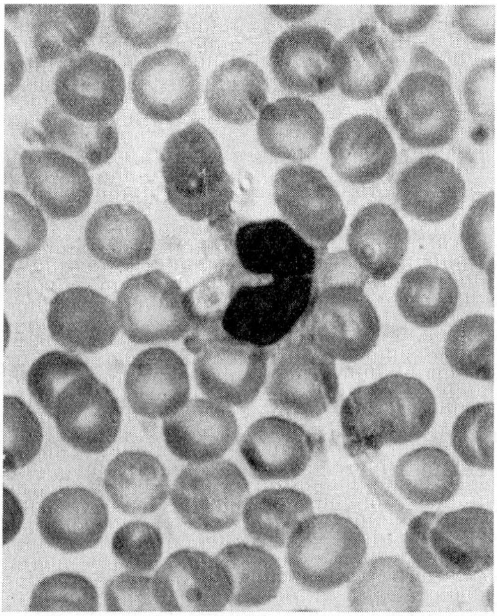

Abb. 1. Fall 1, Zwilling Nr. I. Phagozyte im strömenden Blut. 14.5.1935.

Erythroblastose und der Prognose ist auch nicht vorhanden (APPELBERG-ULFSPARRE). Die Erythroblastämie kann ferner sowohl bei Anaemia neonatorum (BROWN-MORRISON-MEYER, COHEN u. a.) als bei Hydrops foetalis (DE LANGE) und Icterus gravis (THOENES) fehlen. Erythroblasten können im Blut in vermehrter Menge auch bei Sepsis, kongenitaler Syphilis und kongenitalem Vitium angetroffen werden (WHITAKER). Unter solchen Verhältnissen scheint es, dass YLPPÖS Ansicht, wonach die Vermehrung der Erythroblasten einfach die uniforme Reaktionsart des fötalen Organismus und Blutes (oder des Blutes und des Organismus von Neugeborenen) gegen allerlei Schädlichkeiten ist, die beste Erklärung für das launenhafte Auftreten der Erythroblastämie bei den fraglichen Krankheiten gibt.

ABT und andere Forscher (WYATT-COOPER-GROAT) haben darauf aufmerksam gemacht, dass bei Anaemia neonatorum einkernige Zellelemente mit phagozytierten roten Blutkörperchen im Blut vorkommen. Trotz eifrigem Suchen ist es uns nicht gelungen, diese Erscheinung festzustellen, ausser möglicherweise bei einer einzigen Gelegenheit (Fall 1, am 14. 5. Abb. 1). Die oft ausgeprägte Erythrophagozytose, die im retikuloendothelialen System der Leber und Milz bei der Mehrzahl der Früchte vorliegt, die in die Geburt eingetreten sind, dagegen nicht bei Föten im 4.—6. Monat in utero (Schultz), pflegt man als ein Zeichen des bei der Geburt einsetzenden regen Abbaues der Erythrozyten anzusehen, doch wird ein solcher Erythrozytenzerfall von andern Forschern bestritten. Das Vorkommen von Phagozyten wahrscheinlich endothelialen Ursprungs im zirkulierenden Blut der Neugeborenen kann indes unter solchen Umständen nicht überraschen, und ich habe sie auch in dieser Altersperiode im Blut gesunder Kinder gefunden (vgl. Fall 6, Tab. 5).

Das weisse Blutbild ist in unsern Fällen ebensowenig wie in den meisten früher beschriebenen von besonderem Interesse. Die von einigen Autoren beobachtete Leukozytose konnte in unsern Fällen nicht festgestellt werden, wenigstens nicht in den ersten Tagen. Wenn höhere Leukozytenwerte im weiteren Verlauf auftraten, waren sie vorübergehender Natur. Eher war in unsern Fällen während der ersten Tage die relative Leukopenie zu bemerken, welche die nichtausgetragenen Kinder gegenüber den ausgetragenen kennzeichnet.

Ein überraschender und interessanter Befund sind die ausserordentlich hohen Thrombozytenwerte in unsern beiden Fällen. Sie wurden nach Kristensons Methode bestimmt. Die Anzahl der Blutplättchen wird ja sonst so gut wie immer als normal bei dieser Krankheit angegeben. Ich konnte in der Literatur nur folgende Fälle finden, in denen eventuelle Abweichungen nach oben vom Normalen vorlagen. Gelston-Sappington konstatierte am 13. Tage 750 000 Thrombozyten je mm^3, Mannheimer am 11. Tage 497 000 und Vahlquist (Fall 1) am 8. Tage 668 000. Für den letzten Fall kann ich mitteilen, dass das Kind noch im Alter von 1 Monat 674 000 Thrombozyten je mm^3 hatte. Ferner sagt Pasachow-Wilson (2) in einem Fall (Nr. 4), dass »platelets were abundant» am

20. Tage, nennt aber keine Ziffern. Gemeinsam ist diesen Fällen auch, dass die Anämie sehr früh auftrat. In NORDGRENS Fall, welcher auf schwedisch veröffentlicht ist (ausgetragener Knabe, am 11. Tage blass, am 14. Tag Hb 13 %, rote Blutkörperchen 460 000 je mm^3, weisse 94 000, 49 Normoblasten auf 350 weisse; starb an demselben Tag; Sektion: Milz 18 g, sonst keine krankhaften Prozesse ausser der Anämie), wird angegeben, dass »reichlich» Thrombozyten vorhanden waren, jedoch wurden sie nicht gezählt. Dasselbe gilt für die Fälle von DONALLY und SÜSSTRUNK. In weiteren zwei Fällen, welche bei uns in Schweden beobachtet wurden und nachstehend beschrieben werden sollen, wurden hohe Thrombozytenwerte verzeichnet.[1]

Fall 3. Mädchen, geboren 5. 8. 1940. Eltern gesund, der Vater ist jedoch immer blass gewesen. Meinickesche Reaktion bei der Mutter negativ. Eine 1926 geborene Schwester gesund. Zwei Brüder, geboren 1931 bzw. 1935, waren bei der Geburt tot; die näheren Umstände sind unbekannt.

Das Mädchen wog bei der Geburt 3 100 g. Ob es in der ersten Zeit nach der Geburt besonders blass war, kann die Mutter nicht sagen. Keine Zeichen von Blutungen. Erbrach ziemlich viel. Da das Kind elend auszusehen begann, wandte man sich an den Arzt, der es nach dem Krankenhaus überwies.

Bei der Aufnahme am 19. 8. Gewicht 2 930 g. Extreme, wachsgelbe Blässe. Trotzdem ziemlich munter und lebhaft. Innere und äussere Organe o. B. Keine Blutungen, keine Ödeme, normale Stühle mit negativer Benzidinreaktion. Im Harn nichts Pathologisches. Blut: Hb 21 %, 820 000 rote und 14 300 weisse Blutkörperchen je mm^3. Ausstrichpräparat: 51 % Neutrophile (darunter 9 % Stabkernige), 2 % Eosinophile, 41 % Lymphozyten, 6 % Myelozyten. 10—15 kernhaltige rote auf 200 weisse Blutkörperchen. Aniso- und Poikilozytose. Polychromasie. 697 000 Thrombozyten je mm^3. Senkungsgeschwindigkeit der roten Blutkörperchen (Mikromethode) 5 mm in der ersten Stunde. Blutungszeit 45 Sek.

Das Kind erhielt an zwei aufeinander folgenden Tagen eine intraperitoneale Blutinjektion von 15 bzw. 19 ccm und schien

[1] Für liebenswürdige Mitteilung von Fall 3 spreche ich Herrn Chefarzt Dr. med. PER SELANDER, Kristianstad meinen Dank aus. Fall 4 wird später in anderem Zusammenhang von VAHLQUIST näher beschrieben werden.

Tab. 3. Fall 4. Mädchen, geb. 16. 11. 1941.

Tag	Hämoglobin in %	Erythrozyten in Millionen	Leukozyten in Tausenden	Thrombozyten in Tausenden
26/11	39	1,20	23,0	458,0
29/11	49	2,59	18,3	637,0
1/12	46	1,93	13,5	505,0
3/12	38	1,85	7,8	525,0
5/12	46	1,85	9,5	667,0

sich in gutem Allgemeinzustand zu befinden. Am 22. 8. trat indes plötzlich der Tod ein. Die Sektion ergab nichts Bemerkenswertes, abgesehen von der Anämie. Mikroskopische Untersuchungen fanden nicht statt.

Fall 4. Mädchen, geboren 16. 11. 1941. Eltern und zwei Geschwister gesund. Wassermanns Reaktion bei der Mutter negativ. Normale Verhältnisse beim Partus. Die uterine Fläche der Plazenta war grosslobiert. Geburtsgewicht 3 040 g. Am 21. 11. trat leichter Icterus auf, und Pat. war etwas stumpf. Am 25. 11. wurde Blässe beobachtet. Am 26. 11. wurden folgende Blutwerte festgestellt: Hämoglobin 39 %, 1 200 000 rote und 23 000 weisse Blutkörperchen je mm^3. 2 Erythroblasten auf 200 weisse. Polychromasie. 7,4 % Retikulozyten. 458 000 Thrombozyten je mm^3. Meulengracht (Icterusindex) 34. Keine Blutungen. Osmotische Resistenz der roten Blutkörperchen normal. Bluttransfusion am 26. 11. und 28. 11. Allgemeinzustand gut. Am 27. 11. wurde eine leichte Cystopyelitis bei dem Mädchen konstatiert. Die Thrombozytenzahlen schwankten in der aus Tab. 3 ersichtlichen Weise. Der Fall steht zur Zeit noch unter Behandlung.

Merritt-Davidson geben folgenden Mittelwerte für die Thrombozyten normaler Säuglinge an: im Alter von 1 Woche (69 Fälle) 233 000 ($\sigma = 45\,000$) und im Alter von 4 Wochen (48 Fälle) 277 000 ($\sigma = 51\,000$). Berechnet man $M + 3\,\sigma$, so erhält man für das Alter von 1 Woche den Wert 368 000 und für das von 4 Wochen 430 000, welche Ziffern also in den betreffenden Lebensabschnitten der oberen Grenze der Variation entsprechen, die als zufallsbedingt angesehen werden kann.

Bei sämtlichen in dieser Arbeit beschriebenen vier Fällen von Anaemia neonatorum liegen also die Werte zu hoch, und dies gilt auch für die oben aus der Literatur angeführten Fälle, soweit Ziffern mitgeteilt sind. In allen andern Fällen, wo die Thrombozytenzahlen angegeben werden, waren sie normal, aber in einigen Fällen niedrig (z. B. KIRIMLIDIS: 32 000). Es ist klar, dass verschiedene Zählmethoden in hohem Grade für den Unterschied zwischen den Werten verantwortlich gemacht werden können, und die Proben können auch in verschiedenen Phasen der Krankheit entnommen sein. Ein der posthämorrhagischen Thrombozytose gleichartiger Mechanismus könnte in den oben aus der Literatur angeführten Fällen mit hohen Thrombozytenwerten eventuell durch die Leukozytenzahlen wahrscheinlich gemacht werden, welche in den einzelnen Fällen den Thrombozytenzahlen parallele Verschiebungen nach oben aufwiesen. Dieser Parallelismus ist jedoch in unsern eignen Fällen nicht zu beobachten. Die Thrombozytenzahlen erreichten in den Zwillingsfällen ganz bedeutend höhere Werte als in den andern. Zu bemerken ist, dass den Thrombozytenvermehrungen in diesen Fällen keine Adrenalininjektionen in gefässtimulierender Absicht vorhergingen; das Adrenalin erhöht ja die Thrombozytenzahlen, indem es, wie man annimmt, Milzkontraktionen herbeiführt, die eine Plättchenausschwemmung zur Folge haben (HITTMAIR). Von mehreren Fällen weiss man, dass experimentelle Erstickungsversuche und Luftverdünnung (Hochgebirge) eine Vermehrung der Plättchen im Blut bewirken; ob ein Sauerstoffmangel in den Geweben von der Art, wie er in unsern Anämiefällen vorgelegen haben muss, eine gleichartige Wirkung haben kann, ist mir unbekannt. Wenn das Retikuloendothel, in Übereinstimmung mit dem oben Gesagten, in unsern Fällen aus dem einen oder andern Grunde stark in Mitleidenschaft gezogen war, so könnte dies möglicherweise mit der Thrombozytose zusammenhängen, da eine Blockade des Retikuloendothels (z. B. durch Tusche) eine Plättchenzunahme verursachen zu können scheint (Literatur bei HITTMAIR). Inwieweit endlich das die Thrombozytenzahlen regulierende vegetative Nervensystem und andere mehr oder minder bekannte Faktoren in diesem Zusammenhang eine Rolle gespielt haben, lässt sich hier nicht beurteilen. — Von Interesse in diesem Zusammenhang ist, dass HAWKSLEY-LIGHTWOOD eine Vermehrung der Megakaryozyten im Knochenmark bei einem Fall von Icterus gravis gefunden haben, der nach Icterus und Anämie genas und auf der Höhe der Krankheit niedrige Thrombozytenwerte hatte.

Die Knochenmarkpunktionen in unseren Zwillingsfällen zeigten ein Mark, welches Zeichen von Hyperplasie aufwies, wenigstens was die Myelopoese betrifft, bei der man auch auffallend viele unreife Formen sah. Die Befunde stimmten indes mit den Verhältnissen überein, die nach LICHTENSTEIN-NORDENSON bei prämaturen Kindern im allgemeinen vorliegen.

Wenn wir nun zu den beiden Zwillingsgeschwistern der anämischen Kinder übergehen, so begegnen wir bei ihnen dem überraschenden Bilde einer Polyzytämie. Dass man wirklich von einer solchen sprechen kann, zeigt ein Vergleich mit einem Normalmaterial. So gibt MAGNUSSON bei gleicher Methodik der Probeentnahme für frühgeborene Kinder einen mittleren Hämoglobingehalt des Blutes während der ersten Woche (80 Fälle) von 125,1 % an ($\sigma = 16{,}35$), und im Alter von drei Wochen (75 Fälle) einen solchen von 102,8 % ($\sigma = 19{,}29$). Die entsprechenden Werte für die roten Blutkörperchen sind: in der ersten Woche (79 Fälle) 5 230 000 ($\sigma = 720\,000$) und im Alter von drei Wochen (72 Fälle) 4 440 000 ($\sigma = 620\,000$). Bei ausgetragenen Kindern liegen die Werte ungefähr auf derselben Höhe, der Hämoglobinwert möglicherweise etwas höher. Bei den beiden hier in Rede stehenden Zwillingen liegen die Blutwerte während der angegebenen Altersperioden in der Regel über dem Wert $M + 3\sigma$ oder wenigstens über $M + 2{,}5\,\sigma$ und also oberhalb der Variationsgrenze, die als vom Zufall bedingt angesehen werden kann. Die Veränderungen sind bei dem Kinde am ausgesprochensten, dessen Zwillingsgeschwister die exzessive Erythroblastämie aufwies (Fall 2). Bei diesem Kinde waren die polyzytämischen Blutwerte noch bei der Entlassung aus dem Krankenhaus nicht normal geworden, aber eine bleibende Polyzytämie scheint in diesem Fall ebensowenig vorgelegen zu haben wie in dem andern, wo das Blutbild während des Krankenhausaufenthalts normal wurde. Im übrigen bot das Blutbild der Kinder nichts von besonderem Interesse. Die bei Polyzytämie sonst vielfach bestätigte Thrombozytenvermehrung lag hier nicht vor.

Eine späte Abnabelung kann man in diesen Fällen nicht für die Polyzytämie verantwortlich machen (siehe oben), was ja vielleicht auch daraus hervorgeht, dass die letztere ziemlich lange bestehenblieb. Die Kinder hatten, speziell in einem der Fälle, die rötlich zyanotische Hautfarbe, die in den sehr wenigen früher beschriebenen Fällen als charakteristisch für den Symptomkomplex auch in diesem Alter angegeben wird. STRANSKY-WITTENBERG deuten ihren Fall als ein längeres Verbleiben bei embryonalen Verhältnissen ohne bekannte Ursache.

Das Skrotalödem, welches während der ersten Tage in einem der Fälle (»Fall 1», Zwilling Nr. II) beobachtet wurde, könnte in diesem Zusammenhang, entsprechend früheren Mitteilungen in der Literatur, als Äquivalent eines Hydrops foetalis aufgefasst werden. Indes erscheint mir eine solche Deutung hier kaum berechtigt, da keine ausgesprocheneren ödematösen Veränderungen und keine Erythroblastose vorliegt; jedoch verdient der Befund natürlich Beachtung. Dass Anaemia neonatorum und eine gutartige Form von Hydrops foetalis bei je einem von zwei eineiigen Zwillingen vorkommen kann, ist indes beobachtet worden (SHAPIRO-COHEN).

Dass bei unsern beiden Zwillingspaaren wirkliche Monozygotie vorliegt, darf man wohl als sicher ansehen, da die Zwillinge beidemal monochoriotisch waren. In dem Fall, wo beide Zwillinge am Leben blieben, war die Eineiigkeit auch an ihrer Ähnlichkeit erkennbar. Sie unterschieden sich zwar etwas in Länge und Gewicht (siehe oben), sahen sich aber sonst zum Verwechseln ähnlich. Die Ohrenkonfiguration war bei beiden so gut wie genau dieselbe, und in der Augenfarbe unterschieden sie sich nicht im geringsten voneinander.

Dass diese für das Alter seltenen Symptombilder, Anämie

einerseits, Polyzytämie andererseits, bei je einem von zwei eineiigen Zwillingen vorliegen, spricht ja für eine gemeinsame Ursache beider Erscheinungen in unsern Fällen. Es könnte sich um einen schädigenden Faktor handeln, der bei den beiden Zwillingen verschieden wirkte, oder bei beiden uniform war, aber verschiedene Reaktionen bei ihnen auslöste. — In welchem Umfang sich eineiige Zwillinge überhaupt hinsichtlich der Blutwerte bei der Geburt voneinander unterscheiden, scheint noch nicht zum Gegenstand hinreichender Untersuchungen gemacht worden zu sein.

Zufällige Verhältnisse in der Decidua basalis, mechanische und andere Faktoren, welche die Gefässentwicklung in der Plazenta beeinflussen, können sowohl bei dizygotischen als bei monozygotischen Zwillingspaaren bewirken, dass der eine Zwilling besser ernährt wird als der andere. In der Tat unterscheiden sich eineiige Zwillinge in bezug auf Länge und Gewicht bei der Geburt ebensosehr voneinander wie zweieiige, obgleich die ersteren dieselbe Erbmasse haben. Eineiige Zwillinge haben ferner nicht — wie die zweieiigen — einen ganz getrennten Blutkreislauf, sondern ihre Gefässe anastomosieren in grösserem oder geringerem Umfang in dem gemeinsamen Mutterkuchen miteinander. Dies kann zur Folge haben, dass die Zirkulation und damit die Ernährung des einen Zwillings gestört wird und er in der Entwicklung hinter dem andern zurückbleibt. In manchen Fällen kann man geradezu sagen, dass sich der eine Zwilling auf Kosten des andern entwickelt. Schatz hat eine asymmetrische Blutverteilung bei monozygotischen Zwillingen nachgewiesen, wobei Blut von dem einen Zwilling durch das Kapillarsystem der Plazenta in Venen fliesst, die in den andern Zwilling gehen. Es ist natürlich denkbar, dass ein gleichartiger Mechanismus den Störungen bei unsern beiden Zwillingspaaren zugrunde liegt. Zu bemerken ist, dass die Anämie bei jedem Paar den kleineren der Zwillinge betraf. Was hier Ursache und was Wirkung war, falls nun überhaupt ein Kausalzusammenhang besteht, dürfte sich indes unmöglich entscheiden lassen. In diesem Zusammenhang ist der Befund der blassen Plazentahälfte bemerkenswert. Mehr als dass die Anämie sich im vorliegenden Fall auch auf das Trophoblast erstreckt hat, kann man aus der hier gemachten Beobachtung jedoch kaum ablesen. Leider wurde niemals nach dem eventuellen Vorkommen von Erythroblastose in der Plazenta geforscht, die früher einigemal beobachtet worden ist (vgl. BROWN-MORRISON-MEYER, COHEN).

Sollten den Störungen in unseren Zwillingsfällen zirkulatorische Plazenta-Asymmetrien zugrunde gelegen haben und der eine Zwilling sozusagen langsam in den andern ausgeblutet sein, so wäre es interessant, dass sich die Reaktion des Ausgebluteten in starker Erythroblastämie und Thrombozytämie geäussert hätte, und nicht zum mindesten, dass die Blutwerte (Hb und rote Blutkörperchen) ihren tiefsten Stand erst ziemlich lange nach der Geburt erreicht haben. Ob man hierbei mit einer Ermüdung der Erythropoese, einer frühen »physiologischen» Frühgeborenenanämie oder lediglich mit einer fortschreitenden Verdünnungsanämie zu rechnen hat, ist (unter anderm wegen des Fehlens von Serumproteinbestimmungen) schwer zu entscheiden. In diesem Zusammenhang ist es von grossem Interesse, wie sich die Blutwerte in den ersten Wochen nach der Geburt bei Neugeborenen verhalten, die frühzeitig einen grossen Blutverlust erleiden, ohne eine Blutkrankheit zu haben. Nachstehend werden zwei solche Fälle mitgeteilt, in denen es sich beidemal um eine Insertio velamentosa des Nabelstrangs mit Abreissung der Gefässe, blutiges Fruchtwasser und ein bei der Geburt anämisches Kind handelt.

Fall 5. Knabe, geboren 23. 8. 1935. Geburtsgewicht 4 180 g. Mutter Zweitgebärerin, gesund (Wassermanns Reaktion negativ). Sprengung der Fruchtblase am 23. 8., wobei 1 Liter Fruchtwasser von normalem Aussehen abfloss. Partus 10 Min. später. Nach dem Fötus flossen 2—300 ccm stark blutiges Fruchtwasser aus. Der Nabelstrang inserierte in den Eihäuten, und seine Gefässäste teilten sich in der Randpartie der Plazenta. Unmittelbar an der Eintrittsstelle, wo eine Ruptur der Eihäute vorlag, waren sie sämtlich abgerissen. Die Plazenta zeigte nichts Bemerkenswertes, ihr Gewicht betrug 780 g. Das Kind schrie sofort und war leicht zyanotisch, wurde aber bald etwas blass. Sahli betrug 80, die Zahl der roten Blutkörperchen 4 Millionen. Wegen der weiteren

Tab. 4. Fall 5. Knabe, geb. 23. 8. 1935.

Tag	Hämoglobin in %	Erythrozyten in Millionen	Leukozyten in Tausenden	Thrombozyten in Tausenden	Weisses Blutbild						Erythroblasten in Tausenden
					My+Jug	Neutro	Eo	Bas	Lympho	Mono	
23/8	80	4,04	25,9		2	31,5	1	1	46	18,5	0
29/8	75—80	3,78		148,0							
30/8	70	3,70	14,2		0	63	2	0	27	8	0
3/9	65	2,99		670,0							
4/9	60	2,70									
11/9	75	3,31	10,5	430,0	0	33	1,5	0	53,5	12	0

hämatologischen Entwicklung siehe Tab. 4. Innere Organe o. B. Die Milz war niemals deutlich tastbar. Unbedeutender und rasch vorübergehender Icterus neonatorum. Keine Blutungen. Keine Therapie.

Fall 6. Mädchen, geboren 26. 3. 1940, gestorben 14. 4. 1940. Geburtsgewicht 2 410 g. Mutter Erstgebärerin, gesund. Die Eihäute rissen am 26. 3., das Fruchtwasser zeigte nichts Bemerkenswertes. Partus 10 Min. später. Gleichzeitig mit der Geburt des Kindes spritzte eine ziemlich grosse Blutmenge nach allen

Tab. 5. Fall 6. Mädchen, geb. 26. 3. 1940, gest. 14. 4. 1940.

Tag	Hämoglobin in %	Erythrozyten in Millionen	Leukozyten in Tausenden	Thrombozyten in Tausenden	Weisses Blutbild						Erythroblasten in Tausenden	Bemerkungen
					My+Jug	Neutro	Eo	Bas	Lympho	Mono		
26/3	90	4,04	13,7		0,5	32,5	0,5	0	58	8,5	1,4	Polychromasie
27/3	60	2,37	21,1	104,0	3	64,5	0,5	0	28,5	3,5	6,2 (=2,6 ‰)	
28/3	70–75	2,95	13,5	105,0	1	69	0	0	26	4	1,2	Vereinzelte Phagozyten
30/3	65–70	2,81										
1/4	70	2,32	8,3	290,0	0	30,5	1,5	0	57,5	10,5	0,04	
4/4	70	3,09										
8/4	65–70	3,04	49,0	775,0	0	85	0	0	12	3		
12/4	55	2,59	41,2									

Seiten. Es stellte sich dann heraus, dass der Nabelstrang in den Eihäuten inserierte und dass ein grosses Nabelstranggefäss an einer Eihautruptur dicht am Plazentarand abgerissen war. Das Kind war bei der Geburt blass und atmete schlecht. Nach Wechselbad und Lobelin bessere Atmung, aber noch immer sehr blass. Der Hämoglobingehalt (Sahli) betrug am ersten Tag 90 %, die Zahl der roten Blutkörperchen 4 040 000. Wegen der hämatologischen Entwicklung siehe Tab. 5. Innere Organe o. B. Die Milz war niemals tastbar. Keine Blutungen. Seit dem 2. 4. bekam das Kind Ferrum reductum in kleiner Dosis. Nach einer Periode von verbessertem Allgemeinzustand trat am 12. 4. eine Verschlechterung ein, man konstatierte eine Kapillarbronchitis, und Pat. starb am 14. 4. Die Sektion ergab ausser der Kapillarbronchitis unter anderm anämische Infarkte in Leber, Milz und Nieren, die zum Teil inveteriert waren.

Abgesehen von der starken Abnahme von Hämoglobin und roten Blutkörperchen am zweiten Tage in Fall 6, die wohl als eine Verdünnungsanämie zu deuten ist, zeigen die Blutwerte in diesen Fällen im ganzen denselben allmählichen Rückgang während der ersten Wochen wie bei normalen Neugeborenen. Wenn die Kinder die Fähigkeit gehabt hätten, auf gesteigerte Regenerationsansprüche sofort mit erhöhter Hämatopoese zu antworten, so hätte man vielleicht erwarten können, dass diese Kinder, die gleich bei der Geburt Anämie hatten, dieser wenigstens in den ersten Wochen die Stange hätten halten können. Dies war jedoch kaum der Fall. Indes lassen sich ja lediglich aus diesen zwei Fällen keine Schlüsse in dieser Hinsicht in der einen oder anderen Richtung ziehen. Die Hauptsache ist, dass die Blutungsfälle im grossen und ganzen dieselbe postnatale hämatologische Entwickling zeigen wie unsere anämischen Zwillinge.

Indes gibt es andere Möglichkeiten, das gleichzeitige Vorhandensein von Anämie bei einem Zwilling und Polyzytämie bei dem andern zu erklären. Wenn auch der Fötus sein eigenes Blutleben führt, ist es nicht ausgeschlossen, dass Hormone von der Mutter bei seiner Blutneubildung mitwirken. Sollte nun infolge des einen oder andern schädigenden Faktors der eine von zwei eineiigen Zwillingen höhere Forderungen an die Hämatopoese stellen, so wird gesteigerte hormonale

Stimulanz die Folge sein. Es liegt dann nahe, sich die Wirkung hiervon auf den andern Zwilling, der diesem schädigenden Faktor nicht ausgesetzt ist, aber gleichfalls diese gesteigerte Stimulanz erhält, als eine Polyzytämie zu denken. Auch wenn die erhöhte hormonale Stimulanz von dem von der Schädigung betroffenen Zwilling selbst ausgeht, kann man erwarten, dass durch die Plazenta-Anastomosen ein polyzytämischer Effekt bei dem andern Zwilling herbeigeführt wird (vgl. die Entstehung eines hermaphroditischen Zwillingskalbes, sog. »freemartin», bei Rindern).

Verschiedenheiten zwischen einem Paar monozygotischer Zwillinge können bisweilen auf genotypischen Asymmetrien beruhen. Wenn wir in unsern Krankheitsfällen mit erblichen Faktoren rechnen, dürften wir indes kaum Grund zu der Annahme haben, dass die Eigenschaft in diesem Fall, nämlich die Anämie, bei ihrem Träger asymmetrisch verteilt war. Natürlich ist es denkbar, dass die Krankheitsursache in einem unpaaren Organ, z. B. der Leber oder Milz, liegt, aber wahrscheinlicher ist es wohl, dass die fragliche Eigenschaft hier entsprechend dem oben Ausgeführten in der einen oder anderen Art milieubedingt (intrauterin) war.

Es ist von Interesse, wie oft man bisher Fälle von Anaemia neonatorum bei Zwillingen beobachtet hat. Die in der Literatur mitgeteilten Fälle sind leicht gezählt. Shapiro-Cohens eineiige Zwillinge, von denen der eine Anaemia neonatorum, der andere Hydrops foetalis hatte (welcher heilte), haben wir bereits erwähnt. Footes Zwillingsfall wird von mehreren Forschern ausgeschieden, weil man annimmt, dass es sich hier um eine frühe Prämaturanämie, nicht um eine Anaemia neonatorum handelt. Bahrdt hat über ein Paar Zwillinge berichtet, von denen der eine am dritten Tage an Icterus gravis starb, während der andere im Alter von drei Wochen eine kräftige Anämie mit Erythroblastose, aber nur ganz schwachen Icterus aufwies. Nähere Einzelheiten über diesen Fall sind nicht mitgeteilt. Stalling-Schwab beschreibt zwei Zwillingspaare, ein eineiiges und ein zweieiiges, bei denen sämtliche Kinder Anaemia neonatorum hatten. Ferner hat

Lichtenstein 1917 einen Fall von sehr früher Anämie bei Drillingen mitgeteilt: die Kinder wogen bei der Geburt 1 760, 2 300 bzw. 2 850 g und hatten im Alter von drei Wochen folgende Hämoglobinwerte (Sahli): 40, 65 bzw. 110. Zu bemerken ist, dass der kleinste und am meisten anämische der Drillinge laut Angabe auch von der Geburt an blass war. Derselbe Autor fand bei Zwillingen oft einen Parallelismus zwischen Körpergewicht und Hämoglobinwerten, derart, dass der kleinere der Zwillinge auch einen geringeren Hämoglobingehalt hatte; in andern Fällen dagegen fehlte ein solcher Parallelismus. Bei unsern beiden Zwillingspaaren ist der Parallelismus stark ausgesprochen. — Bei den Anaemia neonatorum nahestehenden Krankheiten Icterus gravis und Hydrops foetalis sind Zwillingsfälle sowohl bei ein- als bei zweieiigen Paaren beobachtet worden, wo die Krankheiten in verschiedener Weise kombiniert waren [Lit. bei Pache (1) und Shapiro-Cohen]. In diesem Zusammenhang ist auch darauf hinzuweisen, dass nach Pache (1) eine mässige Häufung von Zwillingsschwangerschaften in den Erythroblastosefamilien vorliegt. Diese Häufung kann in Paches Material indes zufallsbedingt sein (23 Zwillingspaare auf 1 300 Geburten statt erwarteter 16) und würde einstweilen nur für Familien mit Icterus gravis oder Hydrops foetalis oder beiden Krankheiten gelten.

In der Diskussion über Bahrdts Zwillingsfall wurde es für wahrscheinlich erklärt, dass der Icterus die Ursache der Anämie war. In der Regel sieht man ja, dass schwere Anämien den Icterus gravis begleiten oder ihm folgen. Der hierbei wirksame Mechanismus erscheint indes unklar. Lehndorff (1), der sich unter anderen hierüber geäussert hat, verweist auf zwei von Stransky referierte Fälle, die bereits 5 Stunden post partum eine hochgradige Blutarmut zeigten, welche gleichzeitig mit dem Icterus gravis in Erscheinung trat, und sagt, dass die Anämie in diesen Fällen »unmöglich eine Folge der Gelbsucht sein konnte». — Dass das Bild eines Icterus gravis anfangs von einer Anämie vom Typus Anaemia neonatorum beherrscht werden kann, bevor die Gelbfärbung der Haut eintritt, geht aus folgendem Fall hervor, zu dessen Beobachtung ich Gelegenheit hatte. Es handelt sich um das 15. Kind einer Familie (derselbe Vater und dieselbe Mutter), bei der wiederholte Fälle von Icterus gravis unter den Geschwistern zu spezieller Beobachtung des Kindes bei der Geburt Anlass gaben.

Fall 7. Eltern gesund, nicht verwandt. Wassermanns Reaktion der Mutter bei wiederholten Gelegenheiten negativ. In der übrigen Familie sind keine Fälle von bösartiger Gelbsucht der Neugeborenen bekannt. Mutter 1895 geboren. Partus Nr. I 1912: Kind gesund. Nr. II 1913: Kind gesund. Nr. III 1914 und Nr. IV 1917: Beide Kinder an Icterus gravis gestorben. Nr. V 1918: 1 Monat zu früh geborener, mazerierter Fötus. Nr. VI 1920: Das Kind starb an Icterus gravis. Nr. VII 1922: Kind gesund. Nr. VIII 1924: Das Kind starb im Alter von 1 Woche an Krämpfen, war nicht icterisch. Nr. IX 1925, Nr. X 1927 und Nr. XI 1928: Alle drei Kinder gesund. Nr. XII 1930, Nr. XIII 1931 und Nr. XIV 1932: Alle drei Kinder starben an Icterus gravis. Nr. XV 1934: Der nachstehend beschriebene Fall.

Mädchen, geboren 27.9.1934 0,5 Uhr vormittags. Partus 1—2 Wochen zu früh, sonst ohne Besonderheiten. Geburtsgewicht 3 030 g. Zyanotisch und schlaff bei der Geburt. Zerstreute konfettigrosse Hautblutungen hier und da am Körper. Haut und Schleimhäute blass, die Haut hat einen schwachen Stich ins Gelbe. Conjunctivae nicht gelb. Blutwerte am ersten Tag: Sahli 60 %, rote Blutkörperchen 1 970 000, weisse 12 000, Thrombozyten 74 000. Ausstrichpräparat: Neutro 40, Eo 2,5, Bas 0, Mono 6, Lympho 42, My 6, Metamy 3,5 %. 500 Erythroblasten auf 200 weisse. Meulengracht (Icterusindex) 25. Osmotische Resistenz der roten Blutkörperchen normal.

Am 28.9 wurde eine eigentümliche zitronengelbe Tönung der Hautfarbe beobachtet, aber erst am 29.9 begann die Haut, gelber zu werden. Am 30.9. war Sahli auf 40—50 und die roten Blutkörperchen auf 1 700 000 gesunken. Die Zahl der Thrombozyten betrug 34 200, die der Erythroblasten 47 auf 200 weisse. Am 1.10. trat der Tod ein. Die Sektion zeigte das Bild eines Icterus gravis ohne Kernicterus.

In diesem Fall kann man also von einer Anaemia neonatorum sprechen, wo das klinische Bild in das eines Icterus gravis überging. Ein leichter Icterus, wie ihn dieser Fall zuerst aufwies, welcher früher beginnt als der physiologische, ist in ungefähr der Hälfte der bekannten Fälle von Anaemia neonatorum beschrieben worden [PASACHOW-WILSON (2)]. Hautblutungen sind ja auch nicht allzu selten bei der Krankheit [DIAMOND-BLACKFAN-BATY, PASACHOW-WILSON (2), MANNHEIMER u. a.]. Der Fall ist von Interesse teils für die Frage nach dem Zusammenhang zwischen den Symptomen Gelbsucht und Anämie bei diesen Krankheitszuständen, teils für die nach der Zusammengehörigkeit der beiden Krankheitsformen Anaemia neonatorum und Icterus gravis. Was die erstere Frage anlangt, sei an die von mehreren Seiten festgestellte Tatsache erinnert, dass nicht einmal ein starker Blutzerfall den Serumbilirubinspiegel erheblich zu erhöhen braucht, wenn nur die Leber gut Bilirubin abzusondern vermag.

Die Frage nach der Zusammengehörigkeit der verschiedenen Formen der »Neugeboreneneryhroblastose» (ein nicht recht zutreffender Name, da die Erythroblastose nicht obligat ist und ausserdem bei mehreren anderen Krankheitszuständen sowie unter normalen Verhältnissen vorkommt, siehe oben S. 227), Hydrops foetalis, Icterus gravis und Anaemia neonatorum, ist ausserordentlich viel in der Literatur erörtert worden. Ausser den klinischen Zügen, die ihnen gemeinsam sein können, war das Hauptargument der Unitaristen, dass man sie immer wieder nebeneinander bei verschiedenen Kindern desselben Geschwisterkreises oder desselben Zwillingspaares beobachtet hat. Andere wollen sich nicht über die Zusammengehörigkeit äussern, solange die Ätiologie unklar ist. Dass eine Verwandtschaft irgendwelcher Art zwischen diesen drei Krankheitsformen besteht, die sich, wenngleich sie je für sich sehr selten sind, wechselweise in bestimmten Familien in der oben angegebenen Weise anhäufen, dürfte sich schwer bestreiten lassen. Von einem rein zufälligen Zusammentreffen kann ja unter solchen Verhältnissen und bei wiederholten Beobachtungen nicht gut die Rede sein. Was die Krankheitsform betrifft, welche uns hier in erster Linie interessiert, nämlich die Anaemia neonatorum, so ist sie bei mehreren Geschwistern derselben Familie beobachtet worden (SEGAR-STOEFFLER, BONAR-SMITH,

Veldhuysen), ferner in Familien, wo andere Geschwister Icterus gravis hatten (Diamond-Blackfan-Baty, Miller), sowie in solchen, wo andere Geschwister Hydrops aufwiesen [Pasachow-Wilsen (1), Mainka]. Über Familien, in denen alle drei Formen vorkamen, haben Mackay-O'Flynn sowie Kapteyn berichtet. Wie bereits oben bemerkt, sind zwei Zwillingspaare, wo alle Zwillinge Anaemia neonatorum hatten, von Stalling-Schwab beschrieben worden, ein Zwillingspaar, wo bei dem einen Zwilling Anaemia neonatorum und beim andern Icterus gravis vorlag, von Bahrdt, sowie ein Zwillingspaar, wo der eine Zwilling Anaemia neonatorum und der andere Hydrops foetalis aufwies, von Shapiro-Cohen. Zwischen Anaemia neonatorum und Icterus gravis kommen auch rein klinisch fliessende Übergänge vor, worauf bereits früher in dieser Arbeit und u. a. des Näheren auch von Debler hingewiesen worden ist.

Mit der Kenntnis von dem familiären Auftreten der Krankheitsformen musste sich natürlich auch die Frage nach ihrer Erblichkeit erheben. Man kennt eine geringe Anzahl Familien, in denen die Krankheiten (jedoch nicht Anaemia neonatorum) auch in den Seitenlinien vorgekommen sind. Pache (2) hat 5 solche Familien aus der Literatur zusammengestellt (Fall Honecker, Hoffmann-Hausmann, Fordyce-Mc Afee, Hawksley-Lightwood, Bosler-Weitz) und eine von ihm selbst beobachtete Familie hinzugefügt. Natürlich wäre es für die Erblichkeitsforschung von Wert, wenn mehr solche Stammbäume bekannt würden. Taylor hat 1925 eine Familie beschrieben, wo 4 der Kinder (darunter ein Zwillingspaar) an Icterus gravis starben und die Mutter »several sisters» hatte, die im Säuglingsalter an Gelbsucht mit Konvulsionen gestorben waren. Nachstehend wird ein Fall von Icterus gravis non letalis mit Zeichen von Kernicterus mitgeteilt, wo Icterus gravis auch unter den Kindern einer Schwester der Mutter vorkam.

Fall 8. Knabe, geboren 10.9.1932. Eltern gesund. Wassermanns Reaktion bei der Mutter neg. 9 Geschwister gesund, keines von ihnen wies mehr als eine unbedeutende Gelbsucht in der Neugeborenenperiode auf. Keine Fehlgeburten. Eine Schwester der Mutter hat 5 Kinder geboren, von denen 3 gesund waren, aber 2 am 3. Tage an Icterus gravis starben.

Partus normal. Geburtsgewicht 4 170 g. Am 12.9. trat Icterus auf, der schon am 13.9. sehr stark war und sich allmählich mit Stumpfheit verband. Am 20.9. begann die Gelbsucht etwas abzunehmen, aber noch am 3.10. war Pat. stark gelb. Erst am 15.10. war der Icterus verschwunden. Die Milz war tastbar. Die Fäzes hatten normales Aussehen. Hammarstens Probe im Harn pos. Resistenz der roten Blutkörperchen normal. Schon am 15.9. hatte man beobachtet, dass Pat. mit gestreckten Armen lag; allmählich bildete sich eine allgemeine Rigidität aus, die immer mehr zunahm, und zu der Opisthotonusstellung trat. Über die hämatologische Entwicklung siehe Tab. 6.

Tab. 6. Fall 8. Knabe, geb. 10.9.1932.

Tag	Hämoglobin in %	Erythrozyten in Millionen	Leukozyten in Tausenden	Weisses Blutbild						Erythroblasten in Tausenden
				My + Jug	Neutro	Eo	Bas	Lympho	Mono	
16/9	120	5,22	11,7	0	51	5,5	1	26,5	16	0
26/9	65									
7/10	50	2,20	8,4	0	34	6,5	1	50	8,5	0,3
12/10	55	2,69								
24/10	55	2,80	5,3	0	23,5	3	0	69,5	4	0
5/11	55—60	2,71								
28/11	70	3,44	7,0	0	18,5	5	0,5	71	5	

Die Erblichkeitsverhältnisse in den referierten Fällen sind unklar. MACKLIN hat für jedes der drei Syndrome die Frequenz affizierter Kinder in den Familien mit Neugeborenenerythroblastosen untersucht, soweit vollständige Angaben über das Ergebnis aller Schwangerschaften vorliegen. Ferner hat sie die Frequenz affizierter Eltern und die Häufigkeit von Vetternehen zwischen den Eltern in diesen Familien untersucht. Dabei ist sie zu dem Ergebnis gelangt, dass alle drei Syndrome wahrscheinlich auf einer dominanten Mutation in der Erbmasse eines der Eltern beruhen. Was Anaemia neonatorum oder »congenital anemia» betrifft, wie MACKLIN das

Syndrom nennt, sind ihre Berechnungen für unsere Zwecke nicht brauchbar, weil sie sich nur mit der auf die Mittelmeerrassen beschränkten Cooleyschen Anämie (erythroblastic anemia) zu beschäftigen scheint, die ja zwar mitunter kongenital sein kann, aber irreversibel ist und jetzt scharf von den hier behandelten Krankheitszuständen unterschieden wird [LEHNDORFF (1), FANCONI, COOLEY].

Die Theorie, dass eine dominante Mutation die Ursache von Icterus gravis und Hydrops foetalis ist, kann indes die Probleme kaum lösen. Zunächst wäre es eigentümlich, dass, wenn z. B. die Mutation in der Erbmasse der Mutter erfolgen sollte, so viele (über 50 %) ihrer Eier mutieren würden und nicht nur ein einziges, da die Wahrscheinlichkeit einer Mutation äusserst gering ist. Man kann auch nicht annehmen, dass die Mutation in den Geschlechtszellen ihrer Eltern erfolgt ist, denn da die Anlage dominant ist, müsste sie dann selbst krank gewesen sein. In MACKLINS gesamten Icterus-gravis-Material (134 Familien) wurde nur zweimal ein »severe type of jaundice in infancy» bei den Eltern beobachtet, beidemal bei der Mutter.

Ein dominanter Erbgang erklärt ferner nicht, dass das erste Kind der betroffenen Familien — mit einigen wenigen Ausnahmen — nicht von der Krankheit befallen wird. Dieses Verschontbleiben des erstgeborenen Kindes ist eine wohlbekannte und oft erörterte Tatsache bei allen drei Syndromen. MACKLIN hat, wie erwähnt, 134 Familien mit Icterus gravis. Die Gesamtzahl der Kinder in diesen Familien beträgt 648. Von diesen 648 sind also 134 erste Kinder. Wenn nun ein dominanter Erbgang vorläge, müssten 50 % der erstgeborenen Kinder krank sein. Bei Berücksichtigung des mittleren Fehlers $\left(\pm\sqrt{\frac{50 \cdot 50}{134}}\right)$ müssten also in MACKLINS Material mindestens 37 % der erstgeborenen Kinder krank sein (50 minus dem dreifachen mittleren Fehler). Dem widerspricht ja indes alle Erfahrung.

Es scheint auch, dass die Frequenz kranker Kinder in den betroffenen Familien über den 50 % liegt, die man bei dominantem Erbgang bei diesen seltenen Krankheiten zu erwarten hätte. MACKLINS 134 Familien hatten 648 Kinder, von denen 394 krank waren. Dies ist mehr als die erwarteten 50 %. Zu beachten ist auch, dass die Verfasserin alle Fehlgeburten und Totgeborenen nicht in die Gesamtzahl der Kinder in den 134 Familien eingerechnet hat. Es ist aber wahrscheinlich, dass besonders viele dieser Fehlgeburten und Totgeborenen in utero an derselben Krankheit gestorben sind, die bei den lebend Geborenen als Icterus gravis in Erscheinung getreten ist. Ist dies der Fall, so kann ja der Prozentsatz der kranken Kinder wesentlich steigen.

Da es eine ganze Anzahl Fälle von Icterus gravis gibt, welche am Leben bleiben und völlig gesund werden — und solche gab es ja auch vor der Zeit der Bluttransfusion —, müsste man bei dominantem Erbgang auch häufiger, als es tatsächlich geschieht, auf Icterus-gravis-Fälle stossen, in denen die Mutter (oder der Vater) als Kind Icterus gravis hatte. In Wirklichkeit aber kommt dies ja nur äusserst selten vor (vgl. die obigen Ziffern von MACKLINS Material).

Dass die erstgeborenen Kinder so gut wie konsequent verschont bleiben, hat mehrere Forscher veranlasst, die Möglichkeit der erblichen Bedingtheit der Krankheiten abzulehnen. Dies ist indes nicht ohne weiteres notwendig. Es ist nämlich denkbar, dass die erbliche Krankheitsanlage bei der Mutter, nicht bei den Kindern, manifest ist. Solchenfalls äussert sich die Krankheit darin, dass die Generationsorgane nach Überstehung einer Schwangerschaft (durch hormonale, uterine oder andere Faktoren) in der einen oder anderen Weise geschädigt werden, so dass die folgenden Kinder minderwertig werden. Rechnet man in MACKLINS Material alle erstgeborenen, 134 Stück, von denen bloss ein geringer Prozentsatz krank gewesen sein kann, von der Gesamtsumme der Kinder ab, so bekommt man unter 514 Kindern 394 kranke, d. h. 77 %. Nichts hindert ja, dass in einer Familie auf eine Reihe kranker Kinder eine Reihe gesunder folgen kann, wenn Erholungsmöglichkeiten für die Generationsorgane bestehen. Eine gewisse Neigung zu Anhäufung der kranken Kinder in einer zusammenhängenden

Reihe, unterbrochen durch eine Reihe gesunder Kinder in demselben Geschwisterkreis, ist auch bei Icterus gravis zu bemerken, worauf bereits andere Forscher hingewiesen haben (vgl. oben Fall 7). So sagt Fanconi, dass in der Reihenfolge die mittleren Kinder bevorzugt sind. Pache (1) fand jedoch eine deutliche Zunahme der Krankheitsfälle bei steigender Geburtennummer. Eine nähere Untersuchung dieser Verhältnisse mit exakter statistischer Methodik an dem vollständiger untersuchten Material der letzten Jahre wäre zu wünschen.

Falls die Mutter Merkmalsträgerin sein sollte, müssten die Untersuchungen über konsanguine Ehen in der Aszendenz der kranken Kinder in erster Linie positive Resultate ergeben, wenn es sich um die Eltern der Mutter handelt. Bemerkenswerterweise zeigt die Sippentafel in dem einzigen Fall von Icterus gravis in der Literatur, in dem Macklin gefunden hat, dass die Eltern verwandt (Geschwisterkinder) waren, nämlich dem von Hawksley-Lightwood, dass auch die Eltern der Mutter Vetter und Base waren. Der letztere Umstand lag auch in Peters Fall vor. Eine dritte Mitteilung über Verwandtschaft in der Aszendenz von Kindern mit Icterus gravis findet man bei Hoffmann-Hausmann. Es handelt sich um zwei Familien, wo die Eltern der kranken Kinder miteinander verwandt waren, in dem einen Fall »im 4. oder 5. Grad», im andern »im 8. Grad». Die letzteren Familien stammten indes beide aus einer Gebirgsgegend in den Alpen, die eugenisch den Charakter eines Isolats zu haben scheint, wo Verwandtenehen möglicherweise nicht ungewöhnlich sind. Überhaupt dürfte die Forschung auf diesem Gebiet — über die eventuelle Überrepräsentation konsanguiner Ehen zwischen Eltern (bzw. den Eltern der Mutter und des Vaters) von Kindern mit Icterus gravis — auf unübersteigliche Hindernisse stossen, weil es ausserordentlich schwer ist, die ziffernmässigen Resultate mit der Normalfrequenz konsanguiner Ehen zu vergleichen, die ja von Ort zu Ort und von Zeit zu Zeit ausserordentlich variiert. Eine Möglichkeit wäre, wenn es sich um Vetternehen zwischen den Eltern der Mutter handelt, die ja hier aktuell werden können, die Frequenz von solchen auf der Seite der Mutter mit der auf der väterlichen Seite zu vergleichen, vorausgesetzt, dass man über genügend zahlreiche Stammbäume für Kinder mit Icterus gravis verfügte. An dem letzteren Punkt strandet indes diese Möglichkeit. — Aussichtsreicher wäre es vielleicht auf die Dauer, festzustellen, ob in den Fällen, wo die Krankheit in mehr als einer Linie des Stammbaums bekannt ist, zwei Schwestern die kranken Kinder zu bekommen pflegen, wie in den bisher beschriebenen Fällen, und im allgemeinen, ob der Vater oder die Mutter die Rolle des Konduktors spielt, falls man überhaupt annehmen darf, dass Erblichkeit vorliegt.

Über die Ursache der drei Syndrome Hydrops foetalis, Icterus gravis und Anaemia neonatorum sind viele Theorien aufgestellt worden [Lit. u. a. bei Thorling, Peters, Hawksley-Lightwood, Lehndorff (1)]. Für das Verständnis der Krankheitsursache ist es u. a. von Wichtigkeit, den Mechanismus der für alle drei Syndrome charakteristischen Anämie (die jedoch wenigstens bei Icterus gravis nicht obligat ist) näher zu studieren. In diesem Punkte gehen die Meinungen bei Anaemia neonatorum stark auseinander. Es ist bekannt, dass in den meisten Fällen der Krankheit die Anämie erst 1—2 Wochen nach der Geburt »aus voller Gesundheit» auftritt. Mehrere Beobachtungen bestätigen auch, dass sie sich sehr rasch, im Verlauf eines oder einiger Tage, einstellen kann. Die Frage ist nun, wie eine solche rasch eintretende Anämie zu erklären ist. Nach Lehndorff (2), der sich eingehend mit dem Problem der Anaemia neonatorum beschäftigt hat, handelt es sich um eine vorübergehende Störung der Erythropoese infolge eines allergischen Knochenmarkschocks, mit Reifungshemmung oder Ausschwemmungsdrosselung der roten Blutkörperchen. Andere Forscher (Parsons-Hawksley-Gittins u. a.) halten eine primäre Hämolyse für die Ursache. Es ist nicht meine Absicht, hier näher auf diese beiden Ansichten einzugehen oder Stellung zu ihnen zu nehmen. Folgende Tatsachen sollen jedoch in diesem Zusammenhang hervorgehoben werden.

Da unter normalen Verhältnissen der Gehalt des Blutes

an roten Blutkörperchen je Volumeneinheit konstant ist, muss ihre tägliche Destruktion durch eine entsprechende Neubildung aufgewogen werden. Die Destruktion kann man sich entweder so denken, dass die roten Blutkörperchen eine bestimmte Lebensdauer haben, infolge Alters oder Abnutzung sterben und in ein Destruktionsorgan von passiver Natur aufgenommen werden (theory of longevity, SCHIØDT), oder auch so, dass das Destruktionsorgan aktiv ist und täglich eine gewisse Anzahl rote Blutkörperchen unabhängig von ihrem Alter zerstört. SCHIØDT, der sich der Alterstheorie anschliesst, schätzt wegen verschiedener Umstände die Lebenslänge der roten Blutkörperchen unter normalen Verhältnissen auf ca 30 Tage. — Mag man nun die eine oder andere dieser beiden Theorien für richtig halten, so besteht jedenfalls die einzige Möglichkeit zur Erklärung einer plötzlich entstandenen starken Anämie darin, einen stark vermehrten Zerfall der roten Blutkörperchen anzunehmen, da es ja hier nicht gut denkbar ist, dass sie dem Kreislauf in anderer Weise entzogen werden. Man kann sich ja dann sehr wohl vorstellen, dass die roten Blutkörperchen infolge einer defekten Hämatopoese eine stark verkürzte Lebensdauer, z. B. nur von einem einzigen Tag, haben. Bei einer plötzlichen Ausschwemmungsdrosselung könnte dann eine starke Anämie in sehr kurzer Zeit in Erscheinung treten, aber solchenfalls müsste schon früher ein gesteigerter Blutzerfall stattgefunden haben, der aber durch eine entsprechend erhöhte Regeneration ausgeglichen worden wäre. Ohne die Annahme einer gesteigerten Hämolyse ist deshalb das plötzliche Auftreten einer erheblichen Anämie bei Anaemia neonatorum nicht zu erklären. Andererseits ist es, wie erwähnt, keineswegs ausgeschlossen, dass dieser vermehrten Hämolyse ganz oder teilweise eine geschädigte Hämatopoese zugrunde liegt. Es ist auch denkbar, dass die erhöhten Anforderungen an Blutneubildung, welche die Folge einer primären Hämolyse sein würden, in einem Ermüdungszustand des hämatopoetischen Apparats resultieren können, der sich als ein Schock äussern kann. Beide Erscheinungen können also in jeder von beiden Richtungen abhängig voneinander sein, und Spuren von beiden sind auch nebeneinander bei Anaemia neonatorum zu beobachten. Was dann das Primäre ist, die Hämolyse oder die ungenügende Hämatopoese, dürfte sich bei unserer jetzigen Kenntnis von Anaemia neonatorum nicht endgültig entscheiden lassen.

Ein interessanter Befund sind die kürzlich von VAHLQUIST nachgewiesenen hohen Serumeisenwerte in zwei Fällen von Anaemia neonatorum. Indes darf man hieraus nicht ohne weiteres schliessen, dass eine gesteigerte Hämolyse stattgefunden hat, denn auch eine mangelhafte Knochenmarksfunktion dürfte bei normaler Abnutzung der roten Blutkörperchen infolge eingestellten Eisenverbrauchs im Knochenmark eine Vermehrung des Serumeisens herbeiführen. Mit einer Erklärung in u. a. dieser Richtung rechnet VAHLQUIST selbst für die eigentümliche Tatsache, die er bei Blutungszuständen in der Neugeborenenperiode beobachtet hat, dass nämlich keine Hyposiderämie nach der Blutung auftritt, was sonst bei Erwachsenen die Regel ist, sondern dass sogar im Gegenteil in gewissen Fällen die Serumeisenwerte eine Erhöhung über die Grenzen des Normalen erfahren.

In einer Reihe Fällen von Hydrops foetalis, Icterus gravis und Anaemia neonatorum haben in neuerer Zeit DAM-TAGE-HANSEN-PLUM eine ausgesprochene Hypoprothrombinämie konstatiert. Dieser interessante Umstand müsste jedoch an einem grösseren Material beobachtet werden, damit ihm allgemeine Gültigkeit beigemessen werden könnte. Was Anaemia neonatorum betrifft, ist die Koagulationszeit in so gut wie allen Fällen, wo sie untersucht wurde, (einschliesslich unserer eigenen Fälle) normal, und in dem oben beschriebenen Fall 4, wo die Prothrombinzeit bestimmt wurde (nach QUICK), war auch diese normal (22 Sek.). Die zwei Fälle der oben genannten Autoren von Anaemia neonatorum, wo deutliche Hypoprothrombinämie vorlag, waren auch kaum reine Fälle, sondern zeigten eher den Typus von Icterus gravis (der eine war »deutlich», der andere »stark» icterisch bei der Geburt; Icterusindex am 6. Tage 50 bzw. 60). Sollte indes eine Hypoprothrombinämie bei der Krankheit gewöhnlich sein, so müsste man natürlich erwarten, dass eine Anzahl Fälle von Anaemia neonatorum Blutungen aufgewiesen haben, als hämorrhagische Diathesen aufgefasst worden sind und sich aus diesem Grunde der Forschung über Anaemia neonatorum entzogen haben.

Zusammenfassung.

Im Anschluss an zwei Fälle von Anaemia neonatorum, die je den einen Zwilling eines eineiigen Zwillingspaars betrafen, während der andere Zwilling ein polyzytämisches Blutbild aufwies, wird der Mechanismus der Störungen besprochen. Es wird dargelegt, dass wahrscheinlich Plazenta-Anastomosen eine Rolle bei der Entstehung der Polyzytämiebilder in diesen Fällen gespielt haben. Weitere zwei Fälle von Anaemia neonatorum werden beschrieben.

Die Blutveränderungen bei Anaemia neonatorum werden erörtert. Unter anderm wird darauf hingewiesen, dass das Vorkommen von Phagozyten (grosse mononukleäre Zellelemente mit im Protoplasma aufgenommenen roten Blutkörperchen) im kreisenden Blut eine physiologische Erscheinung bei Neugeborenen sein kann. Alle vier Fälle von Anaemia neonatorum zeigten über das Normale erhöhte Thrombozytenwerte. Im Anschluss hieran wird die Thrombozytose als Teilerscheinung des Krankheitsbildes besprochen. Es wird auseinandergesetzt, dass ein plötzlicher Eintritt der Anämie bei Anaemia neonatorum nur durch einen stark gesteigerten Blutzerfall zu erklären ist. Die klinische Bedeutung der Veränderungen des Blutgehalts an Serumeisen und Prothrombin bei Anaemia neonatorum wird besprochen.

Zum Vergleich werden zwei Fälle von wirklicher kongenitaler Anämie bei Neugeborenen ohne Blutkrankheit (Abreissung der Nabelstranggefässe während der Entbindung) mitgeteilt, und anschliessend das einfache posthämorrhagische Blutbild bei Neugeborenen geschildert.

Die Frage nach der Zusammengehörigkeit der drei Syndrome Anaemia neonatorum, Icterus gravis und Hydrops foetalis wird behandelt. Ein Fall von Anaemia neonatorum, wo das klinische Bild in das eines Icterus gravis überging, wird beschrieben. Die Erblichkeitsverhältnisse bei den drei Syndromen werden im Anschluss an einen Fall von Icterus gravis erörtert, wo die Krankheit auch in einer Seitenlinie des Stammbaums vorkam. Es wird hervorgehoben, dass die Verteilung der kranken Kinder auf gewisse Geburtennummern in den betroffenen Geschwisterkreisen nicht der Annahme zu widersprechen braucht, dass die Krankheit erblich bedingt ist, dass man aber solchenfalls annehmen muss, dass die Mutter, nicht die Kinder, die Merkmalsträgerin ist.

Summary.

The mechanism of the origination of the disturbances is discussed in connection with two cases of anemia of the new-born. Each case concerns one of the twins in a monozygotic pair, the blood picture of the other twin being polycytaemic. The fact that placenta anastomoses have, in all probability, played a part in the origination of the polycytaemic pictures in the present cases is emphasized. Two additional cases of anemia of the new-born are reported.

The blood changes in anemia of the new-born are considered. Inter alia, it is pointed out that the occurrence of phagocytes in the circulating blood. i. e. big mononuclear cells with red blood corpuscles absorbed in the protoplasm, may be a physiological phenomenon in the new-born. All the four cases of anemia of the new-born disclosed values of the platelet count, over and above the normal ones. Thrombocytosis as a constituent part of the morbid picture is, in this connection, subjected to examination. A strong increase in blood destruction is shown to be the only possible explanation of a sudden setting-in of anemia of the new-born. The clinical significance of the variations in the blood content of serum iron and prothrombine in anemia of the new-born is considered.

For the sake of comparison, two cases of real congenital anemia of the new-born, without blood disease (the tearing of the umbilical cord vessels during childbirth) are reported. In this connection, the simple posthæmorrhagic blood picture in the new-born is demonstrated.

Attention is directed to the question of the relationship between the three syndromes of anemia of the new-born, icterus gravis and hydrops foetalis. One case of anemia of the new-born, in which the clinical picture was transformed into that of icterus gravis, is described. The hereditary conditions in the three above-mentioned syndromes are studied in relation to a case of icterus gravis, in which this disease occurred also in a side-branch of the genealogical tree. Stress is laid on the fact that the distribution of the sick children in certain birth numbers in the families concerned does not, necessarily, contradict the assumption that the disease is hereditary but that the mother, from a hereditary point of view, is, most likely, in that case the trait-carrier, and not the children.

Literaturverzeichnis.

Abbott-Abbott: Am. J. Dis. Childr. *49,* 724 (1935). — Abt: Am. J. Dis. Childr. *43,* 337 (1932). — Appelberg-Ulfsparre: Acta Pæd. *24,* 30 (1939). — Bahrdt: Mschr. Kinderheilk. *69,* 336 (1937). — Bonar-Smith: Am. J. Dis. Childr. *45,* 594 (1933). — Bosler-Weitz: zit. Pache (2). — Brown-Morrison-Meyer: Am. J. Dis. Childr. *48,* 335 (1934). — Buchan-Comrie: J. Path. and Bact. *13,* 398 (1909). — Calder: Canad. M. A. J. *41,* 484 (1939). — Cohen: J. Pediatr. *7,* 220 (1935). — Cooley: Brennemanns Practice of Pediatrics, Vol. III, Chapter 16. Hagerstown 1938. — Dam-Tage-Hansen-Plum: Ugeskr. f. Laeger 1939, p. 896 (dänisch). Auch erschienen in Lancet *2,* 1157 (1939). — Debler: Z. Kinderheilk. *59,* 199 (1937). — Diamond-Blackfan-Baty: J. Pediatr. *1,* 269 (1932). — Donally: Am. J. Dis. Childr. *27,* 369 (1924). — Fanconi: Mschr. Kinderheilk. *68,* 129 (1937). — Foote: Am. J. Dis. Childr. *39,* 1302 (1930). — Fordyce-McAfee: zit. Pache (2). — Gelston-Sappington: Am. J. Dis. Childr. *39,* 807 (1930). — Gyllenswärd: Nord. Med. Tidskr. *16: 2,* 1158 (1938) (schwedisch). — Hawksley-Lightwood: Quart. J. Med. *3,* 155 (1934). — Hittmair: Fol. haemat. *59,* 50 (1938). — Hoffmann-Hausmann: Mschr. Kinderheilk. *33,* 193 (1926). — Honecker: zit. Pache (2). — Kalbak-With: Nord. Med. Tidskr. *12,* 1921 (1936) (dänisch). — Kapteyn: Maandschr. voor Kindergeneesk. *6,* 397 (1937) (holländisch). — Kirimlidis: Z. Kinderheilk. *61,* 111 (1939). — de Lange: zit. Hawksley-Lightwood. — Lehndorff (1): Erg.

Inn. Med. *52,* 611 (1937). — LEHNDORFF (2): Mschr. Geb. und Gyn. *108,* 264 (1938). — LICHTENSTEIN: Hämatologiska studier å för tidigt födda barn (schwedisch). Stockholm 1917. — LICHTENSTEIN-NORDENSON: Fol. haemat. *63,* 155 (1939). — LOMMEL: Münch. med. Wschr. *52: 1,* 904 (1905). — MACKAY-O'FLYNN: Proc. roy. Soc. Med. *26,* 1360 (1933). — MACKLIN: Am. J. Dis. Childr. *53,* 1245 (1937). — MAGNUSSON: Acta Pæd. *18,* suppl. 1 (1935). — MAINKA: Arch. Kinderheilk. *120,* 40 (1940). — MANNHEIMER: Acta Pæd. *18,* 237 (1935). — MERRITT-DAVIDSON: Am. J. Dis. Childr. *46,* 990 (1933). — MILLER: Yale J. Biol. and Med. *11,* 363 (1939). — NORDGREN: Hygiea *90,* 981 (1928) (schwedisch). — OPITZ: PFAUNDLER-SCHLOSSMANNS Handb. d. Kinderheilk. Bd. I, p. 887. Berlin 1931. — PACHE (1): Z. Kinderheilk. *59,* 73 (1937). — PACHE (2)) Z. Kinderheilk. *61,* 86 (1939). — PARSONS-HAWKSLEY-GITTINS: Arch. Dis. Child. *8,* 159 (1933). — PASACHOW-WILSON (1): Am. J. Dis. Childr. *49,* 411 (1935). — PASACHOW-WILSON (2): Am. J. Obstr. and Gyn. *29,* 415 (1935). — PETERS: Beitr. path. Anat. *92,* 531 (1934). — POLLMAN: Münch. med. Wschr. *45,* 44 (1898). — SALOMONSEN: Acta Pæd. *18,* 357 (1936). — SANFORD: Am. J. Dis. Childr. *30,* 19 (1925). — SCHATZ: zit. DAHLBERG: Twin births and twins from a hereditary point of view, Stockholm 1926. — SCHIØDT: Acta med. scand. *95,* 49 (1938). — SCHLEUSSING: Verh. d. deutsch. path. Ges. *21,* 371 (1926). — SCHULTZ: Z. Geb. und Gyn. *94,* 793 (1929). — SEGAR-STOEFFLER: J. Pediatr. *1,* 485 (1932). — SHAPIRO-COHEN: Am. J. Dis. Childr. *58,* 1050 (1939). — STALLING-SCHWAB: Maandschr. voor Kindergeneesk. *6,* 487 (1937) (holländisch). — STRANSKY: Z. Kinderheilk. *51,* 239 (1931). — STRANSKY-WITTENBERG: Z. Kinderheilk. *43,* 742 (1927). — SÜSSTRUNK: Z. Kinderheilk. *38,* 587 (1924). — TAYLOR: Brit. Med. J. *1,* 1127 (1925). — THOENES: Mschr. Kinderheilk. *65,* 225 (1936). — THORLING: Upsala läkareförenings förhandl. *28,* 1 (1922). — VAHLQUIST: Acta Pæd. *28,* suppl. 5 (1941). — VELDHUYSEN: Maandschr. voor Kindergeneesk. *4,* 197 (1935) (holländisch). — WHITAKER: Illinois Med. J. *74,* 134 (1938). — WYATT-COOPER-GROAT: Am. J. Dis. Childr. *56,* 1319 (1938). — YAGUDA: zit. LEHNDORFF (1). — YLPPÖ: Mschr. Kinderheilk. *65,* 174 (1936). — ÅKERRÉN: Acta Pæd. *13,* 142 (1932).

FROM OSLO MUNICIPAL HOSPITAL, DEPARTMENT I. HEAD: P. M. HOLST M. D., AND FROM THE STATE INSTITUTE OF PUBLIC HEALTH, BACTERIOLOGICAL DEPARTMENT, HEAD: M. TESDAL M. D., CHIEF STATE EPIDEMIOLOGIST.

Epidemiology of scarlet fever illustrated through typing of hemolytic streptococci in a primary case and its return cases.

By

Dr. H. F. LANGE and Dr. V. GAUSTAD.

At the beginning of the school term in August 1939, a six year old boy, Tore (case 1), caught scarlet fever and was sent to the department of epidemic diseases of Oslo Municipal Hospital at Ullevaal. Before his admission he probably infected his younger sister, Berit (case 2). She was admitted to the hospital three days later. Both were isolated during the period stipulated by the Local Board of Health, viz. 6 weeks and then dismissed to their home.

A week after their discharge a cousin of Tore's, Knut (case 3), was admitted. It is stated that he had been playing with Tore. 3 weeks after Tore's discharge his mother (case 4) was admitted to the hospital with a fulminant scarlet fever.

As a consequence of his mother's going to hospital, Tore, with his father and sister, went to stay with relatives. They had been there a couple of days only when another cousin of Tore's, Svein (case 5), fell ill. He was admitted 4 weeks after Tore's discharge.

Tore and his sister were now sent to relatives at Raanaasfoss. Their stay there did not remain without consequences. Some time after their arrival, two of the children in the house where they stayed, named Berit and Sigmund (cases 6 and 7) fell ill and were sent to Stensby Hospital 6 weeks after Tore's discharge from Ullevaal. On inquiry, the Local Medical Officer at Soerum, dr. Bj. Alstad, stated that no other case of scarlet fever occurred in the district at the time. In all probability, therefore, Tore was the source of infection. The latter had, moreover, at this juncture, developed an acute otitis media. He was secured and re-admitted to hospital as a suspected source of infection.

With a view to elucidating, if possible, the epidemiological circumstances, the throats of all the above-mentioned cases were sampled, to be examined for hemolytic streptococci. The examination was carried out at the Bacteriological Department of the State Institute of Public Health. It must be added that one could, of course, not expect to isolate hemolytic streptococci from all the patients, as many of them had reached an advanced stage of convalescence. The results of the examination will appear in fig. I.

It will be seen that the same type of streptococci, Gr. A, type 8, was isolated from Tore and from 3 of the 6 cases infected by him. From Tore's sister, who fell ill 3 days after Tore, hemolytic streptococci Gr. A, type 25 were cultivated. The sample was taken 10 weeks after her discharge from hospital. During this time, she had probably lost the original type and had been re-infected with another type instead. This happened also in case 4, Tore's mother. Samples were taken twice. In the first instance no growth of hemolytic streptococci occurred. The second examination disclosed Gr. A, type 27. In case 7 no growth occured. The patient had been sent to Stensby Hospital in Eidsvoll, and the sample was sent from there on an ordinary ox serum tube, which is far from being an ideal medium for isolating hemolytic streptococci. It is, however, worth noting, that case 6 had the same type as case 1. This case should therefore be a typical return case, and it occurred no less than 12 weeks after the primary case fell ill, and 6 weeks after the conclusion of the stipulated period of isolation. Return cases which arise as

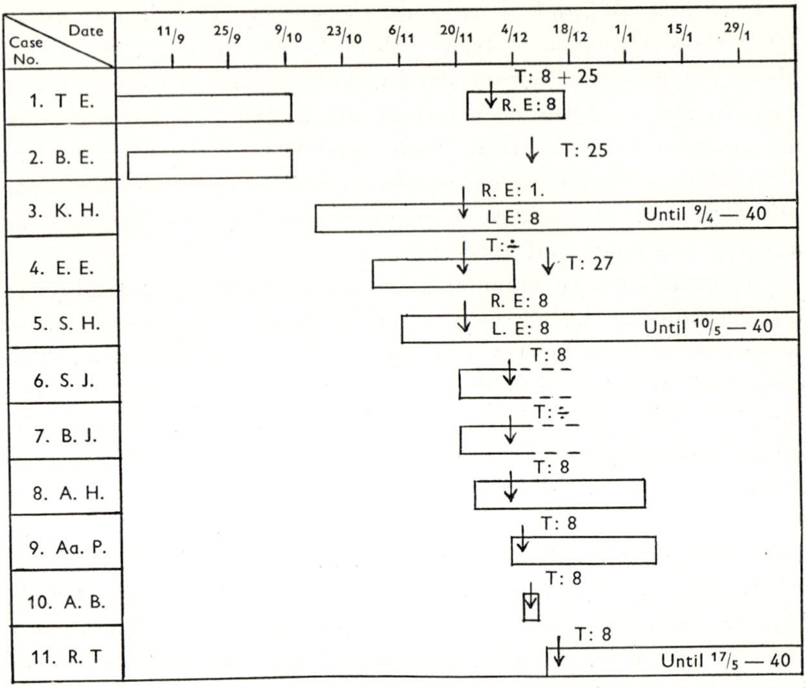

Fig. I. Shows the period of isolation in hospital, and the result of typing of streptococci in the 11 cases mentioned.
T.: Throat. R. E.: Right Ear. L. E.: Left Ear.

late as this are no doubt rare, but they are occasionally seen. Thus NIKELBERG, (quoted by E. MANCHOT) (1), has seen a return case 103 days after the discharge from hospital of the primary case. In LICHTENSTEIN's material (2) from Stockholm, out of 98 scarlet fever convalescents, all causing return cases after their discharge, 7 were isolated in hospital from 10 to 18 weeks.

It has been stated above what happened in Tore's environment until he was re-isolated in hospital. In fig. I, however, are included 4 nurses who attended case 5 or Tore himself during his second stay in the department. In their case, the epidemiological and clinical data are as follows:

Case 8: This nurse had not been in contact with any scarlet fever patient before she started nursing patient No. 5 on November 20th. The latter was at this date very ill and lay with pus flowing from nose, mouth and ears. That very night, the nurse got dysphagia, and she was admitted to the department four days later with a magnificent scarlet fever rash.

Case 9: Nursed the same patient from November 30th. She had a transient dysphagia the same day and after three days a heavy scarlet fever.

Case 10: Nursed the same patient from the 23rd November till the 2nd December. From December 2nd till 6th, she suffered from a tonsillitis without rash and was thereafter admitted to the department for a couple of days for observation. With her, no rash was observed.

Case 11: Nursed patient No. 1 (Tore) during his second stay in hospital. At this date he had otorrhea. The nurse was admitted on the 11th December with a heavy, nearly toxic scarlet fever.

The throats of these 4 nurses were sampled, and from all of them were isolated hemolytic streptococci, Gr. A, type 8.

We have been discussing a patient who, after the end of the period of isolation, caused a series of secondary cases both outside hospital and inside. In a majority of these cases we have isolated an identical type of hemolytic streptococci. We found this so interesting that we took up the problem of typing hemolytic streptococci also in the other return cases occurring during this epidemic, which lasted from the summer of 1939 till the spring of 1940. For various reasons these inquiries were not pushed as far as might have been desirable, but typing of streptococci was carried out in 8 return cases, caused by 4 different primary cases. The samples were taken on the patients' admission to hospital, and the primary cases came up for examination the next day. The results of this inquiry are set out i Table I, which reveals the interesting feature that in all the primary cases examined was found Gr. A, type 8, and this type was also found in 7 return cases. In the 8th case no growth of hemolytic streptococci occurred.

Before discussing further the data presented here, a brief

Table I. Shows the result of typing of streptococci in the primary cases and the corresponding return cases.

Primary case No.		Return case No.	
1.	Throat type 8. Nose type 1.	1, 2.	Throat type 8.
2.	Throat type 8. Nose —	3, 4, 5.	Throat type 8.
3.	Throat type 8.	6.	Throat — Nose —
4.	Throat type 8. Nose —	7, 8.	Throat type 8. Nose type 8.

mention should be made of modern streptococci serology. In 1928 and 1933 R. C. Lancefield (3, 4) published her grouping of hemolytic streptococci by means of a precipitation reaction. She originally posited the groups A, B, C, D, and E. Later on, the groups F, G, H, and K have been added. Each group is characterised by its group-specific antigen, the so-called »C-substance». Of these various groups, group A is the most important in human pathology.

In 1926, 1927 and 1934 F. Griffith (5, 6, 7) published his typing of hemolytic streptococci by means of agglutination with absorbed, type-specific sera. The type-specific antigen has been named the »M-substance». Most of the serological types posited by F. Griffith have proved to belong to Lancefield's group A. A few new types have been added later. Today, some 30 different types are allowed for within group A.

British authors especially have made a series of studies of scarlet fever, where the streptococci isolated have been typed according to Griffith's method. These studies have elucidated many facts relating to the epidemiology of scarlet fever. Among other things, it is no longer possible to maintain the opinion which prevailed until lately, viz. that a special streptococcus, often named strept. scarlatinosus, was the cause of scarlet fever. It has been shown that a series of different types within group A can cause scarlet fever. The factor which, more than anything else, determines the ability of a streptococcal strain to cause scarlet fever, seems to be its toxin-producing properties. The serological types of streptococci most frequently found in cases of scarlet fever have, moreover, been shown to vary according to time and place.

Typing has been of great value also in determining return cases. In our material, group A, type 8 streptococci were isolated in 7 out of 8 return cases. In the 8th case, no hemolytic streptococci were isolated. The same type was isolated from the 4 primary cases. Brown and Allison (8) have examined 30 primary cases. In 4 of these cases, no hemolytic streptococci were isolated on their discharge. In spite of this they were probably infective. The remaining 26 primary cases had caused 36 return cases. In all the return cases except one, they isolated the same type of streptococci from the primary case and the corresponding return cases. The one case where the same type was not found, probably is no return case at all — the patient having supposedly caught the infection otherwise.

As will be known, return cases are those cases of scarlet fever which occur in the immediate environment of the convalescent when discharged at the end of the period of isolation. Otherwise, the definitions given by different authors vary considerably. Lichtenstein (2) includes all who have lived in contact with the convalescent and who have fallen ill within 2 weeks of his discharge. Brown and Allison (8) adopt the following definition: »A case of infectious disease occurring in the same house within 28 days of a patient's discharge from a fever hospital». They moreover recommend the use of »infecting case rate» as being a more adequate notion. The »infecting case rate» denotes the number of discharged patients, stated in percent of the total number of cases, causing new cases of the disease within a definite period after their discharge. As one patient may cause more than one return case, the »infecting case rate» will always be somewhat lower than the frequency of return cases.

The stated frequency of return cases varies with the different authors, among other things because they use different time limits in their definition of a return case. The most usual figures given are from 1 to 5 percent. BROWN and ALLISON (8) found 4,9 percent. LICHTENSTEIN (2), in his material from Stockholm, gives the rate of 3 percent return cases among 3783 scarlet fever patients during the period 1925—30. During the scarlet fever epidemic in Oslo from August 10th 1939 till April 10th, 1940, a total of 1560 scarlet fever patients were admitted to hospital. Using the same definition of a return case as LICHTENSTEIN, the frequency of return cases proved to be about 2 percent.

Disagreement seems to exist as to whether the frequency of return cases is dependent upon the length of the period of isolation. Some authors hold, that the longer the period of isolation, the larger is the number of return cases (PARSON, quoted by BROWN and ALLISON (8)). BROWN and ALLISSON found that patients discharged during the 5th to 7th week caused the largest number of return cases. There is no agreement, either, as to whether cases discharged with complications more frequently cause return cases than patients discharged without complications. E. MANCHOT (1) did, however, find that of 71 primary cases, who all caused return cases, 49 had complications. Complications in the upper respiratory tract were of special importance. LICHTENSTEIN has noted that patients discharged with a cured otitis media, and who in their homes have had a relapse of their otitis, often cause return cases. In this connection it may be mentioned that Tore (case 1) developed an otitis media after his discharge from hospital. All authors seem to agree, however, that the cessation or continuance of peeling is of slight importance for the occurrence of return cases. Most authors assume that the contagion is especially conveyed by secretions from the throat, the nose and the ears. It is, therefore, safe to assume that complications are of special importance for the occurrence of return cases.

Another question which is of some importance in this connection is whether return cases generally are of a more serious nature than other cases of scarlet fever. There is little information on this point in the usual literature. Rolleston (9) does, however, state that A. C. R. Cameron and also Soerensen have observed a higher fatality rate among return cases than in a control group. E. Manchot (1) found that in his own material return cases were not more serious than other cases of scarlet fever.

We ourselves had the impression that the return cases during the Oslo epidemic mentioned here, were of a somewhat more serious character than the epidemic as a whole. In order to verify this, if possible, we have taken all return cases during this epidemic, totalling 35, and compared them with 35 scarlet fever patients chosen at random. In choosing we made the reservation that the control case should be a patient of the same sex and age-group, and approximately the same date of admission (the same phase of the epidemic), in order thereby to obtain the best possible basis of comparison. For the 35 return cases and the 35 control cases we have noted all complications. The results are set out in Table II. It appears from this table that there is a preponderance of complications in the return case material. Disregarding the cases of adenitis which, probably, within the symptomathology of scarlet fever, is the most difficult to place either as a part symptom of the main illnes or as an independent complication, we find that complications occur twice as frequently among the return cases as in the control group.

The return case group would have been larger still, and the difference in the frequency of complications probably still more evident, if we had not used a time limit of 14 days in the definition of a return case (following Lichtenstein) but had included the other cases where there was a strong presumption of an epidemiological connection. If we had done so, the above-mentioned case 5 — one of the most serious cases of the

Table II. Shows the frequency of complications in the return cases and in the control cases.

Nature of Complication	Frequency of Complication in	
	Return cases	Control cases
Adenitis	11	12
Rhinitis	2	0
Tonsillitis	4	2
Catarrhal otitis media . .	2	0
Unilat. purulent otitis . .	3	4
Bilat. » » . .	2	1
Bilat. purulent otitis + mastoiditis	1	0
Doubtful myocarditis . .	3	3
Certain » . .	1	1
Nephritis	5	0
Arthralgia	3	1
Bronchopneumonia	0	1
Panaritium	1	0
Sum	38	25
Less adenitis	11	12
Rest	28	13

whole epidemic — would have been included. Likewise, one of the two deaths which occurred during the epidemic would have been included.

As mentioned above, streptococci group A, type 8, were isolated from all return cases in this material in which typing of streptococci was undertaken. An obvious question is, whether this type was specially potent in causing scarlet fever, so that patients having this type in their upper respiratory tract after their discharge, caused ever new cases. We know that scarlet fever patients very frequently have hemolytic streptococci in their throats at the end of the isolation period. In the epidemic discussed here, throat samples were taken on discharge from 156 patients during the period from October 16th till November 20th. From 105 (70 per cent) of these patients, hemolytic streptococci were isolated by a single examination. This agrees with the result arrived at by BROWN and ALLISON (8), viz. 80 per cent.

Even though as many convalescents as this have hemolytic streptococci in their throats when discharged, a very few percent of them only will cause return cases. The streptococci of these cases must, therefore, possess special properties which make them a danger to their surroundings. In this connection it seems natural to think of the toxin-producing properties of the strains in question. It is now held that the scarlet fever rash is provoked by a streptococcal toxin, the so-called erythrogenic toxin. When an individual catches tonsillitis, it depends upon the antitoxic immunity of the person in question, and on the toxin-producing properties of the streptococcal strain, whether or not the patient develops a rash. The above-mentioned case 10 only caught a tonsillitis without rash. This patient must have possessed a sufficient anti-toxic immunity to prevent the eruption of the toxic exanthema.

We are of the opinion that the streptococcal strain which provoked the return cases discussed here, had strong toxin-producing properties, and that, therefore, case 1 (Tore) for this reason was the primary case of many new cases of scarlet fever both outside the hospital and inside the hospital among the nurses attending him and his victims.

In this connection it is interesting to inquire what were the other types of streptococci found during this epidemic. It might be that group A, type 8 was completely dominating, so that no sure conclusions could be drawn from the data presented above. The control material is regrettably scant, consisting merely of 6 patients picked at random, from whom samples were taken on their admission to hospital, and of 10 patients from whom no samples were taken until the patients had been removed to the isolation wards.

The results set out in table III show that group A, type 8 was not the dominating type in this control material chosen

Table III. Shows the result of typing of streptococci in 16 control cases.

Type	No. of cases
1	2
2	1
3	6
7	1
8	3
14	1
No growth	2
Sum	16

at random. Because of the low numbers, the inquiry gives little information about the epidemic as a whole. It is, however, permissible to draw the conclusion that the epidemic was caused by various types, and that possibly type 8 was the most strongly toxin-producing of these types.

The question arises as to whether it would be possible to contribute towards the solution of the question of isolation through the typing of hemolytic streptococci in scarlet fever patients during an epidemic. It is well known that a lively discussion is carried on everywhere on the value of isolation as a prophylactic measure against scarlet fever. There is no agreement as to how long the patient should be kept isolated. There is no agreement either as to whether the patient should be isolated at home or in hospital. All agree that there is no guarantee that the patients are not infective when discharged at the end of the period of isolation, whether they be then clinically cured or have complications. In this connection, it does not matter whether the period of isolation has lasted 2, 4 or 6 weeks.

The results discussed here may possibly suggest a solution If typing of hemolytic streptococci were carried out consistently and it were discovered that some type or other in a marked degree caused the spreading of the disease, it would seem logical to deal sternly with these cases, isolating them apart in hospital, so that there was no possibility of their infecting scarlet fever patients with other serological types (cross-infection) — and if necessary prolonging the isolation beyond the usual period. Following this line of action, cases caused by other serological types might be dealt with more leniently and possibly be isolated at home.

Summary.

A scarlet fever convalescent was isolated for 6 weeks in hospital. After his discharge he was causing several return cases, one of them occurring 6 weeks after his own discharge. The patient was re-isolated. In the hospital he and one of his return cases infected 4 nurses, 3 of them with scarlet fever and 1 with tonsillitis without rash. Both from the primary case, from most of the return cases and from the 4 nurses hemolytic streptococci, Group A, type 8 were isolated. In the scarlet fever epidemic in Oslo 1939—40 several of the »return cases» were seriously ill. By comparing the return case group (35 cases) in this epidemic with a control group the return case group showed a higher frequency of complications.

References.

1. E. Manchot. Jahrbuch f. Kinderheilk. 150, p. 332, 1938. — 2. A. Lichtenstein. Acta. Pæd. 12, p. 100, 1931. — 3. R. C. Lancefield. J. Exp. Med. 47, p. 481, 1928. — 4. —— J. Exp. Med. 57, p. 571, 1933. — 5. F. Griffith. J. Hyg. Camb. 25, p. 385, 1926. — 6. —— J. Hyg. Camb. 26, p. 363, 1926. — 7. —— J. Hyg. Camb. 34, p. 542, 1934. — 8. W. A. Brown and V. D. Allison. J. Hyg. Camb. 35, p. 283, 1935. — 9. J. D. Rolleston. Acute Infectious Dieseases, London 1925.

AUS DEM EPIDEMIEKRANKENHAUS DER STADT STOCKHOLM. VORSTAND: DOZENT R. BERGMAN.

SCHARLACHSTUDIEN XXIII.

Zweiterkrankung an Scharlach.

Von

FOLKE THURESSON.

Obgleich die meisten Forscher heutzutage darüber einig sind, dass Zweiterkrankungen an Scharlach vorkommen, sind doch ziemlich wenig Untersuchungen angestellt worden, um die Frequenz diesbezüglicher Fälle in Erfahrung zu bringen. Erheblich mehr Aufmerksamkeit hat man den sog. Scharlachrezidiven gewidmet, d. h. Neuerkrankungen während der Zeit, in welcher sich die erste Scharlacherkrankung noch im Gange befindet, oder während der Rekonvaleszenz nach derselben.

Soweit ich finden konnte, ist es nur BIRK (zit. n. OPITZ 24), welcher das Vorkommen von Zweiterkrankungen bestreitet. Andere Autoren betonen jedoch die grosse Seltenheit derselben. OPITZ (24) sagt: »Denn Zweiterkrankungen sind so enorm selten, dass sie praktisch keine Rolle spielen. Das verpflichtet uns aber auch, nur dann eine derartige Diagnose zu stellen, wenn der Nachweis einwandfrei zu erbringen ist.»

Als eine besondere Schwierigkeit bei der Beurteilung der Rezidivfrequenz — eine Schwierigkeit, welche natürlich auch in bezug auf die Zweiterkrankungen Geltung haben muss — heben OPITZ (25) und BESSAU (4) die Unzuverlässigkeit des Symptoms der Schuppung hervor. BESSAU ist der Ansicht, ein Rezidiv, welches bei einem Kinde auftritt, das auf eine Scharlachabteilung aufgenommen worden war, müsse stets den Verdacht wachrufen, dass die erste Diagnose falsch gewesen wäre. Bei den Zweiterkrankungen in Verf.s Untersuchung liegen doch die Verhältnisse zum Teil anders; diese Patienten wurden unter den übrigen Scharlachpatienten stationär behandelt, ohne in der Regel ein Rezidiv zu bekommen.

Zappert (35) erörtert das Verhältnis zwischen Scharlach und Erythema scarlatiniforme desquamativum recidivans und meint, die Schwierigkeit, diese Erkrankungen in gewissen Fällen voneinander zu unterscheiden, habe zur Unsicherheit bei der Diagnose geführt, »in dem Missverhältnis zwischen den geringen Allgemeinerscheinungen sowie der wenig ausgeprägten Beteiligung der Mund- und Rachenschleimhaut gegenüber dem sehr starken, scharlachähnlichen Hautausschlag und der lange dauernden, heftigen Schuppung liegt vielmehr der Unterschied zwischen Erythema scarlatiniforme und Scharlach». Z. steht ferner auf dem Standpunkt, dass, wenigstens im Kindesalter, ein überstandener Scharlach zur Entstehung des Erythema scarlatiniforme disponiert, doch brauchen nicht alle Fälle der letzteren Erkrankung früher Scharlach gehabt zu haben. Er beschreibt ferner zwei eigene Fälle von Zweiterkrankung, von welchen der eine dann noch zwei weitere Erkrankungen aufwies, welch letztere Z. für Erythema scarlatiniforme hält (Pat. erkrankte im Alter von 3, bzw. 11, 15 und 16 Jahren).

Eine Reihe von Autoren haben über einzelne Fälle von Zweiterkrankung berichtet. So beobachtete Reh (27) 1924 einen typischen Scharlach bei einem 6jährigen Mädchen, welches 1921 wegen dieser Erkrankung stationär behandelt worden war. Bei keiner der beiden Erkrankungen traten irgendwelche Komplikationen auf; klinisch unterschieden sie sich dadurch, dass die zweite Erkrankung fieberfrei verlief (was, wie R. betont, früher auch von anderen Autoren konstatiert worden war). Er ist der Ansicht, der fieberfreie Verlauf der Zweiterkrankung sei zweifelsohne als eine Folge der ersten Krankheit zu betrachten, welche wenigstens teilweise immunisierend gewirkt hätte. Bonapace (zit. n. Slawky 29) sah bei einem 4jährigen Knaben 24 Tage nach der Ausheilung eines leichten Scharlachs ein neues, mittelschweres Scarlatinaexanthem, welches in der üblichen Zeit ohne Folgeerscheinungen abheilte.

Schulten (zit. n. Opitz 24) fand unter 4 000 Scharlachfällen nur eine Zweiterkrankung (ausserdem 0,7 % Frührezidive). Auch Herre (10) beschreibt eine Zweiterkrankung (krank 1916 bzw. 1918). Er steht auf dem Standpunkt, dass auch die meisten Rezidive auf einer Neuinfektion beruhen; eine Vorraussetzung für das Zustandekommen derselben sei eine Hyperergie gegen die sekundärtoxische Wirkung des Scharlachs. Hase (zit. n. Gabriel u. Zischinsky 8) gibt an, dass auf ungefähr 1 000 Scharlachfälle eine Zweiterkrankung kommt. Auch Henoch (zit. n. Lämmerhirt 17) hat eine Zweiterkrankung beobachtet.

Lämmerhirt (17) hat selbst über drei eigene Fälle berichtet und sagt, die zweite Erkrankung sei nicht leichter, sondern könne sogar schwerer sein als die erste (einer seiner Fälle verlief tödlich). L.s drei Fälle stammen aus einer 10-Jahrsperiode, während welcher er jährlich 30—50 Scharlachfälle gesehen hatte. Er zitiert ferner Baginsky, der auf dem Standpunkt steht, dass Zweiterkrankungen in seltenen Fällen vorkommen, und Heubner, welcher unter 358 Fällen 6 fand, wo ihm als zuverlässig bekannte andere Ärzte früher Scharlach festgestellt hatten.

Fritz (7) konstatierte im Laufe von 5 Jahren in seiner Privatpraxis bei zwei Fällen sowohl die erste wie die zweite Erkrankung; bei dem einen verlief die Zweiterkrankung erheblich schwerer als die Ersterkrankung. In beiden Fällen war jedoch auch die erste Krankheit eine schwere gewesen, weshalb die Patienten Serum erhielten. Er ist der Ansicht, dass die Serumbehandlung leichter zur Zweiterkrankung Anlass gebe, dass man sich derselben aber doch bei schweren Fällen bedienen solle, da die Prognose dadurch eine viel bessere werde.

Gabriel u. Zischinsky (8) haben in ihrem Krankenhaus 22 sichere Zweiterkrankungen (1,1 ‰) gefunden; sie sagen, dass, da diese Kranken bei beiden Gelegenheiten in demselben Krankenhaus stationär behandelt worden waren, die wirkliche Anzahl der Zweiterkrankungen höher sein müsse. Zischinsky (33) hat später über weitere 9 Zweiterkrankungen berichtet; die längste Zeit zwischen den beiden Krankheiten war 8 Jahre.

Er zitiert ferner CLAUSEN, welcher 31 Zweiterkrankungen gefunden hat, niemals aber einen Patienten, welcher dreimal oder öfters erkrankt wäre.

Schon 1872 konnte TROJANOWSKY (zit. n. WEISSENBERG 34) unter 300 selbst beobachteten Fällen 18 Zweiterkrankungen feststellen (mindestens 1/2 Jahr zwischen den Erkrankungen). KOERNER (14) hat 1876 77 Fälle zusammengestellt; die erste Erkrankung trat in der Regel bei Kindern unter 10 Jahren auf, die zweite 2—6 Jahre später, nur in 6 Fällen betrug die Zeit zwischen den Erkrankungen weniger als 1 Jahr. Die Zweiterkrankung war oft schwerer als die erste. WEISSENBERG (34) beschreibt selbst 7 Fälle, von welchen einer 3 Male erkrankte. Er meint, es gäbe Individuen, bei welchen ein überstandener Scharlach eine gesteigerte Disposition zu der Krankheit schaffe; in W.s sämtlichen Fällen war die Krankheit beim zweiten Mal schwerer.

OPITZ, KLEINSCHMIDT u. SELTER (zit. n. BURGHARD 6) glauben, dass Zweiterkrankungen an Scharlach etwas häufiger sind als an Masern; sie fanden unter 1 000 eigenen Fällen in der Kölner Klinik 3 sichere Zweiterkrankungen.

SLĂTINEANU, BĂLTEANU u. BUTTESCU (zit. n. POPOVICIU 26) haben während 9 Jahren unter im Epidemiekrankenhaus stationär behandelten 5 452 Scharlachfällen 27 (0,49 %) Zweiterkrankungen gefunden (9 Fälle nach 3 Jahren, 3 nach 5, 3 nach 6, 2 nach 7, 2 nach 8 und je einen nach 62 Tagen, 1, 4, 8, 9, 10 und 15 Jahren).[1] Der jährliche Prozentsatz der Zweiterkrankungen war in den letzten 2 Jahren auffallend gestiegen (3,36 % 1934, veröffentl. 1935), obwohl man sich da am Ende einer Epidemiewelle befand und auch die Virulenz abgenommen hatte. Nur in 4 Fällen kamen leichte Intoxikationssymptome vor, ein einziger Fall (eine Mischinfektion von Scharlach, Typhus und Bronchopneumonie) kam ad exitum.

ANDERSON (2) hat in 3,5 % Zweiterkrankungen und in 3,6—4,3 % Rezidive beobachtet. Nach A.s Ansicht beruhen diese hohen Zahlen auf einer relativ leichten Form des Scharlachs,

[1] (Das sind 26 Fälle, obgleich »nach 8 Jahren» an zwei Stellen aufgeführt ist!) Verf.

welche nur eine schwache Immunität zurücklassen soll. Um Rezidive zu vermeiden, impfte der Autor alle beim Beginn der Krankheit Dick-positiven Patienten, nachdem das Fieber aufgehört hatte. Er glaubt, dass eine aktive Immunisierung zur Herabsetzung der Anzahl von Rezidiven führt.

Jochmann-Hegler (12) sagt im Lehrbuch der Infektionskrankheiten, 1924, dass ein überstandener Scharlach in der Regel eine lebenslängliche Immunität verleiht, doch seien eine Reihe einwandfreie Fälle bekannt, in welchen 2- oder 3maliges Erkranken an Scharlach vorlag; Ausnahmen kämen also jedenfalls vor.

Kolle u. Hetsch (15) erwähnen in Experimentelle Bakteriologie und Infektionskrankheiten, 1938, nichts über Rezidive oder wiederholtes Erkranken an Scharlach.

Kolle u. Wassermann (16) sprechen im Handbuch der pathogenen Mikroorganismen, 1938, u. a. von der Häufigkeit der Rezidive, erwähnen aber nichts von späteren Wiedererkrankungen.

Nørby (23) sagt in Nordisk Lærebog i intern medicin, 1939, dass ein durchgemachter Scharlach in den allermeisten Fällen eine Dauerimmunität zurücklässt, aber auch bei Individuen, welche nicht Scharlach bekommen, entwickle sich meistens im Laufe der Jahre eine mehr oder weniger ausgeprägte Unempfänglichkeit für die Krankheit. Das soll wahrscheinlich auf abgewehrten Angriffen wenig virulenter Streptokokken beruhen.

In Nordisk Lärobok i Pediatrik, 1941, schreibt Lichtenstein (22): »Erneutes Erkranken an Scharlach (also nicht Rezidiv während im Gange befindlicher Krankheit) kommt ab und zu vor. An einem Material von ca. 6 000—7 000 Fällen konnte ich etwas weniger als 1/2 % sichere derartige Fälle beobachten, was in Anbetracht dessen, dass sicherlich Fälle vorkommen, bei welchen entweder die erste oder die zweite Erkrankung so abortiv verläuft, dass die Diagnose unsicher wird, bestimmt eine Minimalzahl darstellt. Je leichter der Scharlach ist, desto grösser wird übrigens die Wahrscheinlichkeit, dass die Immunisierung durch die erste Attacke der

Krankheit zum Schutz gegen ein Wiedererkranken irgendeinmal in der Zukunft nicht hinreicht.»

Während die oben zitierten Autoren samt und sonders auf dem Standpunkt stehen, die Zweiterkrankungen kämen verhältnismässig selten vor, was gewöhnlich auf einer bei der ersten Erkrankung geschaffenen Immunität beruhe, bestreitet v. Szontag (30), dass es eine Scharlachimmunität gebe. Als Beispiele hierfür führt er u. a. Fälle an, wo Ärzte, welche früher lange Scharlachkranke behandelt hatten, ohne selbst die Krankheit gehabt oder da bekommen zu haben, später an Scharlach erkranken. Er ist ferner der Ansicht, dass der Scharlach auch nicht besonders ansteckend sei. Er sagt u. a.: »Auch das Gift der Scarlatina gehört zu jenen Krankheitserregern, die an uns und in uns leben. ...... Auch der genuine Scharlach ist, wenngleich kryptogenetischen Ursprungs, nichts anderes als eine Sepsis (Toxinämie) oder Pyämie (Bakteriämie) oder aber eine Kombination von beiden — eine Septikopyämie.» Er führt ferner mehrere Fälle von Wiedererkranken an: »... als ich mich vor einigen Jahren für kurze Zeit in Sopron aufhielt, ein dortiger, inzwischen verstorbener, sehr tüchtiger und glaubwürdiger Kollege, Dr. Manninger, mich darüber versicherte, dass er in dieser Stadt einen Herrn kannte, der im Laufe von mehreren Jahren *neunmal* an Scharlach erkrankte. ... In meiner Patientur gibt es ein Mädchen, das bereits 3mal Scharlach glücklich überstanden hat. Die erste Erkrankung erfolgte am 17. II. 1907, die zweite am 1. V. 1909 und die dritte am 21. IX. 1909.» Ferner berichtet er über ein 3 1/2jähriges Mädchen, welches einmal am 9. I., sodann am 16. XI. 1909 an Scharlach erkrankte.

Im Jahre 1912 äussert sich v. Sz. (31, 32) über Scharlach und Angina, welche er für dieselbe Krankheit hält, wie folgt: »... bloss die Reaktion des Organismus ist eine verschiedene. Sie ist eine andere im Falle einer eitrigen Angina, und sie ist wieder eine andere im Falle einer Scharlacherkrankung. ... Das bösartige Scharlachfieber ist nichts anderes, als die denkbar schwerste Form der gewöhnlichen Angina. ... Das Wesen des Scharlachproblems setze ich also nicht in einem unbekannten Scharlachgift, sondern einzig und allein in der veränderten und gesteigerten Reaktionsfähigkeit des Körpers voraus. Wenn ein Organismus, dessen Reaktionsfähigkeit eine veränderte oder gesteigerte ist, an einer einfachen Angina erkrankt, so entsteht ein Krankheitsbild, das man mit dem Namen der Scarlatina belegt hat.»

Mehrere Forscher haben nachgewiesen, dass die Mehrzahl der Scharlachrezidive auf einer exogenen Infektion beruht hat. Aus von Lichtenstein (18, 19, 20) sowie von Allison u. Brown (1) ausgeführten Untersuchungen geht hervor, dass, wenn Scharlachkranke gänzlich isoliert wurden oder wenn z. B. Geschwister, welche gleichzeitig erkrankt waren, zusammen isoliert wurden, Rezidive in diesen Fällen nicht eintraten. Aus Kiew hat dagegen Reidermann (28) über drei Fälle berichtet, wo die Patienten Rezidive bekamen, obwohl sie nach R. vollständig von der Aussenwelt abgeschlossen waren. Sie wohnten mit ihren Müttern in Separatzimmern mit besonderem Eingang von aussen und wurden von niemand anders als dem behandelnden Arzt besucht. Alle drei Patienten hatten schon bei der ersten Erkrankung ein Exanthem gehabt, und das Rezidiv stellte sich am 15. bzw. 17. und 22. Tage ein. Auf Grund dieser Fälle behauptet R., dass man sehr wohl das Auftreten von Rezidiven bei absolutem Ausschluss jeglicher Ansteckungsmöglichkeit von aussen her annehmen müsse.

Koch (13) fasst die Rezidive als entweder auf einer autogenen Superinfektion beruhend oder als Neuinfektionen mit virulenten Erregern auf. Man kann möglicherweise auch eine familiär bedingte Anomalie des Immunitätsapparats als eine Erklärung für das Auftreten der Rezidive annehmen. Sie sagt ferner bei ihrer Beschreibung einer Anzahl von Rezidiven aus den Jahren 1933—39 im Kinderkrankenhaus Berlin-Lichtenberg, wo unter 1 300 Scharlachfällen 33 Rezidive vorkamen (2,5 %), dass diese bei den in einem grossen Saal liegenden Patienten nicht häufiger waren als bei den in Einzelkabinetten untergebrachten.

Allison u. Brown (1) wollen gezeigt haben, dass sich im

Falle eines Rezidivs ein neuer serologischer Typ von Streptococcus pyogenes bei dem Kranken nachweisen lässt, ein Typ, welcher da in der Regel gleichzeitig bei irgendeinem anderen Scharlachpatienten vorhanden ist, mit dem der Kranke vorher in Berührung gestanden hatte.

Auch GOTTLIEB (9) hält für wahrscheinlich, dass Rezidive durch Infektion von Patienten mit einem anderen Streptokokkentyp als dem zustande kommen, welchen der von dem Rezidiv betroffene Kranke beherbergt, und dass Rezidive bei völlig isolierten Patienten nicht vorkommen.

V. BORMANN (5) geht noch weiter, indem er sagt, »es sei an der Zeit, einzusehen, dass für die Streptokokkenätiologie Beweise vorgebracht worden sind, wie selten bei irgendeiner Infektionskrankheit». Nach v. B. haben ferner SLĂTINEANU, BĂLTEANU, CONSTANTINESCU und FRANCKE Versuche angestellt, welche die Erfahrung, dass der Scharlacherreger nicht filtrierbar ist, weiterhin bestätigen.

Trotz der Anschauungen der oben zitierten und vieler anderer Forscher, welche unleugbar mit schwerwiegenden Gründen für die Streptokokkenätiologie hervorgetreten sind, dürfte die wirkliche Ursache des Scharlachs noch nicht als unbestreitbar festgestellt zu erachten sein. Die obenerwähnten Untersuchungen von LICHTENSTEIN sowie von ALLISON und BROWN sprechen jedoch stark dafür, dass die Ursache der Rezidive in einer exogenen Infektion zu suchen sei. Mit Rücksicht hierauf dürfte sich darüber streiten lassen, ob nicht auch diese bei einer Untersuchung über die Wiedererkrankungsfrequenz mitberücksichtigt werden sollten, d. h. ob nicht die Rezidive als Zweiterkrankungen zu rechnen wären. In der vorliegenden Arbeit soll diese Frage jedoch nicht fernerhin erörtert werden, sondern Verf. wird sich ausschliesslich mit den eigentlichen Zweiterkrankungen beschäftigen, d. h. mit Personen, die nach völliger Genesung von Scharlach von neuem an derselben Affektion erkranken, betreffenden Fällen.

Verf.s Untersuchung gründet sich auf das Material des Epidemiekrankenhauses in Stockholm aus den Jahren 1926—1939. Früher hat LICHTENSTEIN aus demselben Krankenhaus eine Untersuchung veröffentlicht, welche sich auf die Jahre 1924—1933 bezieht und insgesamt 6 028 Scharlachfälle enthält, unter den L. 29 Wiedererkrankungen (0,48 %) fand. Diese waren sämtlich ganz einwandfrei, und LICHTENSTEIN betont, dass es sich um eine Minimalzahl handelt, da es zweifelsohne auch Fälle gibt, wo eine der Erkrankungen mehr oder weniger abortiv verlaufen ist, und die Diagnose daher unsicher wurde. Einer dieser Fälle hatte drei sichere Scharlacherkrankungen, im Alter von 3, 11 und 13 Jahren.

Mein Material wird sich also zum Teil mit dem LICHTENSTEINS decken; dass ich es trotzdem gewählt habe, bis 1926 zurückzugreifen, beruht darauf, dass man in diesem Jahre damit begonnen hatte, das SCHULTZ-CHARLTONsche Auslöschphänomen routinemässig — mit vereinzelten Ausnahmen in den ersten Jahren — bei sämtlichen Patienten durchzuprüfen, welche infolge von Scharlachverdacht in das Krankenhaus aufgenommen wurden. Hierdurch ist es mir auch gelungen, eine verhältnismässig grosse Anzahl Fälle zu erhalten, die bei beiden Erkrankungen neben den rein klinischen Symptomen auch ein positives Auslöschphänomen aufwiesen.

Das Material wurde in vier Gruppen eingeteilt. Von den zu Gruppe I gehörenden Patienten waren 11, von den zu Gruppe II gehörigen 49 bei der Ersterkrankung nicht im Epidemiekrankenhaus von Stockholm behandelt worden, sondern sämtliche in Gruppe I und 29 in Gruppe II in anderen Epidemiekrankenhäusern. Den Herren Kollegen an diesen Krankenhäusern, welche mir die Krankengeschichten freundlichst zur Verfügung gestellt haben, spreche ich an dieser Stelle meinen aufrichtigen Dank aus. In einigen kleineren Epidemiekrankenhäusern für ländliche Bezirke, die ihren Betrieb später eingestellt haben, waren die Krankengeschichten nicht aufzubringen; diese Fälle wurden sämtlich in eine der Gruppen III oder IV eingereiht.

Zu Gruppe I wurden diejenigen Patienten gerechnet, welche bei beiden Erkrankungen positives Auslöschphänomen und sonst typisches Krankheitsbild aufwiesen, sowie die, welche im übrigen bei beiden Erkrankungen ein völlig typisches Krankheitsbild mit Exanthem, Angina, Himbeerzunge und Schuppung gezeigt hatten; da die Ersterkrankung bei einem Teil der Fälle länger zurücklag als 1926, konnte das Auslöschphänomen bei diesen nur bei der späteren Erkrankung geprüft werden.

In Gruppe II wurden einmal diejenigen Patienten eingereiht, welche Exanthem und typische Schuppung hatten, bei den aber das Auslöschphänomen negativ oder zweifelhaft gewesen war (dies kommt normalerweise in 8—18 % vor [1]), oder wo ein charakteristisches Symptom, z. B. die Himbeerzunge, fehlte (in einigen Fällen darauf beruhend, dass ein diesbezüglicher Vermerk in der Krankengeschichte vergessen worden war), sodann Fälle, bei welchen das Exanthem bei einer oder beiden Erkrankungen nicht im Krankenhaus beobachtet worden war, sondern aus der Anamnese hervorging, und wo das klinische Bild sonst völlig sicher war, sowie ferner Fälle mit ganz typischer Schuppung und weiterhin einer Reihe charakteristischer Symptome (Lymphadenitiden u. dgl.), wo aber das Exanthem bei einer oder beiden Erkrankungen nicht beobachtet worden war, und schliesslich einige Fälle, welche bei

[1] Nach Huss (11) wechselt die Frequenz positiver Fälle beim Schultz-Charltonschen Auslöschphänomen in verschiedenen Untersuchungen erheblich; sie beträgt nach H. 82—85 %, bei Untersuchung während der beiden ersten Krankheitstage 91—92 %. Beim Rezidiv wird das Phänomen nach Huss in beträchtlich mehr Fällen positiv, in ca. 93 %, was u. a. darauf zurückzuführen sein dürfte, dass die Untersuchung hier gewöhnlich an frischeren Exanthemen vorgenommen wird. H. hat auch nachgewiesen, dass die Reaktion bei Verwendung antitoxischen Pferdeserums ungefähr ebensooft positiv wird wie mit Rekonvaleszentenserum. Bergman (3) hat später gezeigt, dass die Reaktionen der beiden Serumarten doch einander nicht vollständig decken; in einem Teil der Fälle erhält man gleichzeitig bei demselben Patienten eine positive Reaktion mit Rekonvaleszentenserum und eine negative mit antitoxischem Pferdeserum, in anderen Fällen ist das umgekehrt. Dadurch, dass man stets beide Serumreaktionen gleichzeitig anwendet, erhält man daher eine grössere Anzahl positiver Auslöschphänomene; dieses Verfahren ist im Stockholmer Epidemiekrankenhaus üblich.

der Ersterkrankung nicht in ein Krankenhaus aufgenommen worden waren, aber einen typischen Bericht über ihre Krankheit erstatten konnten, bei der sie zu Hause isoliert und von einem angegebenen Arzte behandelt worden waren.

Zu Gruppe III wurden diejenigen gerechnet, welche angaben, bei der ersten Erkrankung eine sichere Scarlatina gehabt zu haben, bei den man dies aber nicht an Hand von Vermerken in der Krankengeschichte verifizieren konnte; es wird da z. B. angegeben, dass Pat. wegen Scharlachs im Epidemiekrankenhaus behandelt worden sein soll, aber nicht, in welchem Epidemiekrankenhaus, oder aber Pat. berichtete, zu Hause ärztlich behandelt worden zu sein, es fehlt aber eine nähere Beschreibung des Krankheitsverlaufs. Ferner gehören diejenigen Fälle hierher, wo Pat. seine erste Erkrankung ganz typisch schilderte, laut Angabe aber daheim gepflegt worden war, ohne dass ein Arzt gerufen wurde. In allen diesen Fällen war jedoch die Zweiterkrankung völlig typisch.

Schliesslich wurden in Gruppe IV eine Reihe Fälle zusammengestellt, welche zwar angaben, früher Scharlach gehabt zu haben, wo aber keine weiteren Auskünfte hierüber erhältlich waren, oder wo die erstatteten Angaben diese Diagnose weniger wahrscheinlich machten.

Im Hinblick auf die oben aufgeführten Bedingungen dürfte es als sicher zu erachten sein, dass die Anzahl der Zweiterkrankungen mindestens der Gesamtzahl der beiden ersten Gruppen zusammen entspricht, und dass dazu wahrscheinlich auch noch ein nicht geringer Teil der Fälle kommt, die in die dritte Gruppe eingereiht worden waren. Vermutlich liegt die wirkliche Anzahl Zweiterkrankungen zwischen den Summen der Fälle in Gruppe I und II sowie I, II und III, mit der Anzahl der Fälle in allen vier Gruppen als eine absolute Maximalzahl. Es ist selbstverständlich nicht ausgeschlossen, dass es Fälle geben kann, welche früher Scharlach gehabt hatten, ohne dass dies vermerkt worden war, aber das dürfte dadurch kompensiert werden, dass es sich bei der Mehrzahl der Fälle in Gruppe IV und wahrscheinlich auch bei einem

Teil in Gruppe III vermutlich bei der vorausgehenden angegebenen Krankheit nicht um Scharlach gehandelt hat.

Während der vierzehn Jahre, über welche sich die Untersuchung erstreckt, sind 11 969 Scharlachpatienten im Krankenhause stationär behandelt worden. Die Verteilung auf die einzelnen Jahre ist natürlich eine sehr unregelmässige, was aus Tab. 1 unmittelbar ersichtlich wird. In diese Tabelle wurde auch die Anzahl Zweiterkrankungen aufgenommen, auf die verschiedenen Gruppen verteilt; das angegebene Jahr ist stets das der späteren Erkrankung.

Von den Fällen in Gruppe I haben 29 bei beiden Erkrankungen ein positives SCHULTZ-CHARLTONsches Auslöschphänomen aufgewiesen. Wie aus Tab. 1 ersichtlich wird, kamen in Gruppe I 73 und in Gruppe II 110 Wiedererkrankungen vor, d. h. 1,5 %. In Gruppe III findet man 67 Zweiterkrankungen oder 0,6 %, in den drei Gruppen also 250 Fälle, d. h. 2,1 %. In Gruppe IV kommen 19 Fälle hinzu, insgesamt 2,2 %. Mit Rücksicht auf das oben Angeführte dürfte also die Frequenz der Wiedererkrankungen in diesem Material zwischen 1,5 und 2,1 % liegen. Auf Grund der Unmöglichkeit, bei einer derartigen Untersuchung das Vorkommen eventueller Abortivfälle zu berechnen, wurde ein diesbezüglicher Versuch nicht unternommen, man dürfte aber annehmen können, dass solche im Falle ihres Vorkommens proportional gleich oft bei der ersten wie bei der zweiten Erkrankung auftreten würden, weshalb irgendeine grössere prozentuale Verschiebung hierdurch aller Wahrscheinlichkeit nach nicht zu befürchten ist. Es ist eine andere Sache, dass es möglicherweise vorgekommen ist, dass der Arzt durch die Kenntnis davon, dass ein Patient vorher Scharlach durchgemacht hatte, dazu veranlasst wurde, bei einer eventuellen späteren Erkrankung eine andere Diagnose zu stellen, wodurch Zweiterkrankungen bei einer kleineren Anzahl von Fällen diagnostiziert worden sein können, als es der Wirklichkeit entsprechen würde. Im Hinblick auf die relativ grosse Anzahl von Fällen, welche wegen einer typischen Schuppung bei der zweiten Erkrankung ins Krankenhaus eingeliefert worden waren, 33, dürften indessen auch

Tab. 1.

Jahr	Scharlachfälle während d. Jahres	Gruppe I	%	Gruppe II	%	% I u. II	Gruppe III	%	% I, II, III	Gruppe IV	%	% I, II, III, IV
1926	485	2	0,4	3	0,6	1,0	0	0	1,0	0	0	1,0
1927	449	0	0	2	0,4	0,4	1	0,2	0,6	0	0	0,6
1928	656	1	0,2	6	0,9	1,1	5	0,8	1,8	1	0,2	2,0
1929	682	3	0,4	7	1,0	1,5	2	0,3	1,9	0	0	1,9
1930	590	1	0,2	4	0,7	0,9	2	0,3	1,2	0	0	1,2
1931	290	2	0,7	4	1,4	2,1	0	0	2,1	0	0	2,1
1932	340	6	1,8	5	1,5	3,3	1	0,3	3,6	0	0	3,6
1933	489	0	0	7	1,4	1,4	4	0,8	2,2	2	0,4	2,6
1934	1 315	10	0,8	8	0,6	1,4	8	0,6	2,0	0	0	2,0
1935	580	0	0	9	1,6	1,6	1	0,2	1,8	3	0,5	2,3
1936	443	4	0,9	4	0,9	1,8	1	0,2	2,0	2	0,5	2,5
1937	550	1	0,2	4	0,7	0,9	0	0	0,9	2	0,4	1,3
1938	1 706	10	0,6	18	1,1	1,7	12	0,7	2,4	2	0,1	2,5
1939	3 394	33	1,0	29	0,9	1,9	30	0,9	2,8	7	0,2	3,0
Sa.	11 969	73	0,6	110	0,9	1,5	67	0,6	2,1	19	0,2	2,2

derartige Fälle nicht so zahlreich sein, dass sie das Resultat in nennenswertem Grade zu verschieben imstande wären.

Insgesamt enthält das Material 6 206 männliche und 5 763 weibliche Patienten. Die Verteilung der Zweiterkrankungen auf die Geschlechter geht aus Tab. 2 hervor.

Tab. 2.

	Gruppe I	Gruppe II	Gruppe III	Gruppe IV	Summa
männliche Patienten	40	56	36	8	141
weibliche »	33	54	31	10	128

Bei den Zweiterkrankungen finden wir demnach keine grössere Verschiebung zwischen den Geschlechtern im Vergleich zur Gesamtanzahl der Fälle.

In Gruppe I ist das berechnete mittlere Alter bei der Ersterkrankung 5 Jahre 8 Monate und die berechnete mittlere Zeit zwischen erster und zweiter Erkrankung 4 Jahre 11 Monate (kürzeste Zeit 6 Wochen, vom Ende der ersten bis zum Beginn der zweiten Krankheitsperiode gerechnet; längste Zeit 26 Jahre).

Tab. 3.

	mittl. Alter bei der ersten Erkrankung	mittl. Zeit zwischen den Erkrankungen
Gruppe I	5 Jahre 8 Monate	4 Jahre 11 Monate
Gruppe II	6 » 8 »	5 » 11 »
Gruppe III	6 » 5 »	10 » 11 »
Gruppe IV	6 » 2 »	10 » 9 »

Im Hinblick auf die Einteilung des Materials ist die obige Verschiebung gegen eine längere Zeit zwischen den Erkrankungen in den letzteren Gruppen ganz erklärlich. Für Gruppe I und II zusammen wird das mittlere Alter bei der Ersterkrankung 6 Jahre 3 Monate und die mittlere Zeit zwischen erster und zweiter Erkrankung 5 Jahre 6 Monate.

Weissenberg fand bei seinen sieben Fällen, dass die Krankheit stets beim zweiten Mal schwerer war. In meinem Material glaubte ich zur Beurteilung dieses Sachverhalts nur die Länge der Krankheitszeit (nicht der Behandlungszeit!) bei der ersten bzw. zweiten Erkrankung sowie das Vorkommen eventueller Komplikationen untersuchen zu brauchen. Mit Rücksicht auf das sehr häufige Vorkommen von Lymphadenitis acuta bei beiden Erkrankungen (siehe Tab. 4) habe ich jedoch diese Komplikation hierbei ausgeschlossen. Da bei einigen Fällen die Angaben über die Krankheitsdauer allzu unsicher waren, sind diese Fälle bei der Berechnung derselben nicht mitberücksichtigt worden.

In Gruppe I war bei 32 Fällen die Krankheitsdauer bei der zweiten Erkrankung länger als bei der ersten (durchschnittlich 12,5 Tage), bei 34 Fällen kürzer (durchschnittlich 11,8 Tage) und bei 3 Fällen gleich lang. In Gruppe II war sie bei 26 Fällen länger (17 Tage) und bei 34 Fällen kürzer (14 Tage).

In Gruppe I kamen während der ersten Krankheit Rezidive 2 Male und Komplikationen 14 Male vor, während der zweiten Erkrankung Rezidive 3 Male und Komplikationen 17 Male. In Gruppe II waren die entsprechenden Zahlen: Rezidive 3 Male und Komplikationen 14 Male, bzw. Rezidiv 1 Mal und Komplikationen 11 Male.

Diese Zahlen sprechen kaum dafür, dass die Krankheit beim zweiten Male schwerer gewesen wäre als beim ersten, sondern eher dafür, dass der Grade der Schwere bei beiden Erkrankungen ungefähr derselbe gewesen ist. Eine exakte Beurteilung in dieser Beziehung wird jedoch u. a. dadurch erschwert, dass die therapeutischen Möglichkeiten während der Zeit, über welche sich die Untersuchung erstreckt, in gewissem Masse besser geworden sind.

Ebensowenig lässt das Material eine grössere Ähnlichkeit der Komplikationen bei den beiden Erkrankungen erkennen, oder dass gewisse Patienten eine besondere Neigung zu Komplikationen hätten. Wie bereits erwähnt, bildet die akute Lymphadenitis hier eine Ausnahme; da diese in der Regel schon im Beginn der Krankheit auftritt und ausserdem in der Mehrzahl der Fälle vorhanden ist, dürfte es aber als zweifelhaft zu betrachten sein, ob sie zu den Komplikationen zu rechnen oder ob sie nicht vielmehr unter die Scharlachsymptome einzureihen sei. Tab. 4 gibt eine Übersicht über die Komplikationen.

Die Fallzahl ist in den Gruppen der Tabelle 4 nicht vollständig, da die Angaben über die erste Erkrankung in der Regel bei denjenigen Fällen lückenhaft sind, welche da nicht im Stockholmer Epidemiekrankenhause stationär behandelt worden waren, und da derartige Fälle daher ausgeschaltet wurden.

Bei einem der Fälle in Gruppe I bestand bei der einen Erkrankung Verdacht auf Wundscharlach, ein Fall in Gruppe II und 2 in Gruppe IV waren als Wundscharlach diagnostiziert worden.

Ein in Gruppe II eingereihter Fall mit 3 Erkrankungen mag mit einigen Worten näher beschrieben werden: Ein 6jähriges Mädchen erkrankte etwa am 15.X. 1932 an leichten Schluckbeschwerden; etwas anderes wurde da zu Hause nicht bemerkt. Auf Grund von Scharlachfällen in der Schule wurden die Kinder am 17.XI. ärztlich untersucht, und das Kind wurde wegen Scharlachschuppung in das Epidemiekrankenhaus überwiesen. Bei der Aufnahme typische fein- und groblamelläre Schuppung. Rachen leicht gerötet. In den Kieferwinkeln ca. dattelgrosse, unempfindliche Lymphdrüsenschwellungen. Hämolytische Streptokokken im Rachen positiv. Dick-Test negativ. Am 7.XII. 1932 geheilt entlassen.

Am 8.II. 1933 erkrankte sie von neuem unter leichtem Husten, Temperatur etwa 40°, am 13.II. fieberfrei. Bei Untersuchung am 20.II. ausgesprochene fein- und groblamelläre Schuppung an den Füssen sowie kleienförmige Abschuppung in der Leistengegend. Hämolytische Streptokokken im Rachen positiv. Dick-Test negativ. Am 4.III. geheilt entlassen.

Am 14.II. 1935 erkrankte das Kind von neuem, während

Tab. 4.

Komplikation	Lymphadenitis		Otitis		Myokarditis		Nephritis		Synovitis		Sinusitis	
	Anzahl	%	Anzahl	%	Anzahl	%	Anzahl	%	Anzahl	%	Anzahl	%
Gruppe I (von 68 Fällen)												
Kompl. bei beiden Erkr.	45	66,2	1	1,5								
Kompl. bei einer Erkr.	18	26,5	18	26,5	3	4,4	5	7,4	5	7,4	2	2,9
Gruppe II (von 59 Fällen)												
Kompl. bei beiden Erkr.	36	61,0	3	5,1								
Kompl. bei einer Erkr.	16	27,3	13	22,0	4	6,8	2	3,4	1	1,7	1	1,7

es in einem anderen Krankenhaus wegen Scabies stationär behandelt wurde, weshalb es nun von Anfang an beobachtet werden konnte. Am 16.II. typisches Scharlachexanthem, Angina, Himbeerzunge, kleine Lymphadenitiden am Halse, subjektiv ziemlich unbeeinflusst. Die Schuppung begann schon am 18.II. (infolge der Scabiesbehandlung?). Am 29.III. wurde das Mädchen geheilt aus dem Epidemiekrankenhause entlassen.

Zusammenfassung.

Während der Jahre 1926—1939 sind im Stockholmer Epidemiekrankenhause 11 969 Scharlachfälle stationär behandelt worden.

Unter diesen kamen Zweiterkrankungen in zwischen 183 und 250 Fällen vor, d. h. zwischen 1,5 und 2,1 %, wahrscheinlich näher am höheren Wert.

Aus dem Material scheint ferner hervorzugehen, dass der Schweregrad bei den beiden Erkrankungen ungefähr derselbe gewesen ist, und dass eine Neigung zu gleichartigen Komplikationen nicht vorkam.

Das berechnete mittlere Alter (für Gruppe I und II) bei der ersten Erkrankung war 6 Jahre 3 Monate, die berechnete mittlere Zeit zwischen erster und zweiter Erkrankung 5 Jahre 6 Monate.

Literaturverzeichnis.

1. Allison and Brown. J. of Hyg. 37: 153 1937. — 2. Anderson, J. S. Arch. Dis. Child. IX: 373 1934. — 3. Bergman, R. Nord. Med. Tidskr. 9: 510 1935. — 4. Bessau. Arch. f. Kinderh. 117: 211 1939. — 5. v. Bormann, F. Mon.schr. f. Kinderh. 76: 107 1938. — 6. Burghard. Zentr.bl. f. Kinderh. 29: 482 1934—35. — 7. Fritz, S. Jahrb. f. Kinderh. 144: 42 1935. — 8. Gabriel und Zischinsky. Jahrb. f. Kinderh. 127: 253 1930. — 9. Gottlieb. Ugeskr. Læg. S.: 1054 1936. — 10. Herre, E. Mon.-schr. f. Kinderh. 58: 293 1933. — 11. Huss, R. Acta Pæd. XIV suppl. III 1933. — 12. Jochmann-Hegler. Lehrbuch der Infektionskrankheiten, 1924. — 13. Koch, E. Arch. f. Kinderh. 117: 211 1939. — 14. Koerner, R.

Jahrb. f. Kinderh. 9: 362 1876. — 15. KOLLE, W. und HETSCH, H. Experimentelle Bakteriologie und Infektionskrankheiten, 1938. — 16. KOLLE, W. und v. WASSERMANN, A. Handbuch der pathogenen Mikroorganismen, Bd 4: II: 859 1938. — 17. LÄMMERHIRT. Med. Kl. IX: 1499 1913. — 18. LICHTENSTEIN, A. Acta Pæd. X: 379 1930—31. — 19. ——. Acta Pæd. XII: 75 1931—32. — 20. ——. Acta Pæd. XII fasc. 4: 181 1931—32. — 21. ——. Kinderärztl. Praxis 5: 207 1934. — 22. ——. Nordisk lärobok i pediatrik Bd 2: 135 1941. — 23. NØRBY, G. Nordisk Lærebog i intern medicin Bd. 1: 32 1939. — 24. OPITZ, H. Zentralbl. f. Kinderh. 29: 37 1934—35. — 25. ——. Arch. f. Kinderh. 117: 211 1939. — 26. —. POPOVICIU, G. Zentralbl. f. Kinderh. 31: 372 1935—36. — 27. REH, TH. Arch. de Méd. des Enfants 30: nr 12 1927. — 28. REIDERMANN, I. Wien. klin. Wchnschr. 45: 1477 1932. — 29. SLAWYK. Zentralbl. f. Kinderh. 30: 274 1934—35. — 30. v. SZONTAG, F. Jahrb. f. Kinderh. 72: 661 1910. — 31. ——. Jahrb. f. Kinderh. 76: 654 1912. — 32. ——. Jahrb. f. Kinderh. 76: 1 (Erg.heft) 1912. — 33. ZISCHINSKY, H. Jahrb. f. Kinderh. 142: 53 1934. — 34. WEISSENBERG, H. Arch. f. Kinderh. 52: 17 1910. — 35. ZAPPERT. Wien. klin. Wchnschr. 29: 795 1916.

AUS DEM SACHS'SCHEN KINDERKRANKENHAUS, STOCKHOLM. VORSTAND: DOZENT CURT GYLLENSWÄRD.

Über die tuberkulotoxische Meningitis beim Kinde.

Von

BERTIL HAMNE.

Fall 1. Am 30. Dez. 1939 wurde ein 11 1/2 Monate alter Knabe (Bo S., geb. 15.1.39, Journ. Nr. 528/39) wegen Erythema nodosum in das Krankenhaus aufgenommen.

Aus der Anamnese erfahren wir, dass der 31jährige Vater während des Wehrpflichtalters eine Pleuritis exsudativa gehabt hat, später aber nicht ärztlich untersucht wurde. Er fühlte sich gesund und frisch, hatte aber im letzten Jahre mehrmals Erkältungen durchgemacht und ist jetzt seit mehreren Monaten mit einem hackenden Husten beschwert gewesen. Der Vater hat einen guten Allgemeinzustand, bei einer näheren Untersuchung wird aber eine linksseitige Spitzenkaverne und kleinfleckige Verdichtungen im linken Lungenfeld sowie im rechten I_2 und I_3 festgestellt. S.R. 40 mm/1 Std. Im Sputum reichlich Tbb. Nach fünfmonatigem Sanatoriumsaufenthalt (kein Pneumothorax) war die Kaverne ausgeheilt und der Prozess befand sich in seiner Gänze in beträchtlichem Rückgang. Der Mann war dann in der folgenden Zeit gesund und arbeitsfähig.

Die Mutter, 32 Jahre alt, war gesund und ohne Zeichen für Tuberkulose. Lungenröntgenbild negativ (4.1.40). Bei der Untersuchung im Oktober 1941 ist sie tuberkulinpositiv (Mantoux 0.10 = 15 × 15 mm, Moro schwach positiv) und auf der Röntgenplatte sind kleine Kalkflecken im linken Unterlappen zu sehen. Beim Vergleich mit der Platte vom 4.1.40 werden sie auch dort wiedergefunden und die Infektion, die keine subjektiven Beschwerden verursacht hat, dürfte zeitlich relativ lange zurückliegen.

Ein einziges Geschwister, eine dreijährige Schwester, wurde Mitte Dezember 1939 zu Hause wegen einer Pyelitis behandelt. Im Zusammenhang damit bekam sie rote, druckempfindliche

Flecken an den Unterschenkeln, da sie aber relativ bald fieberfrei und gesund wurde, wurde der Hausarzt hierüber nicht informiert. Eine Untersuchung des Kindes am 10.1.40 zeigte, dass es stark tuberkulinpositiv war und einen frischen Primärkomplex im Zwischenlappen der rechten Lunge aufwies. M.S.R. war 28 mm/1 Std. und die Magenspülflüssigkeit enthielt Tbb. von humanem Typus. Der Nachverlauf war unkompliziert.

Der Patient selbst war einen Monat vor der berechneten Zeit geboren worden. Geburtsgew. 2370 g. Reine Brusternährung 5 Monate lang, im Alter von 7 Monaten entwöhnt. Rachitisprophylaxe seit dem Alter von 3 Wochen durch periodenweise Zufuhr von Adol. In den letzten Tagen hat Patient Schnupfen gehabt und unbedeutend gehustet; zwei Tage vor der Aufnahme in das Krankenhaus, d.h. am 28.12. war plötzlich der Ausschlag auf den Unterschenkeln aufgetreten. Die Temp. betrug während der beiden Tage, die er zu Hause gelegen war, zwischen 39—40°.

Aus dem Status am 30.12.1939: Normales, etwas schlaffes Fettpolster. Kräftiges Schreien und kräftige Bewegungen. Keine Dyspnoe. Keine Zeichen für Meningitis. *Haut*: Leichte exsudative Dermatose der Wangen. Auf der Aussenseite des linken Oberschenkels eine halb-erbsengrosse Papel mit zentraler, schuppender Nekrose. Ähnliche Papeln jüngeren Datums auf der linken Rumpfseite ebenso einige an den Armen und am Hals (Tuberkulide). An der Vorderseite beider Unterschenkel mehrere 1 bis 2 Öre grosse, teilweise konfluierende, blaurote, druckempfindliche Hautinfiltrate, deren Typus mit Eryth. nodosum übereinstimmt.

Rachen: Lebhaft gerötet, schleimig belegt.

Lymphdrüsen: einige halb-erbsengrosse am Hals, sonst keine zu palpieren.

Skelett, Nervensystem, innere Organe o. B., insbesondere war die Milz nicht palpabel.

Pirquet (Ritz): intensiv pos. Reaktion.

Temperatur: beträgt die ersten 5 Tage um 40° und geht im Verlauf der folgenden 10 Tage allmählich auf den Normalwert zurück. Der Verlauf stimmt also mit dem eines Primärfiebers gut überein.

Mikrosenkungsreaktion: hoch, 40 mm/$^1/_2$ Std., 58 mm/1 Std. Verbleibt während der ersten 3 Wochen wenigstens ebenso hoch, Noch nach 3 $^1/_2$ Monaten betragen die Werte 16 bzw. 34 mm (Pat. wird in diesem Zeitpunkt zur weiteren Pflege in das Heim auf dem Lande entlassen).

Röntgenbild Nr. 1 der Lungen (2.1.40), am 6. Krankheitstag, zeigt nichts Besonderes. Klinisch wird aber doch an diesem

Tage angezeichnet, dass das Atmungsgeräusch links interskapulär stärker und rauher als auf der rechten Seite ist (vgl. den späteren Röntgenbefund).

Röntgenbild Nr. 2 (19.1.40); am 23. Tage nach dem Auftreten des Eryth. nodosum lautet der Befund: Möglicherweise ist eine Volumenzunahme der Weichteile im linken Lungenhilus vorhanden. Augenblicklich wird aber der Röntgenbefund doch als negativ angesehen.

Röntgenbild Nr. 3 (23.2.40), am 58. Krankheitstag: Verdichtung im linken Hilus mit abgerundeter lateraler Kontur. Im übrigen neg. Röntgenbefund der Lungen. Diagnose: linksseitige Hilusadenitis.

Röntgenbild Nr. 4 (5.4.40), 100. Krankheitstag; der Befund lautete: lateral nach oben vom linken Hilus tritt jetzt deutlich eine kleine homogene Parenchymverdichtung hervor. Im übrigen unveränderter Lungenstatus. Diagnose: linksseitiger Primärkomplex.

Bereits einige Tage nach der Aufnahme wurde aufgezeichnet, dass Pat. merkwürdig apathisch und benommen ist, sich vom Licht abwendet und zur Wand sieht und kein Interesse für die Umgebung zeigt. So bald man ihn berührt, beginnt er unwillig zu werden und bringt ängstliche, quitschende Laute hervor. Es liegt deutlich eine Hypersensibilität vor; bereits am 5. Krankheitstage wird eine ausgesprochene Nackensteifigkeit beobachtet, hingegen fehlen Basalnervensymptome.

Lumbalpunktion Nr. 1 (2.1.40), am 6. Krankheitstage. Nach Ablassen von 2 ccm Liquor liegt Pat. völlig ruhig. Der Druck beträgt da 100 mm. Queckenstedt: freie Passage. Es werden weitere 5 ccm klaren Liquors abgelassen und diese zeigen negative Globulinreaktionen (Pándy, Nonne). Der Zellgehalt ist 19 pro mm^3, nur Lymphozyten. Blutzucker/Liquorzucker 75/40 mg%. Meerschweinchenprobe mit Liquor neg.

Magenspülung: Wurde am 9.1.40, am 13. Krankheitstage ausgeführt und die Meerschweinchenprobe mit dem Spülwasser fiel pos. für Tbb. aus. Eine Typenbestimmung ergab, dass es sich um humane Tbb. handelte.

Am 10.1.40, dem 14. Krankheitstage wurde angezeichnet, dass die klinischen Zeichen der meningitischen Reizung allmählich zurückgegangen sind. Pat. ist psychisch klar, hat wieder begonnen sich für die Umgebung zu interessieren und setzt sich selbst im Bett auf.

Lumbalpunktion Nr. 2 (13.1.40), am 17. Krankheitstage, zeigt einen Initialdruck von über 400 mm., wobei Pat. aber nicht ruhig ist. Nach Ablassen von 5 ccm klaren Liquors ist der

Druck 200 mm, wobei Pat. aber doch etwas presst. Pándy und Nonne neg. Zellgehalt: 11 Lymphozyten pro mm^3. *Der Zuckergehalt ist jetzt deutlich gesenkt:* 26 mg% (Blutzucker unmittelbar vor der Lumbalpunkt. 125 mg%). Die Meerschweinchenprobe mit Liquor fällt neg. aus.

Lumbalpunktion Nr. 3 (29.2.40), 64. Krankheitstag, ergibt einen klaren Liquor mit neg. Globulinreaktionen (Pándy, Nonne), Zellgehalt: jetzt nur 3 pro mm^3; der Zuckergehalt ist wieder normal, Blutzucker/Liquorzucker 90/50 mg%.

Nach einem Krankenhausaufenthalt von 3 1/2 Monaten wurde Pat. Mitte April zur weiteren Pflege in das Heim auf dem Lande entlassen. Sein Gesundheitszustand ist im weiteren Verlauf besonders zufriedenstellend und bei der nächsten persönlichen Kontrolle im Sept. 1940 ist die M.S.R. normal und der Umfang des Primärkomplexes hat angefangen abzunehmen. Bei weiteren Kontrollen im Tuberkulosebureau war alles gut und eine telephonische Nachfrage bei der Mutter am 23. Sept. 1941 ergab folgenden Bescheid: »Der Knabe ist so tüchtig und frisch, dass es eine richtige Freude ist, ihn zu sehen.»

Fall 2. Rolf A., geb. 22.7.37 (Journ. Nr. 419/39). Aus der Anamnese: Mutter 29 Jahre alt, I-para, gesund, auch bei der Kontrolle im Oktober 41 ist sie tuberkulinneg. (Moro, Mantoux 0.10 und 1 mg). Lungenröntgenbild da neg. Eine Schwester ihrer Mutter war an Tuberkulose der Lungen 1910 gestorben. Der Vater des Patienten ist 32 Jahre alt und war 1931 und 1937 wegen Lungentuberkulose im Sanatorium. Beim ersten Sanatoriumaufenthalt wurde ein linksseitiger Pneumothorax angelegt, bei dem zweiten sollen auch Veränderungen in der rechten Lunge festgestellt worden sein. Guter Allgemeinzustand, »Bazillenfrei», völlig arbeitsfähig (Kupferschmied). Täglicher Kontakt mit dem Kinde.

Pat. zur erwarteten Zeit am 22.7.37 geboren. Normale Entbindung. Geburtsgew. 3540 g. Brustkind. Entwöhnung mit 9 Mon.

Am. 18.10.39 begann der Knabe schlecht gelaunt zu sein. Als die Temp. einige Tage später gemessen wurde, betrug sie 38.5°—39.5° und hielt sich bis zur Aufnahme in das Krankenhaus am 28.10.39 ungefähr auf dieser Höhe. In der letzten Woche vor der Aufnahme hatte Pat. gell gehustet und auch einigemale erbrochen. Er klagte über Schmerzen im Nacken und in den Fussgelenken. Nackensteifigkeit oder Gelenkschwellungen wurden aber nicht beobachtet. Nach Aussage des Hausarztes war Pat. im Febr. und Sept. 1939 tuberkulinneg., während eine Tuberkulin-Pflasterprobe am 25. Okt. stark positiv ausfiel.

Aus dem Status am 28.10.39: Normales aber schlaffes Fettpolster (Gew. 12.480 kg). Allgemeinzustand leicht beeinflusst. Leichte Dyspnoe. Am Rumpf und an den Gliedern ein *feinpapulöses Exanthem. Rachen:* gerötet und geschwollen. — Innere Organe, Gelenke und Nervensystem o. B. Keine Nackensteifigkeit.

Temperatur: 38.5°, erreicht innerhalb einer Woche normale Werte. Später stieg sie im Zusammenhang mit einer Verschlechterung des Pat. wieder an.

M.S.R. 34 mm/1 Std. Erst 2 Monate später ging sie auf 10 mm/1 Std. zurück, dann kam es wieder zu einer lange dauernden Steigerung im Zusammenhang mit einem Fortschreiten der Lungenherde sowie rezidivierender Pharyngitiden.

Röntgenbefund Nr. 1 (31.10.39) lautete: Starke Vergrösserung der Weichteile im oberen Teil des rechten Lungenhilus und eine diffuse Parenchymverdichtung in Höhe mit dem medialen Teil von Scl.-I_1. Linke Lunge o. B. Diagnose: Primäre Tuberkulose der rechten Lunge (Lob. sup.).

Röntgenbefund Nr. 2 (17.11.39): Bedeutende Zunahme des Umfanges der Parenchymverdichtung.

Röntgenbefund Nr. 3 (20.12.39): Abnahme des parenchymatösen Teiles der Verdichtung.

Röntgenbefund Nr. 4 (30.1.40): Im oberen Teil des rechten Zwischenlappens ist eine inhomogene Verdichtung hinzugekommen, die nicht mit Sicherheit nur von Atelektasenatur ist. *In der Pleurahöhle ist parietal eine dünne Exsudatschicht vorhanden.*

Röntgenbefund Nr. 5 (20.2. 40): Die Verdichtung im rechten Zwischenlappen ist verschwunden. Keine Zeichen für Pleuritis. Im übrigen seit dem 30.1. unveränderter Status.

Röntgenbefund Nr. 6 (2.4.40): Rückgang des Parenchymprozesses und der Adenitis.

Röntgenbefund Nr. 7 (10.5.40): Weiterer Rückgang des Parenchymprozesses.

Magenspülflüssigkeit (3.11.39) enhält keine im Meerschweinchenversuch nachweisbaren Tuberkulosebazillen.

Nachdem Pat. 14 Tage im Krankenhaus war (= 24 Tage nach der Erkrankung) trat eine Verschlechterung ein. Pat. erbrach mitunter, bekam eine gewisse Obstipation (geht oft 2 Tage ohne Stuhlgang), Temp. und M.S.R. beginnen wieder zu steigen und der Röntgenbefund (17.11) ergibt eine bedeutende Zunahme der Parenchymverdichtungen im Gebiete des rechten Oberlappens. Eine Nackensteifigkeit ist immer noch nicht vorhanden, seit dem 12.11. ist aber ein *konvergenter Strabismus hinzugekommen* (s. auch letzten Absatz der Beschreibung von Fall 2). Dieser ist so ausgeprägt, dass er bei früheren Untersuchungen schwerlich übersehen worden sein kann; die Mutter frug auch anlässlich eines Besuches im Krankenhaus spontan, was mit den Augen des Knaben sei, da sie früher niemals bemerkt hatte, dass er geschielt hat. Es ist jetzt auch eine *Konjunktivitis,* doch ohne abgrenzbare Phlyktäne, vorhanden.

Bereits einige Tage später, 19.11.—21.11., weist die Temperatur einen remittierenden Charakter mit einigen Zacken über 40° auf. Der Allgemeinzustand ist noch mehr verschlechtert, Pat. gibt plötzliche Schreie von sich, sagt, dass er Schmerzen habe an welcher Stelle man ihn auch berührt und ist bei jeder Berührung sehr gereizt (Hypersensibilität). Der Strabismus ist immer noch vorhanden. Starke Schmerzreaktion bei der Untersuchung auf Nackensteifigkeit. Babinski neg. Es wird nun eine *Lumbalpunktion* (21.11.) ausgeführt; um eine zufriedenstellende Druckmessung ausführen zu können, wurde die Punktion in Chloralnarkose ausgeführt. Der Druck ist hierbei erhöht: 130 mm. Der Liquor ist klar, Pándy und Nonne neg. Zellgehalt 18/mm^3 (nur Lymphozyten). Der Liquorzucker wurde in zwei Portionen bestimmt, beide wiesen 27 mg% auf, der Blutzuckergehalt war in zwei unmittelbar vor der Lumbalpunktion entnommenen Proben 85 bzw. 86 mg%. Meerschweinchenprobe mit Liquor neg.

Der Strabismus bleibt bestehen, die meningeale Reizung klingt aber allmählich ab und der Knabe wird lebhafter. Die Reizbarkeit verschwindet und als die Lumbalpunktion nach 25 Tagen wiederholt wurde (16.12.39), wird ein klarer Liquor mit einem Zellgehalt von 3 Lymphozyten, 2 Leukozyten und 6 Erythrozyten pro mm^3 erhalten. Die Globulinreaktionen (Pándy, Nonne) sind negativ und der Liquorzucker ist jetzt wieder normal und beträgt 60 mg% (Blutzucker 95 mg%). Die Meerschweinchenprobe mit Liquor ist immer noch negativ.

Im weiteren Verlauf ist der Allgemeinzustand des Pat. zufriedenstellend. Nach einem Aufenthalt von 3 Monaten im Krankenhaus (28.1.40) steigt aber die Temperatur wieder und es wird über der rechten Lunge eine Dämpfung und ein abgeschwächtes Atemgeräusch festgestellt. Die Röntgenaufnahme (30.1) weist auch das Hinzukommen eines Randexsudates nach. Dies geht indessen schnell zurück und bei der Röntgenkontrolle am 20.2. finden sich keine Zeichen für Pleuritis vor und die Parenchymverdichtung hat abgenommen.

Am 23.2.40 bekam Pat. Varizellen und wurde für eine Zeit nach Hause entlassen. Wurde erneut am 30.3.40 aufgenommen und war bis zum 6.4.40 im Krankenhaus. Der Zustand des Pat. war in diesem Zeitpunkt gut, sowohl der Parenchymherd als auch die Hilusadenitis hatte noch weiter abgenommen. M.S.R. 8 mm/1 Std.

Im Verlaufe der weiteren poliklinischen Kontrolle wurde alles gut befunden und bei der Röntgenaufnahme am 10.6.41 waren bloss kleine *verkalkte* Reste des Parenchym- und Drüsenherdes vorhanden. Der Allgemeinzustand war im Oktober 1941 dauernd sehr gut, Pat. war afebril, M.S.R. 5 mm/1 Std. *Die Röntgenaufnahme des Schädels zeigt keine intrakraniellen Kalkherde.*

Bezüglich des Strabismus wurde am 27.6.41 ein Augenarzt konsultiert, der feststellte, dass es sich um einen Strabismus concomitans conv. dexter handelt, der sich völlig durch die Feststellung einer Hyperopie von + 3 D. auf beiden Augen erklären liess. Sehvermögen rechts 5/40, links 5/5. Unter Lappenbehandlung und Korrektion der Hyperopie war das Sehvermögen auf dem rechten Auge im Sept. 1941 auf 5/7.5 gestiegen.

Zusammenfassung und Besprechung.

Es handelt sich hier also um zwei Fälle mit primärer Tbc. in frühem Alter, die manches Interessante bieten. In beiden Fällen ist die Ansteckungsquelle der Vater und bei Fall 1 ist auch die Schwester infiziert, während Fall 2 das einzige Kind in der Familie ist. Die Mutter des ersten Falles weist kleine Kalkherde in der Lunge und eine positive Tuberkulinreaktion auf, die von einer früher überstandenen, aber für sie unbekannten tuberkulösen Infektion Zeugnis ablegen. Die Mutter des 2. Falles hingegen weist noch im Oktober 41 eine negative Tuberkulinprobe und einen negativen Lungenröntgenbefund auf. Diese Beobachtung beleuchtet die geringere Resistenz der Kleinkinder gegenüber Tuberkulosebazillen im Vergleich zu Erwachsenen.

Beide Fälle weisen zu Beginn der Erkrankung eine lebhafte Rötung des Rachens auf. Es ist ja bekannt, dass im Zusammenhang *mit dem Eintritt einer Allergie die Resistenz für banale Infektionen herabgesetzt wird* (Wallgren u. a.), weswegen es kein Zufall ist, dass wir oft einen Rachenkatarrh im Zusammenhang sowohl mit einer Primärtuberkulose als auch beim Eintreten der Vaccinationsallergie beobachten. *Eine Tatsache, die uns mahnen muss, bei jeder akuten, fieber-*

haften kindlichen Erkrankung fleissig von der Tuberkulinprüfung Gebrauch zu machen, und zwar auch dann, wenn wir eine plausible Ursache nichttuberkulöser Genese für das Fieber finden (die Schwester von Pat. 1 erkrankte als erste von beiden Kindern mit Fieber, das als Ausdruck einer Pyelitis gedeutet wurde. Der weitere Verlauf ergab aber, dass sie auf jeden Fall auch eine Primärtuberkulose gehabt hat).

Fall 1 ist zahlreiche Wochen früher als durch das Röntgenbild der Lungenherd nachgewiesen werden kann, tuberkulinpositiv und in der Magenspülflüssigkeit werden frühzeitig Tbb. gefunden. Wenn man bei einem poliklinischen Material systematisch alle Kinder bei dem 1. Besuch und auch bei jedem Besuch auf Grund eines akuten Fiebers mit Tuberkulin prüft, so ist es nach Erfahrung des Verf. *nicht so selten, dass man es erlebt, dass die Tuberkulinempfindlichkeit das erste objektive Zeichen für eine tuberkulöse Infektion darstellt, während der Röntgenbefund auf sich warten lässt.* Dies stellt einen weiteren Fingerzeig für den Wert der Tuberkulinprüfung dar, wenn es sich wie bei den Kindern um eine Primärtuberkulose handelt, dies um so mehr, da ja, wenigstens nach Überschreiten des ersten Lebensjahres, die einfache Prüfung nach Moro oder die Pirquet-Prüfung bei einer solchen ausreichend ist. — Es muss ja nach dem Eindringen der Bazillen eine gewisse Zeit verstreichen bis der Lungenherd so gross wird und auch so dicht, dass er sich auf der Röntgenplatte abzeichnet. Eine so zu sagen experimentelle Demonstration für die Dauer dieses Zeitintervalles beim Menschen wird in einem Fall gegeben, bei welchem nach einer massiven Tbb.-Invasion, in diesem Falle auf dem Blutwege (2 ccm Bazillenemulsion, intravenös injiziert von einem Arzt mit der Absicht einen Selbstmord zu begehen), es 4 Wochen dauerte, bis auf der Röntgenplatte die ersten kleinen Flecken sichtbar wurden (die Angabe stammt von SIMON).

Bei meinen beiden Fällen traten nun klinisch Symptome einer tuberkulösen Meningitis auf, die das Prodromalstadium von Rominger mit allgemeiner Veränderung des Wesens, Überempfindlichkeit für Licht und Berührung, gesteigertes Schlafbedürfnis, oft Obstipation (Fall 2) und oft unregelmässige Atmung (bei meinen Fällen nicht besonders studiert) umfassen. Es kommen auch Symptome vor, die dem 2. Stadium angehören, nämlich Kopfschmerzen und Nackensteifigkeit, Erbrechen (nur zweimal bei Fall 1 aber im Anschluss an den Meningismus gehäuft bei Fall 2) sowie »Augenmuskelparesen» (Fall 2).

Der Liquor weist einen erhöhten Druck und einen vermehrten Zellgehalt auf. Hingegen sind die Globulinreaktionen negativ während der *Liquorzucker während eines bestimmten Stadiums deutlich bei beiden Fällen herabgesetzt ist,* eine Beobachtung, der die Mehrzahl der Autoren eine grosse diagnostische Bedeutung zumisst, wenn es sich um einen Verdacht auf tuberkulöse Meningitis handelt. — Wiederholte Prüfungen des Liquors im Meerschweinchenversuch fielen hingegen negativ aus und der weitere Verlauf mit einer relativ schnellen Gesundung zeigt auch, dass es sich nicht gut um eine tuberkulöse Meningitis gehandelt haben kann.

Meiner Ansicht nach ist die Koinzidenz mit durch Virus bedingten Meningitiden eine weitgesuchte Erklärung. Da wir hingegen wissen, dass das Auftreten einer Tuberkuloseallergie mit einer Reihe von Haut- und Schleimhautphänomenen verbunden sein kann: Erythema nodosum, Exanthem, Phlyktäne, Gelenkschwellungen u.s.w., wofür auch meine Fälle Beispiele darstellen, dürfte es nicht unangebracht sein, auch allergische (tuberkulotoxische) Reaktionen von Seiten der Meningen zu erwarten.

Seitdem Villaret und Tixier bereits 1905 auf Grund der Beobachtung, dass man bei tuberkulösen Meningitiden nicht immer Bazillen im Liquor nachweisen konnte (direkte Züchtung, Verimpfung auf Meerschweinchen) die Vermutung ausgesprochen haben, dass gewisse Fälle von tuberkulöser Meningitis durch Toxine der Tuberkulosebazillen verursacht werden, ist das Interesse für vorübergehende Meningitiden bei tuberkulösen Individuen in der Literatur allmählich immer mehr hervorgetreten (z. B. in der französischen Literatur: Barbier und Gougelet, Bernhard und Debré, Gougelet, Herman, Lyonnet, Paisseau und Laquerrière, Tinel und

CASTINEL, TROISIER und BOQUIEN, VAJA ferner VINCENTELLI; in der deutschen Literatur: BROCKMANN, FINKELSTEIN, FRISCH, FRISCH und SCHÜLLER, HERSCHMANN, HOFFMAN u. a.).

Wenn auch die Mehrzahl der Autoren damit rechnet, dass es sich wirklich um eine tuberkulöse Meningitis handelt, sind andere aber auf Grund der vom Normalen abweichenden Befunde bei den Züchtungs- und Inokulationsversuchen mit dem Liquor gewisser Fälle der Ansicht, dass diese durch Tuberkulosebazillen mit modifizierter Virulenz bedingt werden (PAISSEAU und LAQUERRIÉRE), während andere hingegen mit der Möglichkeit rechnen, dass die Tuberkulosebazillen mitunter andere und heilbare Reaktionen von Seiten der Meningen hervorrufen können als die klassische Piatuberkulose: »Pourquoi le bacille ne serait-il pas apte, dans certains cas, a soliciter une simple réaction séreuse avec exode leucocytaire, qui serait susceptible de regression complète?» (BERNHARD und DEBRÉ). — Zu diesen theoretischen Überlegungen gesellt sich die Ansicht, dass diese passageren Meningitiden toxisch bedingt sein können (HERSCHMANN, HOFFMAN, KNOPF, LYONNET, PHOTAKIS), worauf auch Sektionsfälle hinweisen (HOFFMAN). Aus einer Polemik zwischen FRISCH und HERSCHMANN ergibt sich, dass der erstgenannte seine und die Meningitisfälle von SCHÜLLER nicht als toxisch bedingt erklärt haben will, sondern dass er, besonders im Hinblick auf spätere eigene Beobachtungen, wo der Liquor bei dem Patienten oder anderen allergischen tuberkulösen Patienten eine positive Impfreaktion ergab (schwächer als Mantoux, aber positiv im Vergleich mit Kontrollversuchen mit dem Liquor nicht Tuberkulosekranker) die Auffassung hat, »dass es sich offenbar um den Einbruch von Tuberkulosebazillen in die Meningen, gefolgt von einer Forme fruste einer Meningitis tuberculosa gehandelt hat». Eine Erklärung, die wohl in Erwägung gezogen werden kann. LYONNET hat bereits früher gezeigt, dass der Liquor ähnlicher Fälle die Reaktion von Merieux gibt (= bei tuberkulösen, nicht fiebernden Meerschweinchen Fieber hervorruft), was auf das Vorhandensein von Tuberkulin deuten soll; LYONNET ist darum der Ansicht, dass unter gewissen Umständen eine

Anhäufung von Tuberkulin im Liquor und dadurch eine meningeale Reizung zustandekommen kann. Der Versuch von FRISCH scheint mir in die gleiche Richtung zu weisen und damit würde die Natur des supponierten Toxines klargelegt sein.

Dass wir von Seiten der Meningen allergische Reaktionen erhalten können, wurde im übrigen experimentell von MORITZ gezeigt. Bei 10 Fällen mit Erythema nodosum findet er meningeale Reaktionen und kann einen erhöhten Liquordruck nachweisen. Der Zellgehalt schwankt zwischen 3—5 in der Fuchs-Rosenthalschen Kammer, der Liquorzucker ist in sämtlichen Fällen normal: MORITZ will in diesem Befund eine meningeale Reizung allergischer Natur sehen; um sichere Anhaltspunkte in der Lösung dieser Frage zu erhalten, führte MORITZ bei jedem von 5 tuberkulösen Kindern gleichzeitig 4 intrakutane Reaktionen mit Tuberkulin in steigenden Dosen aus. Bei 3 Fällen trat 48 Std. nach Ausführung der Injektionen ein allgemeines Unwohlsein, Fieber und meningeale Symptome mit hartnäckigem Erbrechen, Obstipation, positivem Kernig und Babinski auf. Der Liquor stand unter hohem Druck, war klar, Pándy neg., besass normalen Gesamteiweiss und Zuckergehalt, der Zellgehalt war 3—5 in der Fuchs-Rosenthalschen Kammer. Nach einigen Tagen bis zu einer Woche gingen die meningealen Symptome spontan zurück.

ARMAND-DELILLE erhielt bei nicht sensibilisierten Tieren (Meerschweinchen, Hund) bei intracerebraler Tuberkulininjektion toxische Reaktionen (in Kontrollversuchen mit dem Lösungsmittel allein wurden keine entsprechenden Reaktionen erhalten).

Andererseits stösst auch die Diagnose tuberkulotoxische (allergische) Meningitis auf gewisse Schwierigkeiten und kann auf jeden Fall nicht ohne eine relativ lange Beobachtungszeit mit Sicherheit gestellt werden. Es wird nämlich in der Literatur erwähnt, dass tuberkulöse Meningitiden mit Remissionen, die im Verlaufe von einigen Monaten bis zu einem Jahr auftreten, vorkommen (MASSARY und LECHELLE, SIMON, VAJA u. a.). Es kann also vorkommen, dass solche Episoden, wie die von mir hier geschilderten nur die Einleitung einer tuberkulösen Meningitis darstellen (Vincentelli). Die Beobachtungszeit dürfte aber bei meinen Fällen jetzt ausreichend sein, um eine echte tuberkulöse Meningitis ausschliessen zu können.

Gleichzeitig will ich auch die Schwierigkeiten hervorheben, die bei der Stellung der Diagnose tuberkulöse Meningitis vorhanden sind, da nicht einmal ein positiver Bazillenbefund im Liquor beweisend ist. Der Bazillenbefund kann nämlich teils seine Ursache in einer Fehlerquelle haben, teils für etwas anderes als tuberkulöse Meningitis sprechen.

Was die Fehlerquelle betrifft, so kann es vorkommen, wenn man in einem Laboratorium mit einer Menge auf Objektgläsern ausgestrichenen Sputumproben zu tun hat, dass ein Teil derselben nicht angewandt sondern durch Kochen unschädlich gemacht wird. Die gekochten Bazillen können an dem Glase haften. Diese gekochten Tuberkulosebazillen verhalten sich aber gegenüber der Färbung immer noch so wie die frischen. Man muss also mit neuen oder auf jeden Fall mit in Schwefelsäure gereinigten Gläsern arbeiten (eine alte Beobachtung, die nicht immer beachtet wird). — Eine andere Fehlerquelle soll das Vorkommen säurefester Stäbchen in gewöhnlichem Wasserleitungswasser darstellen (Trocmé und Bieto).

Massary und Lechellle sowie Rist und Boudet nehmen auf Grund der Beobachtung, dass Liquor mit säurefesten Stäbchen mitunter für Meerschweinchen nicht pathogen war, an, dass im Liquor andere säurefeste Bazillen als der Kochsche vorhanden sind; dies scheint mir nicht berechtigt zu sein. Derartige Beobachtungen, die in der Literatur oft als ausgeheilte Fälle veröffentlicht werden (z. B. Archangelsky, Hochstetter, Pissavy und Terris, Reichmann und Rauch), können wohl ebenso gut durch die Annahme erklärt werden, dass es sich um avirulente Bazillen im Liquor gehandelt hat, die gerade auf Grund ihrer Avirulenz auch nicht eine echte tuberkulöse Meningitis verursacht haben, d.h. eine Meningealtuberkulose, etwas, was die Heilungsmöglichkeiten dieser Fälle erklärt.

Bemerkenswert ist jedoch die grosse Anhäufung von Bazillen bei dem Fall von RIST und BOUDET, da Tuberkulosebazillen im Liquor sonst nur vereinzelt aufzutreten pflegen. Die Autoren selber halten eine Verunreinigung für ausgeschlossen.

In der Literatur sind gewiss Meningitisbilder mit virulenten Tbb. im Liquor (Verimpfung auf Meerschweinchen) beschrieben worden, wobei die Fälle in Heilung ausgingen (s. eine Reihe von Fällen S. 231—234 in der Zusammenstellung von CRAMER und BICKEL, ausserdem kommen einige Fälle aus der Arbeit von CRUCHET hinzu). Nicht einmal bei diesen Fällen kann man sich aber völlig davon überzeugt fühlen, dass es sich wirklich um eine tuberkulöse Meningitis gehandelt hat. Es kommt nämlich vor, dass auf der Klinik die Diagnose tuberkulöse Meningitis gestellt wird, die spätere Sektion aber ergibt, dass an ihrer Stelle Tuberkulome vorgelegen haben (z. B. bei einem Fall von BLACKLOCK und GRIFFIN, ferner bei dem ersten Fall von BROCKMANN); viele Autoren nehmen an, dass solche Tuberkulome mit einer meningealen Reaktion, die dann ausgeheilt sind, mitunter fehlerhafterweise als geheilte Meningitisfälle aufgefasst wurden. — Es verdient auch erwähnt zu werden, dass E. COTTIN »un cas de méningite tuberculeuse caractérisée avec B.K. dans le liquide céphalo-rachidien» beobachtete, der ausheilte, aber 9 Jahre später an seiner Lungentuberkulose starb. Bei der Sektion konnten aber keine meningealen Veränderungen nachgewiesen werden, es darf aber wohl auf jeden Fall als ausgeschlossen angesehen werden, dass eine meningeale Tuberkulose keine anatomischen Veränderungen zurückgelassen hätte.

Auch BEITZKE erwähnt, dass er Gelegenheit gehabt hat, makroskopisch und mikroskopisch Tuberkulosefälle zu untersuchen, die agonal Zeichen einer tuberkulösen Meningitis aufgewiesen haben; er konnte bei diesen aber keine tuberkulöse Meningitis feststellen. Es handelte sich nur um eine agonale Bazillenaussaat in den Liquor mit klinischen Meningitiszeichen aber ohne anatomische Veränderungen in den Meningen. BEITZKE ist der Ansicht, dass falls sich derartige Patienten von ihrer Grundkrankheit erholen, sie unrichtigerweise als geheilte tuberkulöse Meningitiden bezeichnet werden.

Wenn somit auch die klinische Diagnose tuberkulöse Meningitis, d. h. Tuberkulose in den Meningen, auf so grosse Schwierigkeiten stösst, und man sich der Mehrzahl der als geheilt bezeichneten Fälle gegenüber skeptisch eingestellt fühlt, so kann doch nicht verneint werden, dass unter gewissen Voraussetzungen eine tuberkulöse Meningitis ausheilen kann, wie dies der Sektionsfall von RUMPEL zeigt: Ein 8jähriger Knabe erkrankte plötzlich mit meningealen Symptomen: geringe Nackensteifigkeit, Erlöschen der Patellarreflexe und Hyperästhesie bei Druck auf die Extremitätenmuskulatur, doppelseitige Stauungspapille bei kurzer Pupillenreaktion, später rechtsseitige Externusparese und doppelseitige Ptosis. In der bei erhöhtem Druck entleerten Spinalflüssigkeit wurden Tuberkulosebazillen nachgewiesen (es wird nicht angegeben, ob auch eine Verimpfung auf Meerschweinchen vorgenommen wurde). Der Fall heilte aus und Pat. besuchte die Volksschule bis zum Ende. Er kam mit einer fortgeschrittenen Lungentuberkulose im Alter von 17 Jahren wieder. Der Nervenstatus war in diesem Zeitpunkt gänzlich negativ, Pat. war psychisch normal. Tod an der Lungenphthise. Sektion: »Das Gehirn ist völlig normal; die Gehirnhäute zeigen in beiden Foss. Sylv. Verdickungen, die an der rechten Fossa Sylvii zu derben Verwachsungen geführt haben. Tuberkelknötchen nicht mehr nachweisbar». RUMPEL selbst ist der Ansicht, dass die Ursache dafür, dass nur dieser eine Fall von seinen vielen Meningitisfällen ausheilen konnte, die sein dürfte, dass es sich wahrscheinlich nur um eine wenig ausgedehnte Aussaat von Tuberkeln in den Meningen gehandelt hat.

Schliesslich pflegt man ja auch einem herabgesetzten Zuckergehalt im Liquor bei einer lymphozytären Meningitis eine relativ starke Beweiskraft für deren tuberkulöse Natur zuzuschreiben. Dass der Befund indessen nicht pathognomonisch ist, zeigen u.a. meine eigenen Fälle.

Der Wert einer Untersuchung des Kochsalzgehaltes des Liquors wird von verschiedenen Autoren sehr wechselnd beurteilt. Aus einer vor kurzem erschienenen Veröffentlichung (ALTROCK) scheint indessen hervorzugehen, dass einer Herabsetzung des Kochsalzgehaltes keine entscheidende differentialdiagnostische Bedeutung zugemessen werden kann.

Man muss also etwas vorsichtig sein mit der Prognosestellung, auch wenn im Verlaufe einer Lungentuberkulose Meningitiszeichen auftreten, soweit sie nicht im Anschluss an eine Miliartuberkulose auftreten, da sämtliche derartige Fälle bisher tödlich verlaufen sind (LIEBERMEISTER).

Zusammenfassung.

Es werden zwei Fälle von Primärtuberkulose bei Kindern im Alter von 11 $^1/_2$ Monaten bzw. 2 Jahren und 3 Monaten beschrieben. Im ersten Falle lagen gleichzeitig ein Eryth. nod. und Hauttuberkulide vor, im anderen Falle zu Beginn ein feinpapulöses Exanthem und später eine Pleurareizung mit schnell zurückgehendem kleinem Exsudat. In beiden Fällen traten klinische Zeichen von Seiten der Meningen auf: Nackensteifigkeit, Lichtscheu, Empfindlichkeit für Berührung, Somnolenz, Erbrechen (Fall 2) und Obstipation (Fall 2). Ein bei Vorhandensein der Meningitissymptome auftretender Strabismus bei Fall 2 wurde zuerst fehlerhaft als eine im Anschluss an eine Basalmeningitis aufgetretene Augenmuskelparese gedeutet, erhielt aber seine richtige Erklärung als ein während der allgemeinen Herabsetzung der Kräfte manifest gewordener Strabismus concomitans conv. dx., durch eine Hyperopie von + 3 D verursacht.

Der unter erhöhtem Druck stehende Liquor enthält 19 bzw. 18 Zellen pro cmm, nur Lymphozyten. Globulinreaktionen (Pándy und Nonne) negativ, der Liquorzucker ist aber in beiden Fällen während einer gewissen Zeit deutlich herabgesetzt. Wiederholte Verimpfungen des Liquors auf Meerschweinchen ergeben ein neg. Resultat. Völlige Heilung.

Die Fälle werden als toxisch bedingte (allergische) meningeale Reizung angesehen.

Im Anschluss an die Fälle werden auch die Schwierigkeiten in der Diagnostik einer tuberkulösen Meningitis besprochen und deren Heilungsmöglichkeiten berührt.

Bei der systematischen Tuberkulinprüfung jedes Kindes mit akutem Fieber ergibt sich, dass ein positiver Ausfall der Prüfung nicht selten das erste Symptom objektiver Art für eine tuberkulöse Infektion darstellt, während ein Röntgenbefund erst später zu erheben ist.

Literatur.

ALTROCK, JOHANNA: Ueber die Bedeutung der Kochsalzuntersuchung in der Rückenmarksflüssigkeit für die Diagnose der tuberkulösen Meningitis im Kindesalter. — Arch. f. Khk. 1941, 123, 126. — ARCHANGELSKY (zit. nach CRAMER u. BICKEL). — ARMAND-DELILLE, P. F.: Méningite tuberculeuse. — Thèse, Paris 1903. — BARBIER, H. und GOUGELET: Épisodes tuberculeux méningés curables chez les enfants. — Bull. Soc. med. Hôp., Paris 1911, 32, 440. — GOUGELET, J.: Thèse, Paris 1911. — BEITZKE, H.: Diskussion zu der Arbeit von SIMON. — BERNHARD, L. und DEBRÉ, R.: Relations entre certaines meningites curable et la tuberculose. — Bull. Soc. med. Hôp., Paris 1910, 30, 587. — BLACKLOCK, J. W. S. und GRIFFIN, MARY: Tuberculous meningitis in childrens. — J. Path. and Bact. 1935, 40, 489. — BROCKMANN, H.: Zwei Fälle von Pseudomeningitis bei tuberkulösen Kindern. Jahrb. f. Khk. 1915, 81, 433. — COTTIN, E.: Antwort bei der Enquète von CRUCHET, S. 220. — CRAMER, A. und BICKEL, G.: La méningite tuberculeuse est-elle curable? — Ann. de med. 1922, 12, 226. — CRUCHET, R.: La méningite tuberculeuse est-elle curable? — Congrès francais de med., Paris 1936, 24:e session, 191. — FINKELSTEIN, H.: Zur Entstehung seröser Meningitiden bei tuberkulösen Kindern. — Berl. klin. Wschr. 1914: 1, 1164. — FRISCH, A. V. und SCHÜLLER, A.: Tuberkulöser Kopfschmerz. Wien. med. Wschr. 1921, 71, 2267. — FRISCH, A. V. 1: Über tuberkulösen Kopfschmerz. Beitr. Klin. Tub. 1922, 49, 203. —— 2: Zur Symptomatologie der Meningitis tuberculosa discreta. Wien. klin. Wschr. 1923: 1, 162. — HERMAN, M. E.: Méningite séreuse tuberculosigène. — Rev. neurol. 1930, 1, 661. — HERSCHMANN, H.: Ueber tuberculotoxische Meningitis. — Arch. f. Psych. 1921, 62, 879. — HOCHSTETTER (zit. nach CRAMER u. BICKEL). — HOFFMAN, H. W.: Meningismus bei Miliartuberkulose. — Zschr. f. Tub. 1930, 59, 55. — KNOPF (zit. nach SIMON). — LIEBERMEISTER (zit. nach SIMON). — LYONNET, B.: De l'encephalopathie tuberculineuse. — Rev. de med. 1911, 31, 502 C (Jubilée de Prof. Lépine). — DE MASSARY und LECHELLE: Épisodes méningés bacillaires curables au cours de la tuberculose pulmonaire chronique. — Bull. Soc. med. Hôp., Paris 1920, 44, 377. — MORITZ, D.: Allergische Reaktionen während der Tuberkulose bei Kindern. — Orvosi hetil. 1939, 83, 827 (nicht im Original zu erhalten).

— PAISSEAU, G. und Madame LAQUERRIÈRE: Épisodes méningés bacillaires curables au cours de la tuberculose pulmonaire chronique. — Bull. Soc. med. Hôp., Paris 1934, 58, 215. — PHOTAKIS (zit. nach SIMON). — PISSAVY, A. und TERRIS: Méningite tuberculeuse apparemment guérie depuis cinq mois. — Bull. Soc. med. Hôp., Paris 1923, 47, 304. — REICHMANN und RAUCH (zit. nach CRAMER u. BICKEL). — RIST, E. und BOUDET, G.: Présence de bacilles acido-resistants dans le liquide cérébro-spinal d'un malade atteint de symptômes méningitiques. Guérison. — Bull. Soc. med. Hôp., Paris 1908, 26, 503. — RUMPEL, TH.: Demonstriert ein Gehirn von einem 17-jährigen, an Lungentuberkulose verstorbenen Arbeiter, der vor acht Jahren eine tuberkulöse Meningitis überstanden hat (Verein f. inn. Med. in Berlin). — Deutsche med. Wschr. 1907: 2, 2021. — SIMON, G.: Die tuberkulöse Gehirnhautentzündung. — Beitr. z. Klin. d. Tub. 1939, 93, 285. — TINEL, J. und CASTINEL, P.: Les états méningés des tuberculeux. — XII:e Congrès fr. de méd., Lyon 1911, 166. — TROCMÉ, M. O. und BIETO, H.: Eine wichtige und zu wenig bekannte Fehlerquelle in der bakt. Diagnose der Tbc. (Ref.) Münch. med. Wschr. 1941: 2, 1145. — TROISIER, J. und BOQUIEN, Y.: Les spirochétoses méningées, Paris 1933, S. 138. — VAJA, G.: Épisodes méningés curables au cours de la tuberculose pulmonaire. — Bull. medicale 1939, 53, 817. — WALLGREN, A.: Om primär lungtuberkulos hos barn. — Sv. läkartidn. 1935. ——: Vad en praktiker bör veta om barntuberkulos. — Ugeskr. f. Laeger 1936, 52, 1285. — WALLGREN, A. und MILLER, J. A.: Pulmonary tuberculosis in adults (MILLER) and children (WALLGREN). — Thomas Nelson & Sons. 1939. — VILLARET und TIXIER: Dissociation des réactions cliniques, cytologiques, bactériologiques et anatomo-pathologiques dans certaines formes de méningite tuberculeuse. — La Sémaine med. 1905, 25, 609. — VINCENTELLI, L.: Les phénomènes méningés aigus transitoires et curables et l'état des méninges au cours de la tuberculose pulmonaire chronique de l'adulte. — Thèse, Paris 1919.

FROM ÅKEBERGVEIEN INFANT HOME, HEAD: ALEX. BRINCHMANN, M. D.

Some Remarks on the X-Ray Appearance and Prognosis of Infant Tuberculosis.

By

TORFINN DENSTAD, Oslo.

With a view to gaining an impression of the X-ray manifestations of tuberculosis of the lung in babies and infants and their development and prognosis, I have, with the gracious permission of ALEXANDER BRINCHMANN, M. D., had the opportunity of examining the journals and X-ray pictures of *the tuberculin-positive children* in the Åkebergveien Infant Home from September 1931 till January 1st 1941, i. e. during the period in which the Infant Home has had its own X-ray apparatus.

From a radiographic point of view, the characteristic feature of tuberculosis of the lung in infants is the occurrence of extensive diffuse opacities. In part they are caused by caseous tuberculous pneumonia, in part they are more benign with a pathological-anatomical substratum which so far has not been fully elucidated, but which is designated in a variety of ways: perifocal infection or edema, paratuberculosis, epituberculosis, benign tuberculous pneumonia, splenopneumonia etc.

It would be of special interest to elucidate whether it is possible to draw conclusions for the prognosis from the X-ray pictures. Further it would be of value if it were possible to gain an impression of the pathogenesis of benign opacities, of how frequently they arise around the primary focus or have a different origin, of whether they are primary or secondary.

Before entering upon the discussion of the material, a brief mention should be made of *the normal thorax picture* in infants. The heart is relatively large and transversally situated, the mediastinum is short and broad. This is the case especially when the child is examined lying on its back, which is usually the case. The diaphragm then is pushed upwards and the upper part of the mediastinum broadens on account of increased blood congestion in the large veins. If the child cries, the congestion increases and the width of the mediastinum changes accordingly (EBENIUS). ARMAND-DELILLE and LESTOCQUOY state that when the child is examined in an upright position, the lateral limit of the upper mediastinum normally should not exceed the point of the processi transversi. In studying radiographs of tuberculin-negative infants under 2 years of age, examined when lying down, I have in a couple of cases found the lateral limit of the upper mediastinum 1—2 mm. beyond the processi transversi, but as a rule within them. According to EBENIUS the width of the mediastinum at this point should not exceed half the width of the thorax on a level with the second anterior rib or the third breast vertebra. In children, an increase in width beyond these limits or a more or less convex lateral boundary — normally the boundary is slightly concave — is practically always due to adenitis or enlargment of the thymus. In tuberculin-positive children it is generally a matter of adenitis. One should, however, be aware of the fact that even a widespread adenitis cannot always be established by means of radiography (DALE). The intra-thoracic part of the trachea in children is always situated more or less to the right, sometimes entirely to the right of the median line. This lack of symmetry should not be ascribed to dislocation. In a couple of the tuberculin-negative children, a thin line was observed, corresponding to the interlobular fissure between the right upper and middle lobes, without any indication that the possible cause might be a previous non-specific affection of the lungs. As is the case in adults, the normal inter-lobular pleura is probably sufficient to produce this linear shadow, when its course to some extent coincides with the direction of the rays. It should further be noted that the shadow of the vessels over the apices (subclavia) may be rather broad, its sharp, concave lower limit may be projected just above and parallel the third posterior rib, and must not be mistaken for a thickening of the pleura.

The material consists of 120 infants, 64 boys and 56 girls, aged 0—6 years on admission, averaging 1 year and 7 months. 38 were under 1 year, 84 (70 percent) under 2 years.

The children are X-rayed immediately after admission and generally checked several times during their stay. In some cases the children have stayed upwards of 5 years. On an average, they stayed 1 year and 4 months.

The rough distribution of the X-ray findings will appear from the table.

Table.

X-ray finding	Number	Average age	Dead	Remarks
No examination . .	1	2 years	1	2 year old boy, died of meningitis 3 days after admiss.
Normal	20	2 years 4 months	0	
Adenitis	22	1 year 1 month	2	4 mth. old girl, died of miliary tuberc. and meningitis. 1 year old boy died of meningitis 9 mth. after discharge.
Opacities of the lung: around primary focus 22; appearing later 8; unknown relation to primary focus (most often early) 47	77	1 year 7 months	4 (+2)	$2\frac{1}{2}$ mth. old girl, died of mil. tbc. and meningitis. $4\frac{1}{2}$ mth. old boy died of tub. pneumonia. $1\frac{1}{2}$ year old boy died of tub. pneumonia (+ meningitis?). $2\frac{1}{2}$ year old boy died of meningitis. (5 mth. old girl died of acute appendic. with peritonitis. 9 mth. old girl died of probable croupous pneumonia).
Total	120	1 year 7 months	7 (+2)	Lethality rate 6 per cent (with reservations).

Normal X-ray appearance.

20 children averaging 2 years and 4 months of age. This group includes a patient in whom a calcified primary complex was found on admission. In 4 cases it was doubtful whether the patient suffered from adenitis. In 1, possibly 2 of these cases, calcification of glands was found on discharge. 5 of these patients were re-examined after 4—7 years (ROSENBERG). Calcified glands were found in 2 cases and a calcified primary complex in 2 (of whom one had it on admission). If the others were re-examined, some calcification would probably be found despite the normal X-ray findings during the stay in the Home.

One of the patients was rather seriously ill during the earlier part of the stay. For all the others, the stay was on the whole uneventful. Presumably their tuberculous infection had subsided.

Their average age was, indeed, somewhat higher than the average for the material as a whole.

In one of the patients, who had been lying in another hospital for a month, with a diagnosis of croupous pneumonia, was found a narrow, ribbon-shaped dense shadow with a sharp lower limit just above the inter-lobular fissure between the right upper and middle lobes. The opacity was deemed to be a leaving of the pneumonia, which had been treated with conspicuous success with M & B 693 (tuberculous pneumonias are rather worsened through such treatment (VANNFÄLT)). The differential diagnosis between a tuberculous opacity and a croupous pneumonia in children cannot be made by means of a simple X-ray examination, as pneumonias produce such varied X-ray pictures (DALE, FRIDERICHSEN). HOLM and WINGE have found that the X-ray picture in cases of pneumonia usually becomes normal in the course of 1—3 months — in some cases only after 3—6 months, while a tuberculous opacity as a rule lasts longer. Perihilar infiltrations are due to tuberculosis four times as frequently as to pneumonia.

Adenitis.

22 children, average age 13 months. The adenitis was somewhat more frequently localised to the right than to the

left. This may partly be accidental, due to the limited material, partly it may be due to the fact that both a hilar and a paratracheal adenitis on the right side is more easily visible than on the left. Finally, the cause may to a certain extent be real, as primary foci show a similar distribution.

Especially on the right side where, as mentioned above, it is easier to judge of circumstances, both hilar and paratracheal glands were often simultaneously enlarged. In some cases the adenitis was bilateral.

Whereas the enlarged paratracheal glands gave the upper mediastinum a sharp convex limit — if the limit is not sharp there is always a possibility of pulmonary opacity — the enlarged hilum glands were always surrounded by a more or less extensive opacity without any definite outline, often of the typical triangular shape with the point directed laterally. The perihilar opacity was sometimes so voluminous that the possibility of a lung focus as its cause must be taken into account, especially as generally no lateral pictures, allowing a more accurate localisation, have been taken. It is specially difficult to distinguish in the case of opacities corresponding to the lower part of the right hilum, to the side of the right auricle. It was impossible to establish with certainty any pulmonary opacity in the patients on admission, but during their stay calcified lung foci appeared in 5 cases — 1 of which with 2 and 1 with 3 primary foci, each of them with its calcified regional gland. Later we shall see examples of how little a fresh primary focus asserts itself in the skiagram in proportion to an adenitis. There should, therefore, be no reason to consider these adenites with their perihilar reaction as typical examples of the so-called secondary stage, as done by Simon & Redeker, following Ranke's immune biological classification of stages. The reaction round the primary focus should have subsided. In the great majority of cases it is probable that the infection has taken place a relatively short time before admission. Two of the patients had, for instance, recently suffered from erythema nodosum. Incidentally, the average age in this group is low. When the primary focus in these cases cannot be directly shown, it must be assumed that the reason most often is its small size. The alveolitis with its perifocal exsudate is too small for X-ray demonstration. FRIMANN-DAHL & WAALER also mention an example of how little is seen of a nut-sized focus with a pneumonic border zone (autopsy). It must also be taken into account that in some cases the primary focus is hidden behind the heart shadow, the diaphragm or near the mediastinum. It goes without saying that these findings of adenitis without any visible lung focus cannot be adduced in favour of the theory that adenitis frequently is due to intestinal or other extrapulmonary infection, as maintained i. a. by CALMETTE and WESTERGREEN. PARROT's law (1876) still holds good. »Toutes les fois qu'un ganglion bronchique est le siège d'une lésion tuberculeuse, il y a une lésion tuberculeuse du poumon.»

There is one case where the clinical examination reveals the pulmonary lesion, probably corresponding to the primary focus, while the skiagram only shows dubious changes:

A boy aged 1 year and 3 months, whose father had suffered from tuberculosis of the lung for a couple of months, had on admission sibilant respiration and small râles at the base of the left posterior surface. The skiagram, however, only showed some very dubious spots at the left base. 2 months later was found a serious perihilar opacity on the left side, and at the base a horisontal linear shadow with the appearance of a planiform atelectasis. The latter persisted for more than a year, when a dobtful grain-sized spot appeared just above it — the primary focus? At the same time, the perihilar opacity receded and a calcium deposit appeared in one of the lower broncho-pulmonar glands. Clinically, the case followed a peaceful course.

In 8 cases, calcification in the affected glands could be demonstrated in the course of the period of observation, generally becoming visible only after a year or more. These patients often had fever, specially to start with, but on the whole the clinical course was relatively uneventful. Indeed, the X-ray findings seem to show that despite their low age these patients controlled their infection well. During their stay, the adenitis receded. The clinical recovery, however,

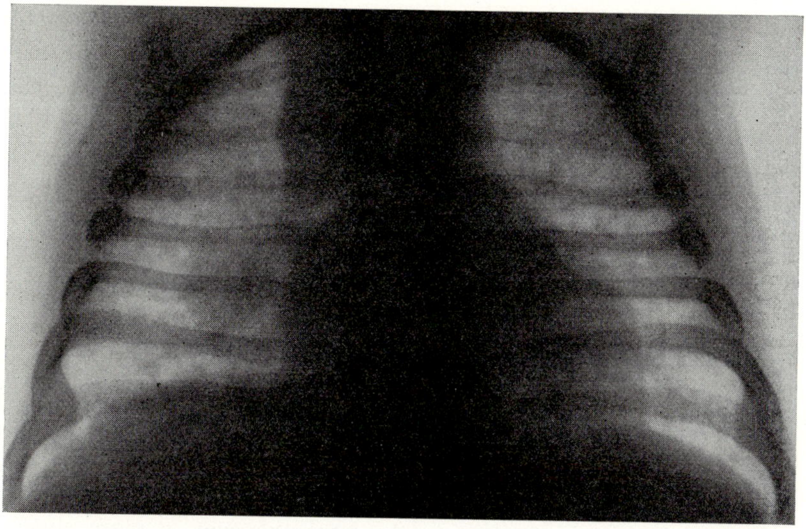

Fig. 1. 4 months old girl. Right-sided paratracheal adenitis. Miliar spread.

cannot always be depended upon. A one year old boy with enlarged paratracheal and hilum glands on the right side was discharged as feeling well after 6 months' stay. 9 months after his discharge he died of meningitis.

In this group is further included a girl of 4 months old with paratracheal adenitis and *miliar tuberculosis.* She died after a short stay in the Home. (Fig. 1.)

Opacity of the lungs.

77 patients, not quite two-thirds of the total. 27 are less than 1 year, 52 ($^2/_3$) less than 2 years of age. Average age on admission: 1 year and 7 months.

Nearly all of them had adenitis which could be radiologically established, in part with a strong perihilar reaction.

Opacity round the primary focus.

In a good quarter (22 cases) of these children with opacities of the lung that could be radiologically established, a calcification of the lung, in all probability the primary focus, could be demonstrated on the site of the opacity after the latter had receded. It must be assumed, therefore, that these opacities are conditioned by the primary focus with its perifocal reaction. The latter may be more or less extensive. In about half these cases it was relatively limited, in part so diminutive that it would hardly have been noticed unless the later calcification had suggested its existence.

As an instance I would mention a girl of 8 months old who was admitted in a state of good health, but had a positive tuberculin test. She had no doubt been infected by her mother who had lately been coughing and whose tuberculosis of the lung had recently been established. A skiagram taken on admission shows a probably bilateral adenitis and a slight shadow in the central region of the left lung. This shadow increases by and by, and 4 months after admission there appears in addition a diffuse spot, the size of a nut kernel at the base of the left side sinus. 1 1/2 months later the spot is more sharply defined, while the opacity in the central part of the lung is more saturated and more extensive — it must be taken as

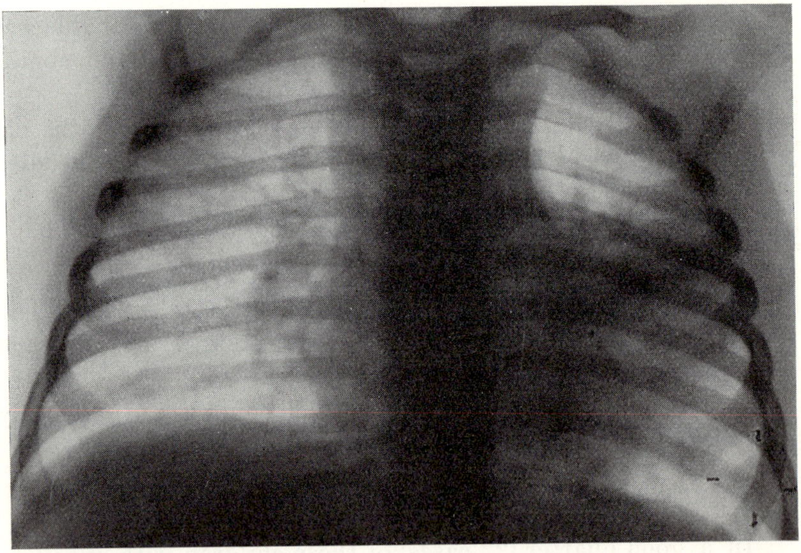

Fig. 2 a. 13 1/2 months old girl (5 1/2 months after admission.) Bilateral paratracheal adenitis. Left-sided hilar adenitis with considerable perihilar opacity. Primary focus the size of a nut kernel at left base.

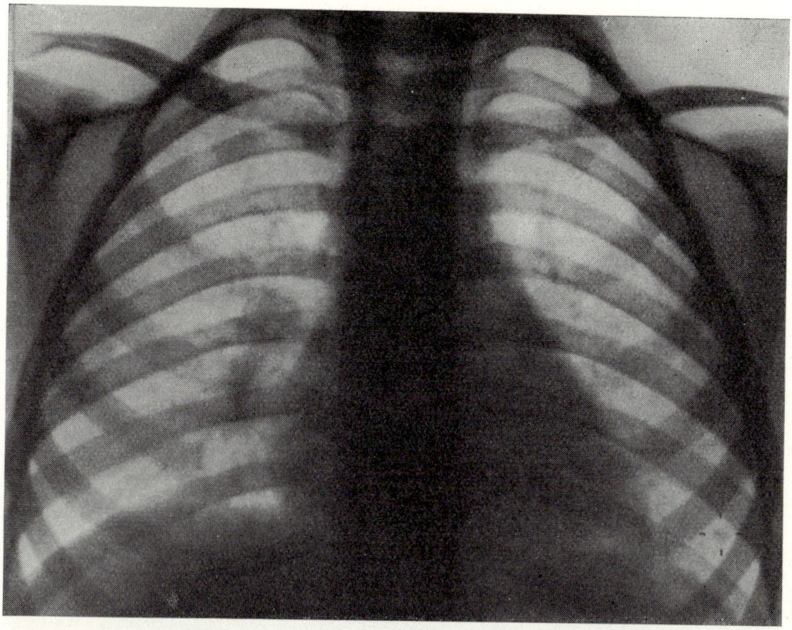

Fig. 2 b. 2 1/2 years later. The primary focus is calcified.

perihilar. (Fig. 2 a.) Little by little, the picture then clears. A good 2 years after admission all that is found is a grain-sized, calcified spot as a remnant of the little shadow at the left base. (Fig. 2 b.)

During the earlier part of her stay the patient was much subject to coughing, put on little weight and had fever. The recovery did, however, set in while the perihilar opacity was still on the increase.

The other cases also definitely give the impression that it is possible to establish the adenitis with its perihilar reaction radiologically a good deal earlier than the primary focus, and that the reaction around the latter is often insignificant. Armand-Delille & Lestocquoy maintain that perihilar opacities generally are only apparently perihilar, being in most cases conditioned by pulmonary opacities which are projected over hilum. Unfortunately, lateral pictures which might settle the question, are rare in our material. The localisation round

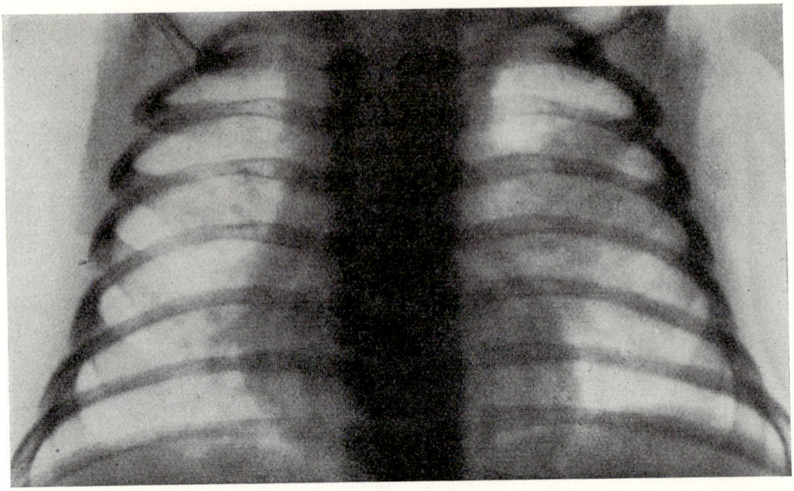

Fig. 3 a. 2 1/2 months old girl. Left-sided perihilar opacity.

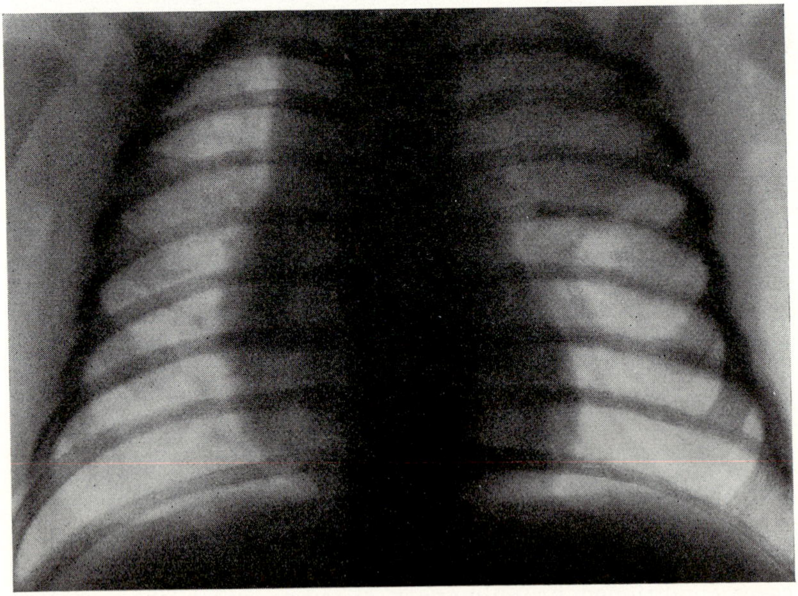

Fig. 3 b. 4 months later. Perifocal opacity over the left top coterminus with the perihilar opacity, which is receding. Right-sided paratracheal adenitis. The heart displaced to the right.

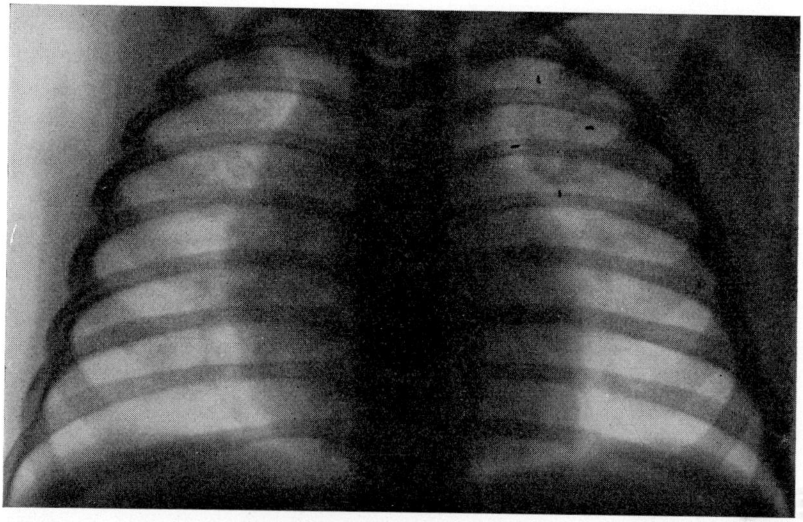

Fig. 3 c. 8 months later. A group of pinhead-sized calcified shadows above the left hilum (conglomeration tubercle). For the rest nearly complete clearing.

hilum of the opacities on the frontal skiagrams, and not least a primary focus which can be pointed out simultaneously in another place do, however, speak forcibly in favour of their adenitic genesis.

In other cases the opacities round the primary focus were more extensive and could cover as much as half the lung. This may partly be explained by the primary focus itself having been voluminous, leaving a calcified conglomeration of tubercles (5 cases).

In one case which is, indeed, also an example of how well even quite small infants may control the infection, the calcification or, more precisely, the shadow of the density of calcium, which may also be caused by chalky deposits (FRIMANN-DAHL & WAALER), disappeared.

A girl, 2 months old, whose father was consumptive and whose mother had just caught erythema nodosum, on her admission looked well, but coughed a little. The first few weeks she suffered from a strong gastro-enteritis. The first skiagram, taken after 2 weeks' stay, showed a homogeneous shadow with an indefinite outline round the left hilum right against the chest

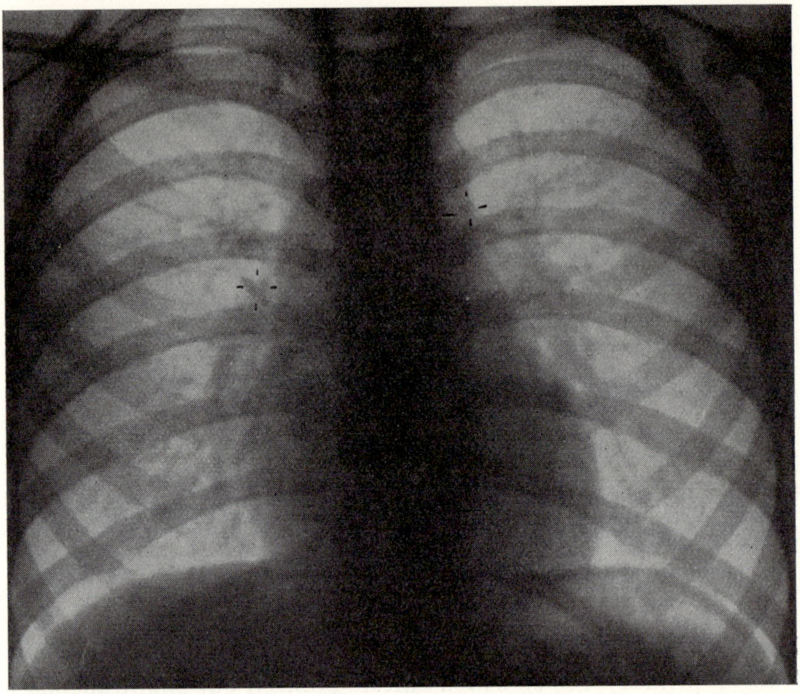

Fig. 3 d. 6 years later. All that is left is a couple of glandular calcifications.

wall (Fig. 3 a). 4 months later, a diffuse, saturated shadow has developed over nearly the whole upper half of the left lung. The mediastinum has a slightly convex upper right limit, revealing a paratracheal adenitis, and the heart seems somewhat displaced to the right (expansive process?) (Fig. 3 b). Meantime, the child has been lively and flourishing, as a rule with a normal temperature. She had, however, passed through an otitis media and had coughed a little, with a hint of toux bitonale. The opacity thereafter began to clear. One year after admission, all that could be seen beyond a slight shadow were a few spots of calcareous density the size of pin-heads in a region the size of a threepenny bit above the left hilum (Fig. 3 c). One year later these spots had also disappeared, all that could now be seen was a small calcification of glands just below the aortic arch and in the right hilum. A control skiagram taken after 7 years showed no change (Fig. 3 d).

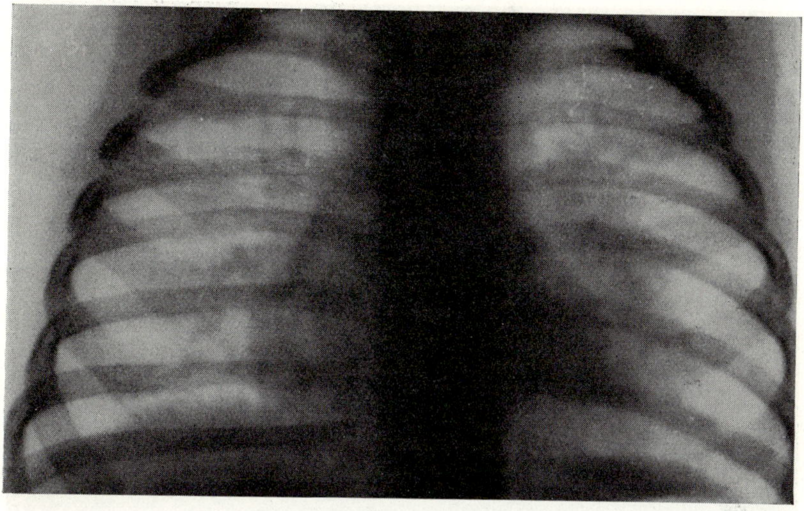

Fig. 4 a. 7 months old boy. Left-sided pirihilar opacity.

In some cases, however, the opacity around the primary focus may gain considerable extension without any evidence — at least in the skiagrams — of the primary focus having been specially voluminous. All that is found as a remnant of it is a small calcified focus.

One example may be quoted. A boy of 7 months who had been coughing for a month was sent to the Internal Medicine Department of Aker Hospital. He had a positive tuberculin test. The source of infection was unknown. X-ray examination revealed a left-sided hilar adenitis with perihilar opacity (Fig. 4 a). One week after his admission he had a high fever for a few days, and was then sub-febrile. A new skiagram a good month after the first showed a diffuse saturated shadow across the lower half of the left lung, merging into the hilar opacity (Fig. 4 b). He recovered satisfactorily. On his admission to the Åkebergveien Infant Home 1 1/2 year after the inception of his illness, all that was found was a mottled shadow in a region the size of a nut-kernel near the apex of the heart, and a little later deposits of calcium in the hilum glands and the lung focus (Fig. 4 c a good 3 years after he fell ill).

All transitions, therefore, may be seen, from such cases where the primary focus does not appear at all or appears

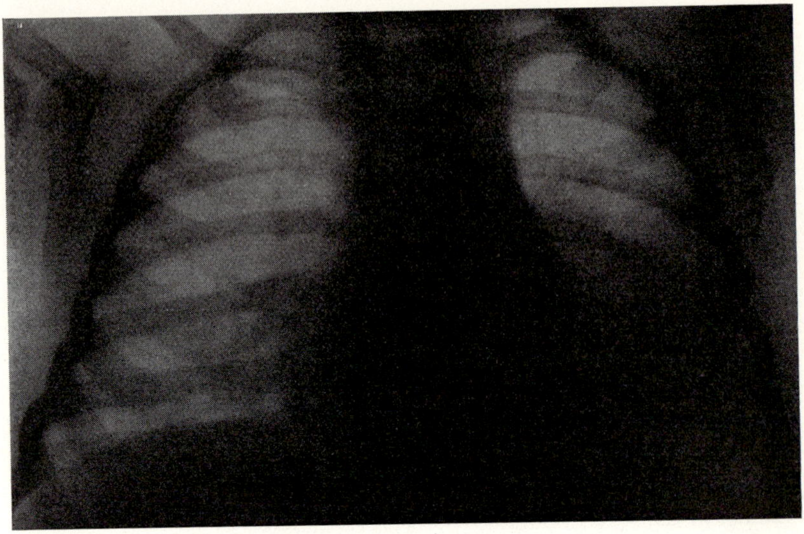

Fig. 4 b. A good month later. Perifocal opacity at the base, coterminous with the perihilar opacity.

only as it calcifies, to such cases which start with an extensive opacity caused by a strong perifocal reaction. In all cases the adenitis first asserts itself. And those cases, which show a normal X-ray appearance before the adenitis and, contingently, the lung focus appear, show that one should not rest satisfied with such a normal appearance but keep the child under continuous and vigilant supervision.

While Armand-Delille and Lestocquoy hold that the pathological-anatomical substratum of benign perifocal pneumonic opacities is a specifically tuberculous tissue, Simon and Redeker, Wallgren and others maintain that we are faced with a non-specific exsudative reaction due to excessive sensitiveness to the toxins of the tubercle bacillus. Wallgren assumes that atelectasis also plays an important part. At any rate the assumption of a specific process does not fit in so well with the mild course and the complete clearing of the opacities. A collateral infection edema which persists as long as the primary focus or the glandular focus remains active, seems a more satisfactory explanation. I have not been able

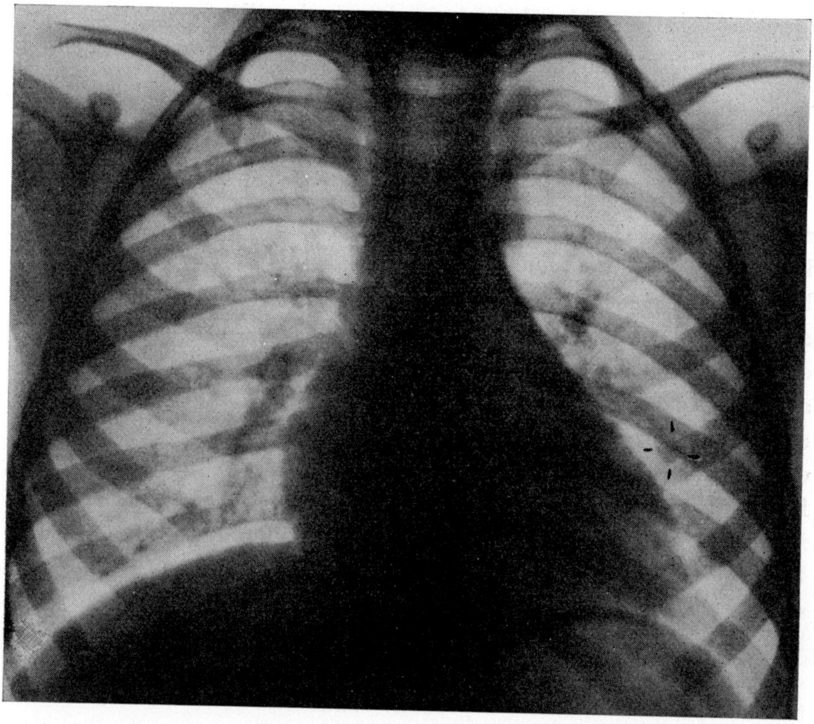

Fig. 4 c. 3 years later. Calcified primary complex.

to show radiologically any atelectatic component in these cases, the process has rather, at times, been of an expensive type.

Whether the opacities were small or large, there was no marked difference in the clinical picture, but the material is, of course, limited. The absence of such differences does, however, to a certain degree tell against the assumption that the opacities consist of specifically tuberculous tissue. In conjunction with the primary infection some of the children have suffered from an acute gastro-enteritis with, in part, sanguiferous diarrheas and vomiting — probably of a toxic nature. The primary focus, however, was in the lung. In a patient who was tonsillectomised, tuberculous tissue was found in the tonsils. This patient had, none the less, his primary lung focus. It is possible that the tubercle bacilli during the pre-allergic period may settle in more than one organ, several primary foci may, indeed, be found in the lungs.

Opacities occurring at a later stage.

In a few cases (8) opacities are found which have developed after the reaction round the primary focus has been completed — both the primary focus and the regional glands may already be calcified. These opacities are diffuse, more or less saturated and of a larger or smaller extent, though most often rather extensive. In a couple of cases they were, however, limited and circular, probably metastases. While the opacities round a primary focus usually persist for 1—2 years, these later-developed opacities seem to be more transient. The general health of the patients is affected to a remarkably small degree, in some cases the patients are completely free from symptoms. In this connection it is natural to think of atelectasis — for some reason or other the glands may swell and compress the bronchi. In some cases the X-ray examination gives a hint of this — in other cases it does not. WALLGREN holds that these opacities partly represent exacerbations of the same nature as the perifocal reaction and partly — with fluctuating transition — acute pulmonary infiltrations which he classes as secondary tuberculosis. In part they are located around or in the immediate vicinity of the primary focus, in part at quite a different place in the lung.

I shall describe some of these cases:

In a boy of 4 months with a consumptive mother are found on admission a left-sided hilar adenitis and tumor of the para-tracheal glands on the right, possibly also on the left side. 5 months later a saturated shadow has developed over the upper half of the left lung (Fig. 5 a). The opacity then clears, 10 months later all that is left is a calcified focus in the left top and calcified glands in the left hilum and near the aortic arch (Fig. 5 b). It seems reasonable, therefore, to explain the opacity as a perifocal reaction round the primary focus. During all this time the boy has been feeling well, has put on weight regularly and on the whole been without fever. A little less than 2 years

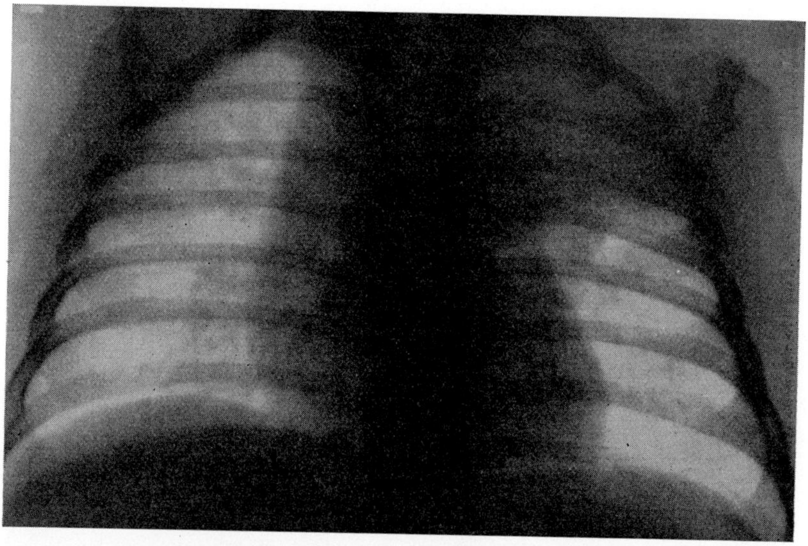

Fig. 5 a. 4 months old boy. Saturated perifocal opacity across the left top. Right-sided paratracheal adenitis. Displacement of the heart to the right?

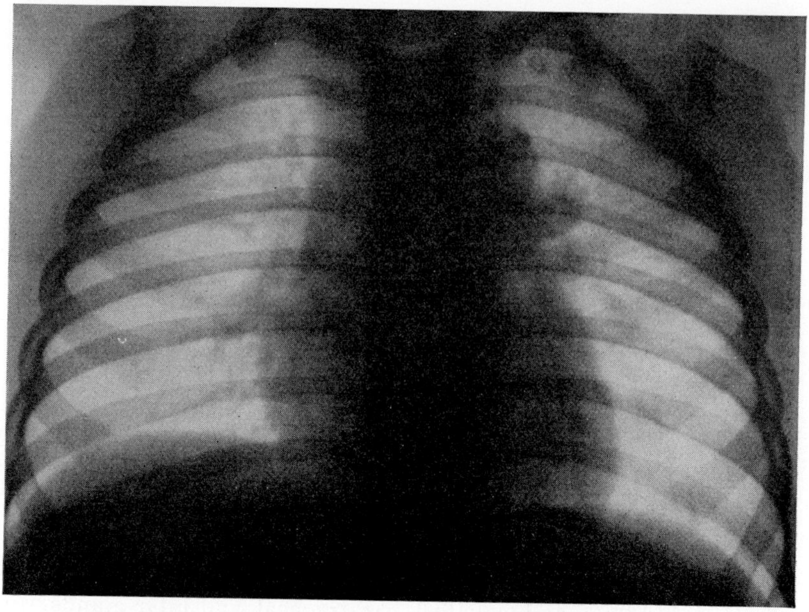

Fig. 5 b. 10 months later. Calcified primary complex.

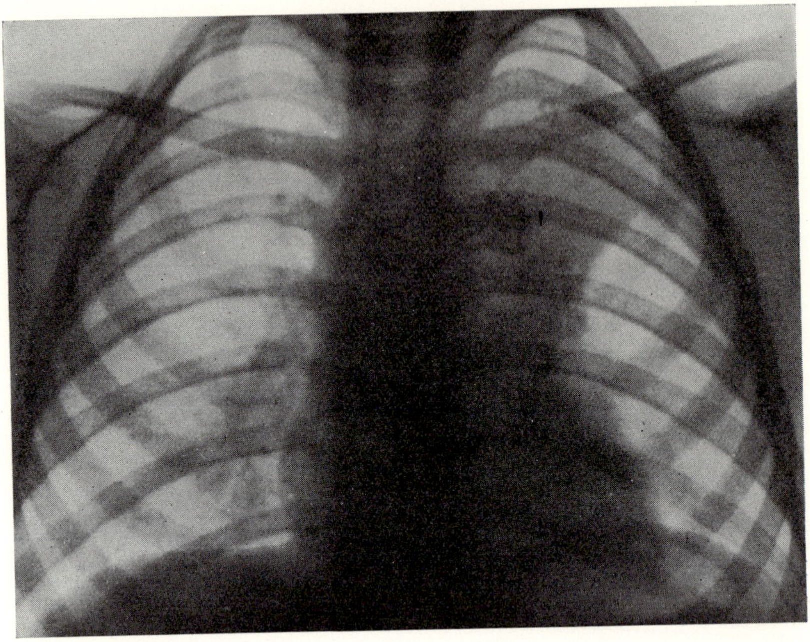

Fig. 5 c. 1 1/2 year later. Once more a diffuse, but less saturated opacity across the left top, now with an atelectatic character. The heart displaced to the left.

after his admission he began to peak and coughed a little. A skiagram reveals a diffuse, but much less saturated opacity in the same place as the first one (Fig. 5 c). While the first opacity was rather expansive, this one is pronouncedly atelectatic with pulling over of the mediastinum and a concave lower edge. It was, moreover, transient, a good month later it had disappeared. At the same time the patient suffered from frequent catarrhs and at times had subfebrile temperature. These symptoms persisted for a time after the opacity had receded and are possibly a sign of a certain lability of his state (with increased tumor of the glands and a compression-atelectasis?).

Another boy with a consumptive mother was admitted at the age of 5 months to Department VIII of Ullevål Hospital, where a left-sided adenitis and opacity of the lung off the hilum were established. He was later transferred to Åkebergveien where — a good year after the first skiagram — was found as a remnant of the primary infection a calcification the size of a nut-kernel off the left hilum and calcified paratracheal aud hilar glands. In

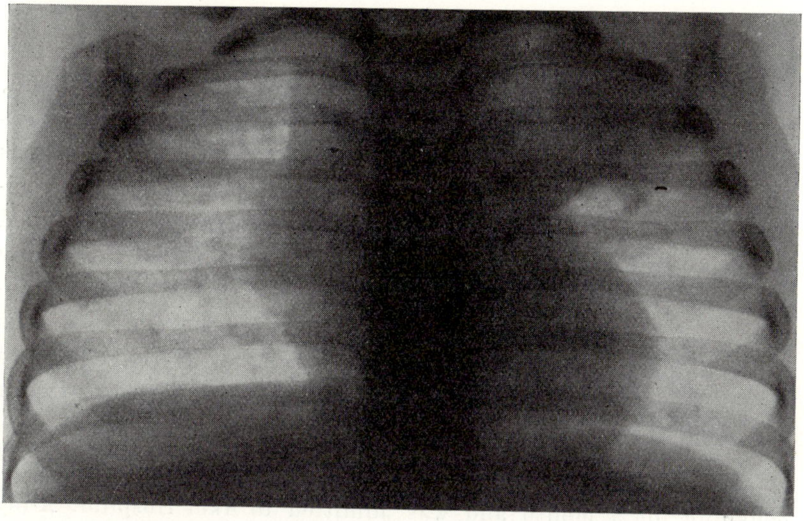

Fig. 6. 1 year and 8 months old boy. Diffuse opacity across the left top. Calcified primary complex (primary focus at the lower edge of the opacity). Hilar and paratracheal adenitis on the right side.

addition, however, is seen a saturated opacity right across the upper part of the left lung, above the primary focus (Fig. 6). The patient is practically without symptoms, the child feels well, a year later the opacity has practically disappeared.

To conclude, one instance where the opacity is not located in the same part of the lung as the primary focus: A 3 year old girl with a consumptive father is admitted on account of a strong tuberculin reaction. A right-sided hilar adenitis is established, in the lower region, especially. It recedes within one year and simultaneously the primary focus appears as it calcifies — it is situated right at the base, partly hidden by the diaphragm. A control examination one year later, 2 years after admission, shows a saturated shadow in the middle region of the right lung above the hilum. The patient has shown no subjective symptoms — an X-ray examination one year later shows that the lung is clear apart from the calcified primary focus.

Opinions vary greatly as to whether such opacities which appear some time after the inception of the illness are occasioned by an exterior cause and, if so, as to what is the nature of that cause. According to Simon and Redeker, the so-called secondary infiltrations are practically a proof of superinfection, and if it persists they soften. ARMAND-DELILLE and LESTOCQUOY, WALLGREN and others, on the other hand, hold with intercurring illnesses as the cause, as such illnesses reduce the power of resistance of the patient. On the basis of the few cases in the present material, I am not in a position to express any opinion on the issue. It must be assumed that the children are exposed to superinfection, and very many of them have tonsillitis, non-specific catharrs, measles, whooping-cough etc. without any apparent effect on the course of the tuberculous infection. In a couple of cases, in the course of measles or whooping-cough, there appeared — post or propter — fresh opacities partly of an atelectatic character.

A boy of 2 1/2 years whose mother was consumptive had been coughing for a month and was admitted to Aker Hospital. X-ray examination reveals a left-sided hilar adenitis with a considerable

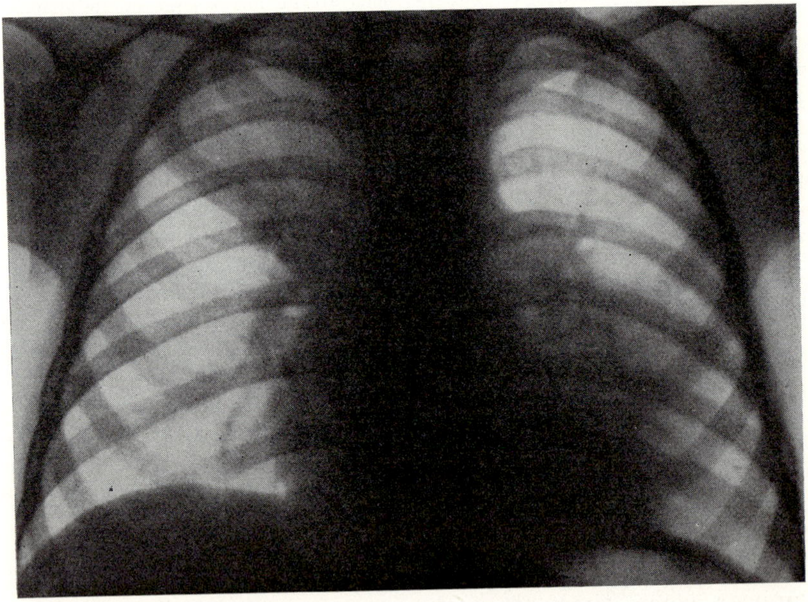

Fig. 7. 2 years and 10 months old boy (2 months after admission). Perihilar opacity coterminous with perifocal opacity on the left side. Opacity across the right top in connection with measles.

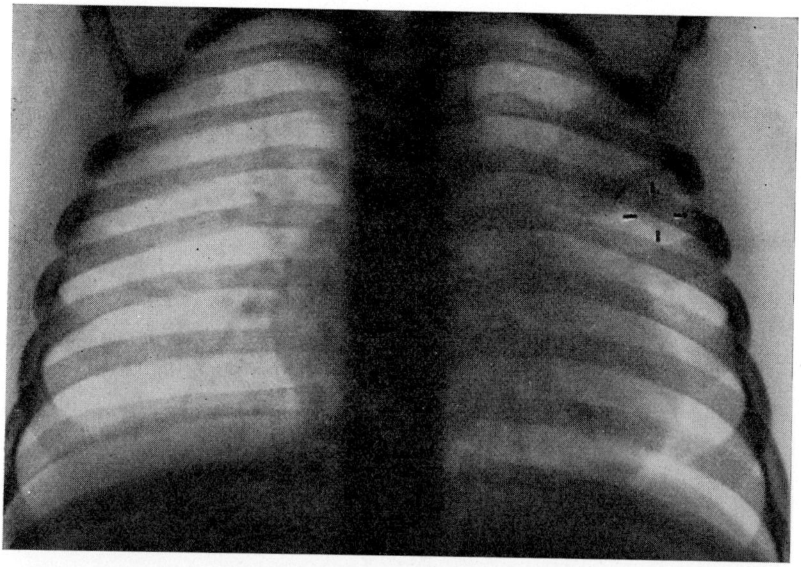

Fig. 8. 2 years and 5 months old girl. Diffuse opacity across upper part of left lung in connection with whooping cough. Calcified primary focus at the sharp lower edge of the opacity.

perihilar opacity, especially in the lower part. 1 1/2 months later — after his removal to the Åkebergveien Infant Home — there has developod a rather extensive opacity of the lung below the left hilum. These opacities recede in 2 years' time and leave a calcified primary complex. The boy had caught measles a short time after his admission, and a skiagram taken 2 weeks after the appearance of the rash showed a slight shadow across the upper part of the right lung, possibly with a slight pulling over of the mediastinum (Fig. 7). 3 1/2 weeks later there was no trace of this last-mentioned opacity.

In a 2 year old girl whose mother was consumptive is found on admission a left-sided hilar adenitis with perihilar opacity which, after 2 months, had cleared a little. 4 1/2 months after admission she catches whooping cough, and a diffuse shadow appears across the upper part of the left lung, densest in its lower part where it is separated from the clear part of the lung by a sharp and slightly convex boundary line. Immediately below this line is found a pea-sized saturated spot, no doubt the primary focus (Fig. 8). 3 months later, the picture is unaltered. The child

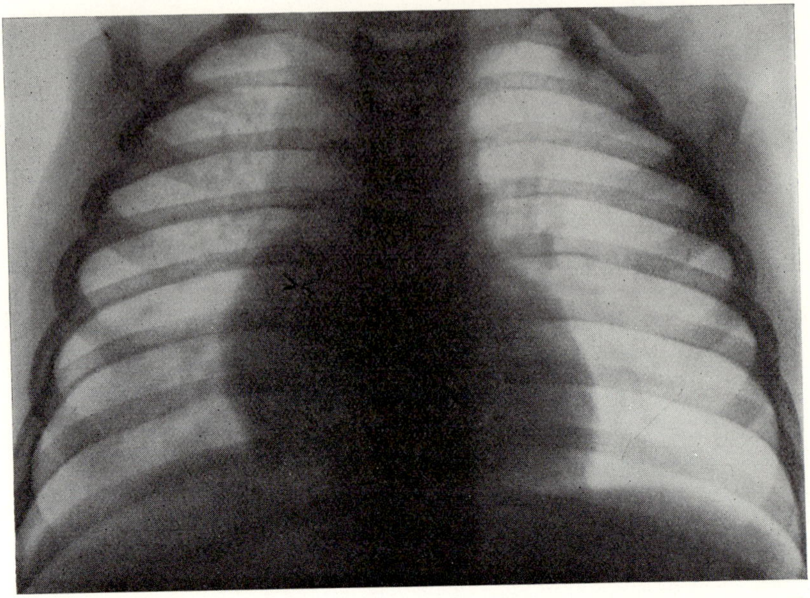

Fig. 9. 1 1/2 year old boy (2 1/2 months after admission). Paratracheal right-sided adenitis and mottled shadow across the upper part of the right lung. Slight shadow at the base of the right side, pulling over of the heart to the right and compression of right main bronchus. Inconsiderable exsudate.

was non-febrile and looked well. Unfortunately no more X-ray pictures were taken.

One gains the impression that the less saturated, slight and comparatively transient opacities may very well represent pure collapses. Autopsies do, indeed, reveal that the bronchial wall which, in children, is rather yielding, is thrust in by the glands which are often much enlarged. Abscesses and secretions in the mucous menbrane may also contribute towards the contraction of the lumen. In skiagrams one sees not infrequently how the right-sided broncho-pulmonary glands contract the right main bronchus — one does not get such a good view of the left main bronchus.

In a boy, 1 year and 4 months old, who had been infected 2 months before admission by his father (a sailor who had been at home a couple of days only before he was sent to Ullevål

Hospital) was found a right-sided paratracheal adenitis. 1 month later there was in addition a diffuse shadow over the whole upper part of the lung. Probably the primary focus is situated here. 2 1/2 months later — the temperature having been a little heightened all the time — the shadow has cleared considerably, but a slight shadow has appeared at the base (Fig. 9). It does, however, recede within half a year. In all pictures the strongly compressed right main bronchus is clearly seen through the heart-shadow, which is displaced to the right. It seems reasonable to explain the latter opacity as an atelectasis.

In some cases, where such an opacity is located above or below the inter-lobular fissure between the right upper and middle lobes, effecting a pulling up or down of the latter, the presence of — at least — an atelectatic element must be assumed.

The more saturated, late-appearing opacities without signs of collapse are not satisfactorily explained as mere atelectases. There must be other factors at work — but as such cases very rarely come up for autopsy little is known of their real nature. One does, at any rate, get the impression that they are generally benign.

Opacities, the relation of which to the primary focus is unknown.

In those cases where no calcified primary focus can be shown during the period of observation (47) — and they are the majority — it is impossible to say with any certainty whether the larger and smaller opacities found represent perifocal reactions round a primary lung focus or opacities which have developed at some other point of the lungs possibly after the lapse of a certain time. In most cases the opacities appear so early — so closely related to the moment of infection where it is possible somehow to determine the latter — that causation by the primary focus and its perifocal reaction or a process derived from it must be assumed.

The opacities of which we have seen examples so far all receded. In order to explore whether it is possible by means of X-ray examination to find any data for the *prognosis*, we shall first examine those cases which ended in death. It is among these cases that we may expect to find the caseous tuberculous pneumonias with their desolate prognosis. As will be seen from the table, 6 children died with lung opacities. One of these, however, died of acute appendicitis with peritonitis, another in all probability died of a croupous pneumonia. Of the 4 who died of their tuberculosis, 2 died of meningitis — one of them had in addition a miliar spread in the lungs — a finding which is a clear warning, but which does not interest us in this connection. Miliar tuberculosis and meningitis may strike like a bolt from a clear sky in connection with a diversity of tuberculous manifestations. Probably only 2 of the children died directly of their pulmonary lesion.

In a boy, 4 1/2 months old, source of infection unknown, who had had a »cold» and a fever before admission, approximately identic changes were found through repeated X-ray examinations during

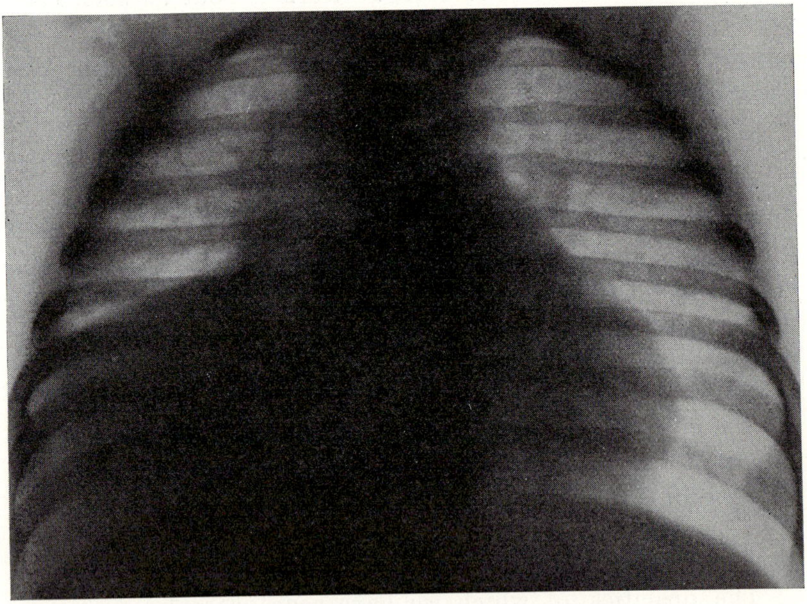

Fig. 10. 10 months old boy (nearly 1/2 year after admission). Saturated opacity, probably of the whole lower right lobe (in case with slight collapse). Taken as tuberculous pneumonia. Perihilar opacity. Mors.

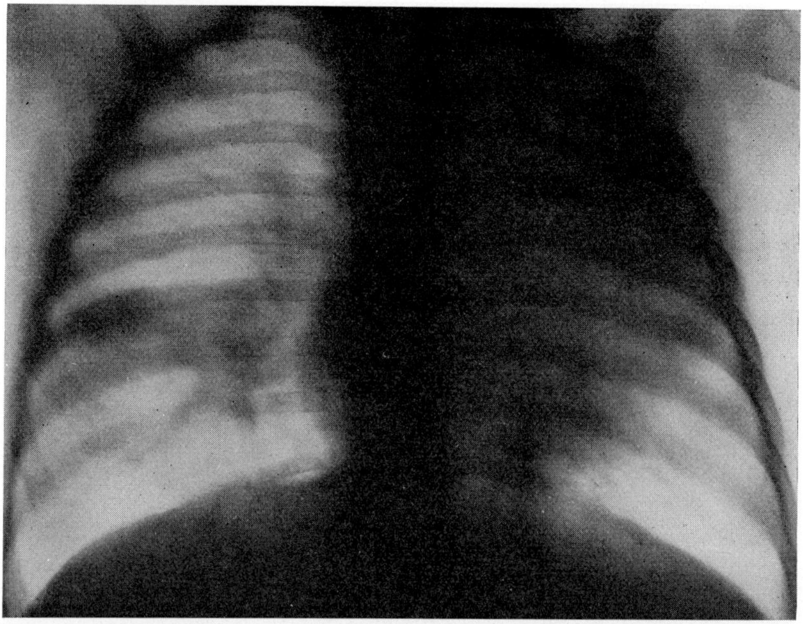

Fig. 11. 1 1/2 year old boy. Saturated opacity over the whole upper left lobe, with a couple of clearings at the top. The heart displaced to the left. Taken for tuberculous pneumonia. Lesser opacity in right middle lobe. Mors.

a stay of 1/2 year's duration. On the lower right side a saturated opacity with a clear-cut upper edge, probably corresponding to the whole lower right lobe. It must be assumed that an atelectatic factor is present, the upper edge of the lobe being pilled downwards a little. In addition, there is a right-sided perihilar opacity (Fig. 10). The latter was more pronounced during the earlier part of the stay. The patient was all the time in a very bad condition, with high fever. He died 5 1/2 months after his admission.

I boy aged 1 1/2 year with a consumptive mother had suffered from »bronchitis» from the age of 4 months. The skiagram reveals a saturated diffuse opacity covering the whole upper left lobe with a couple of distinct clearings in the upper part and a slight pulling over of the heart. In addition a smaller opacity is found in the right middle lobe (Fig. 11). He got constantly worse and died after 3 weeks with increasing sopor (meningitis)?

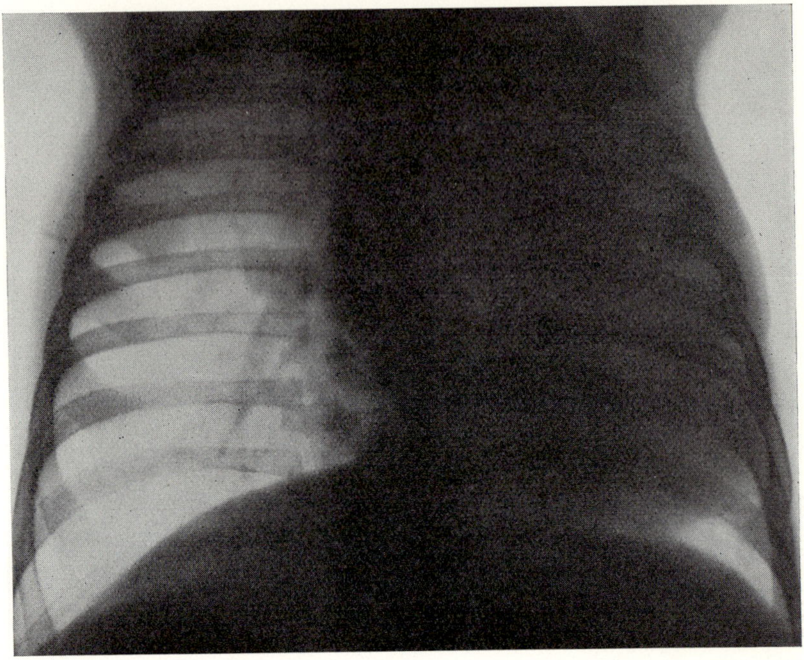

Fig. 12 a. 9 months old boy (2 months after admission). Saturated opacity covering whole upper left lobe, with strong pulling over of the heart. So-called epituberculosis. Slight shadow across right top.

As mentioned above, it is probable that caseous pneumonias are the cause of these opacities which are more extensive and more saturated than the benign opacities we have seen earlier. The hope of having discovered a datum for prognosis is, however, vain, as we have instances of similar opacities clearing up completely.

In a boy aged 7 months whose parents were consumptive, a slight shadow is found on admission, covering the upper lobe on both sides. The heart is displaced to the left. In the course of the next 2 months the opacity grows considerably on the left side and the heart is further pulled over (a lateral picture confirms the localisation in the left upper lobe). On the right side, conditions are unaltered (Fig. 12 a). The opacities then begin to clear, 3 months later there are only remnants left (Fig. 12 b). During the first half year of his stay the child was low, with

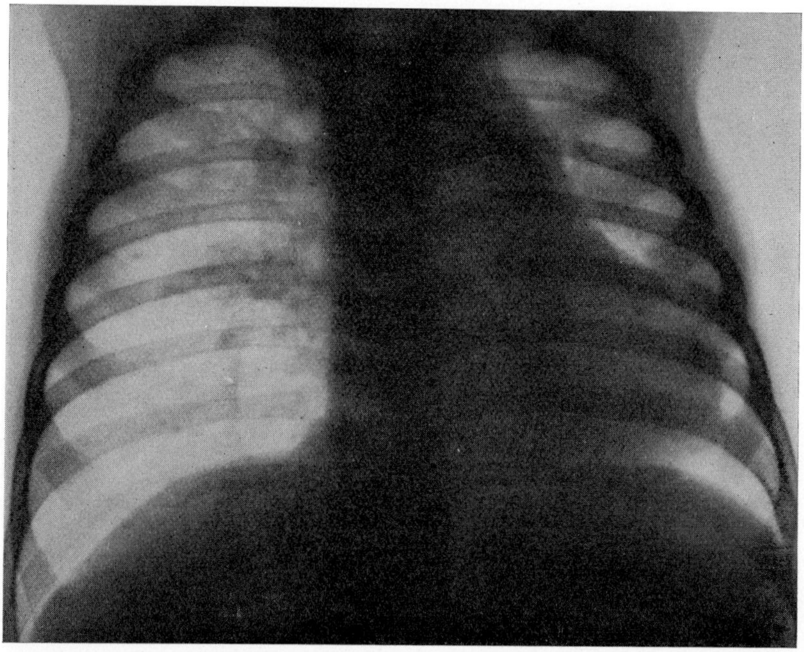

Fig. 12 b. 3 months later. Nearly complete clearing.

dyspnæa and coughing but only slight fever, a condition which prevailed for a considerable time after the opacities, as revealed through X-ray examination, had started receding. Later the child recovered quickly.

A boy of 1 year and 5 months was admitted to the Children's Department of the National Hospital. He had been ill for a good month, with increasing cough, dyspnæa and fever. A cavernous phtisis had been found in his mother a couple of weeks earlier. X-ray examination revealed a right-sided hilar adenitis. 2 weeks later the child was transferred to the Åkebergveien Infant Home. He had tracheal stridor, exspiratory dyspnæa and bi-tonal cough. Coterminous with the perihilar opacity there had now appeared a small opacity in the lower part of the right upper lobe with a sharp lower edge corresponding to the inter-lobular fissure and with the point directed laterally. In addition was found a right-sided paratracheal adenitis and an insignificant amount of fluid in the pleura cavity (Fig. 13 a). A week later, the shadow in the right lung increased considerably both in extent and saturation,

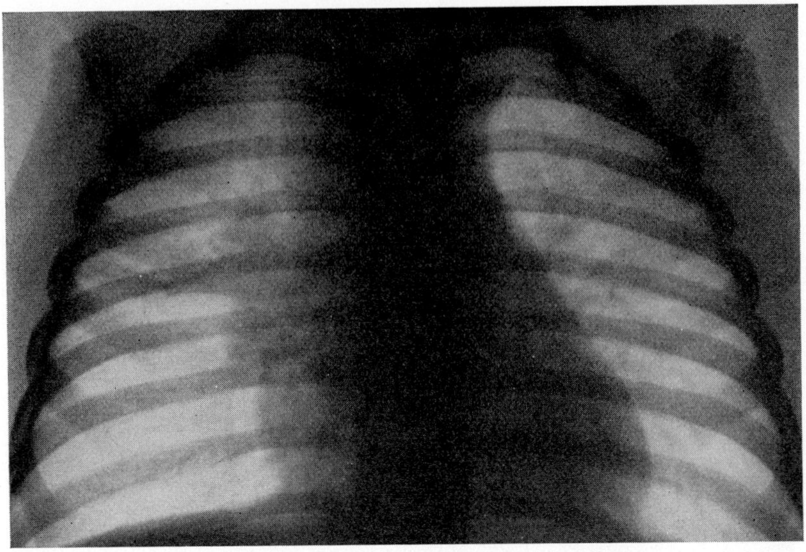

Fig. 13 a. 1 1/2 year old boy. Right-sided paratracheal and hilar adenitis with perihilar opacity. Inconsiderable exsudate.

covering the whole upper lobe with special density in its lower half (Fig. 13 b). There is no displacement of the mediastinum, but the inter-lobular fissure against the middle lobe is situated more caudally than is usually the case, indicating an expansive process. During the period the condition of the patient otherwise remained unchanged, although with less coughing and more changing dyspnæa. The temperature remained at 38—39 centigrades. The opacity then gradually cleared from above (Fig. 13 c, 1 1/2 months after the previous picture). 10 months after admission the picture is practically the same as then, 5 months later the lung is very nearly completely clear. A control examination about 6 years after the inception of the illness reveals merely a small calcification just beyond the right hilum (Fig. 13 d). Along with the recession of the lung opacity as revealed by X-ray examination, the state of the patient went improving. He passed through both whooping cough — which affected him seriously — and measles without his lung affection being noticeably influenced.

As will be seen, a rather homogeneous X-ray appearance of saturated lobal opacities is found in the 4 last-mentioned cases with their widely varying courses. Armand-Delille

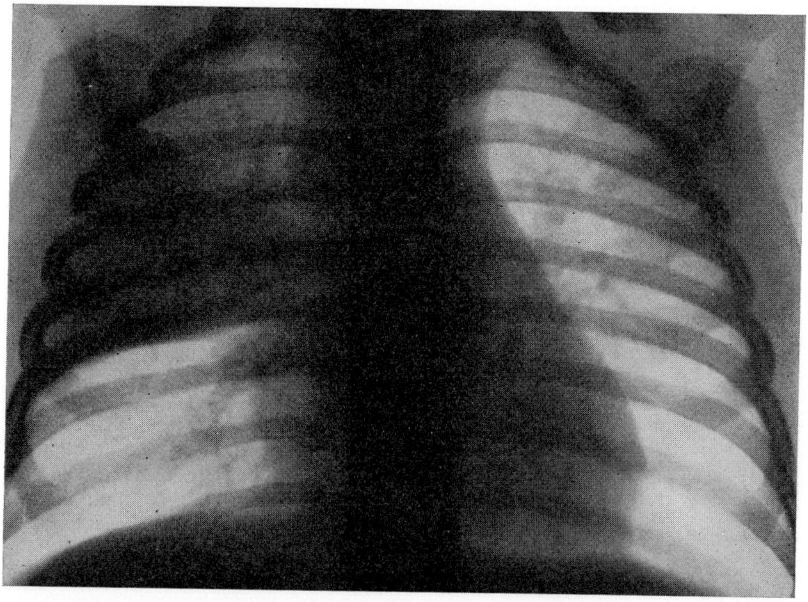

Fig. 13 b. One week later. Opacity covering whole upper right lobe, specially saturated in lower part. Lower edge of lobe pushed downwards — expansive process. So-called epituberculosis.

and Lestocquoy put forward as a means of differential diagnosis that the malignant opacities, the caseous tuberculous pneumonias, are more saturated and expansive than the benign ones. The cases quoted above do not confirm this hypothesis. In the two who died, there was, clearly, an atelectatic component, while one of the benign lobal opacities was atelectatic, the other expansive. The demonstration of cavity-like clearings in the opacities is not decisive either. When the somewhat more extensive benign opacities clear, one or more round and quite well defined clearer spots are not infrequently observed to start with, although there is no clinical evidence of necrosis (pseudo-cavities). The explanation may be interstitial emphysema, or, possibly, certain parts simply clear before the rest. The same phenomenon is sometimes observed in croupous pneumonias in the stage of resolution, especially in children.

On the whole, apart from the demonstration of miliar

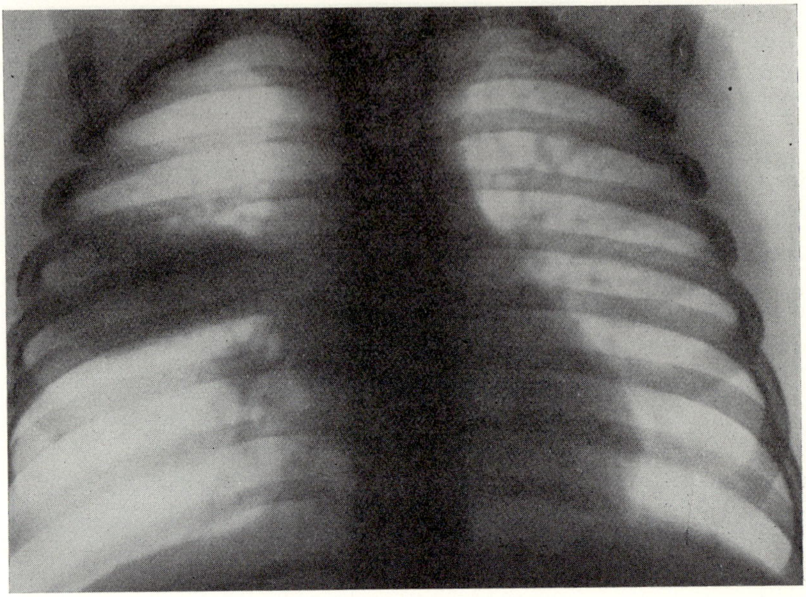

Fig. 13 c. 1 1/2 months later. Clearing from above. (A good year later practically complete clearing).

tuberculosis of the lung, no reliable data for prognosis are found in the skiagrams. Great caution must be shown in drawing any conclusions concerning the pathological-anatomical process from the X-ray findings. But in conjunction with the clinical picture they do in most cases make it possible to form a correct conception of the nature of the process. Especially in cases of saturated lobal opacities one should keep in mind the caseous pneumonias.

The two last cases described, with saturated lobal opacities, with a prolonged but benign course, are typical examples of so-called *epituberculosis* as described by ELIASBERG and NEULAND, who were the first to define this concept clinically and radiologically. This interesting state has recently been elaborately treated by SÖDERLING who, in a material consisting of 900 tuberculin-positive children aged 0—2 years found 12 cases of typical epituberculosis. In addition he has described another 4 cases. As in the case of the perifocal opacities, the pathological-

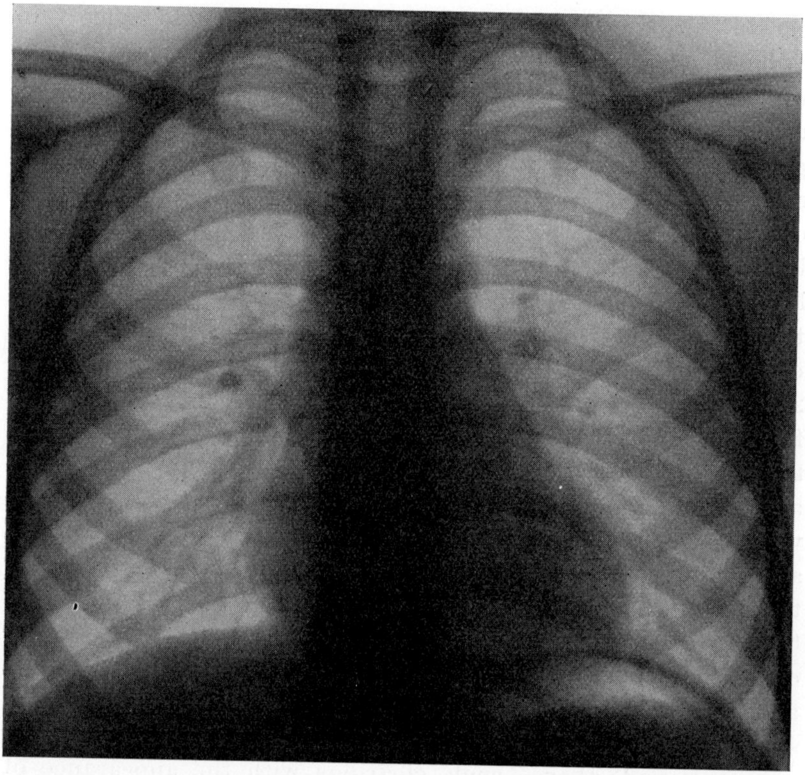

Fig. 13 d. 5 1/2 years after first picture. Small calcification laterally from right hilum.

anatomical substratum is unknown, as these cases rarely come up for autopsy. Söderling discusses the various theories relating to their pathogenesis: tuberculous parenchyme infiltration, massive collapse of the lung and excessive perifocal reaction, and concludes that neither of these alone is a sufficient explanation of the clinical and X-ray appearance. The favourable prognosis, the complete clearing and benign clinical appearance of these cases tell against a tuberculous infiltration as sole cause, and the slow clearing from the periphery, the long duration leading nevertheless to complete clearing, the bronchial blowing and the fact that in most cases no collapse can be shown by X-ray examination speak against the theory of collapse. So far there is every reason for agreement. But when, on account of the long duration (in most cases 6—12 months) he rejects the possibility of causation by a strong perifocal reaction, I cannot agree. There are many examples of extensive — if not lobal (and consequently not epituberculous) opacities around the primary focus persisting for an equally long time. On the basis of his own observations, Söderling holds that 3 components may be distinguished as the foundation of epituberculosis: a tuberculous pneumonia, a perifocal edema round it and a massive collapse of the lung. The first 2 should explain the increase in extent (cp. the last case, fig. 13 b), the last one the mild course despite the pneumonia, the collapse being deemed to have a salutary effect. This last assertion is much disputed, many authorities hold an opposite view. Assuming that the epituberculous opacities consist of an extensive perifocal reaction which in most cases is intrinsically benign, and sometimes complicated by collapses (cp. fig. 12 a), there is no need to recur to the salutary effect of an atelectasis. The demonstration of pseudo-cavities should, according to Söderling, reinforce the theory of atelectasis, some parts becoming filled with air before the others. But, as mentioned above, such clearings with the appearance of cavities are also seen in smaller opacities without any atelectatic character when they begin to recede, and also in non-specific pneumonias. On the whole, the justification for positing epituberculosis as a distinctive facies morbi seems rather dubious — there are all transitions from opacities not demonstrable by X-ray methods via more or less extensive primary opacities to the lobal ones. The so-called epituberculous opacities do, indeed, appear at an early stage of the illness, in close connection with the primary infection. Through careful X-ray examination and bronchography it may prove possible to elucidate further this interesting problem.

In conclusion, I would merely mention that exsudate in the pleura was found i 6 cases only. The pleuresis would appear some months after the inception of the illness and the exsudate was quickly resorbed. In most cases it was scarce, in one case only it was abundant.

Prognosis.

As will appear from the table, a total of 7 out of the 120 tuberculin-positive children died of their tuberculosis, a lethality rate of 6 per cent. Even if we compute the rate of lethality among the 99 cases with a pathological X-ray appearance of the lungs, counting in the one child who died without having been X-rayed, we only find a lethality rate of 7 per cent. And of the 18 children aged 0—6 months, 2 only died of their tuberculosis. It should, however, be noted, that the material is hardly representative in this respect, as children suffering from meningitis or other illnesses with a bad prognosis will generally be sent to hospital (where, consequently, one is apt to form too dark an opinion of the prospects). All the children were, however, really ill on admission, with fever, stagnant weight, reduced tonus and turgor and with cough. In judging of prospects it should further be taken into account that some of the children were discharged on the demand of their parents before their condition was fully satisfactory. On the whole, however, during their stay a fair impression has been gained of the tendency of development of the illness. Control examinations (ROSENBERG) have further confirmed this impression. I should think, therefore, that the prognostic impression given by the material is hardly far from being realistic.

Such a low rate of lethality is, however, in strong contradiction to the prevalent idea of the prognosis for babies and infants infected with tuberculosis. According to ARMAND-DELILLE and LESTOCQUOY, caseous pneumonia dominates in babies, with 58 per cent malignant and 42 per cent benign opacities before the age of one year. The rate of lethality is given as at least 75 per cent in case of infection during the first 6 months of life, 54 per cent in case of infection during following 6 months. And SIMON and REDEKER, in whose material there are, however, very few babies and infants, state that even in babies resorbtion of »primary infiltrations» is *possible* (they mention as an instance of this an 11 months old boy). Through control examinations of infants born of consumptive mothers FALKENFLETH finds a lethality rate of 41 per cent (and a mortality of 7 per cent) in good accordance with YNGVAR USTVEDT, who gives the mortality of infants under 1 year born in consumptive families as 4—8 per cent (twice as high in cases with consumptive mothers as in cases with consumptive fathers). WALLGREN finds a lethality rate of 35,9 per cent in cases of infection during the first year of life and SÖDERLING, who has undertaken control examinations of 917 tuberculin-positive children aged 0—2 years, finds that the rate of lethality for children infected during the first year of life has fallen from 71,1 per cent (for the period 1914—23) via 59,9 per cent (1924—33) to 41,2 per cent (1933—37), and for children infected during the second year of life from 43,8 per cent via 38,7 per cent to 16,3 per cent. In his opinion, the lower lethality figures in later years are due to the fact that more mild cases are taken and sent to hospital now than earlier. This view is supported by his having been unable to trace any effect on lethality rate by factors such as nutrition, social circumstances, different sources of infection, different therapeutics, superinfection or period of exposure. Age is the only relevant factor.

In all probability this is also the reason for the low rate of lethality in the material on which I have worked, the tuberculous infection in the great majority of the infants having been discovered through examinations undertaken on account of evident consumption in the mother or father. BELTLE, who has made a control examination of about 500 children treated for active tuberculosis, finds similarly low figures of lethality rate: 8,3 per cent in cases of infection during the first year of life (20,6 per cent if infected during the first half-year) 6 per cent in cases of infection during the second year and 0,75 per cent only if infected during the 3rd—6th year of life.

Summary.

In the overwhelming majority of cases of babies and infants infected by tuberculosis, X-ray examination reveals changes in the lungs. Paratracheal and hilar adenites, which appear early and may be the only sign of the primary infection of the lungs demonstrable by X-rays, are the most common findings. In the majority of cases opacities of the lung are also found, from minute, hardly visible ones to diffusely saturated lobular ones. Probably, in most cases, these represent the primary focus with its perifocal reaction, as they generally appear early and in some cases leave a calcified lung focus. The somewhat more extensive opacities at times are of an expansive nature, at times an atelectatic component is evidently at work. In two cases of saturated lobal opacity, so-called epituberculosis, the process in one case was expansive, in the other atelectatic. This difference in the X-ray appearance, however, does not enable us to draw any conclusions with regard to prognosis. They nearly all receded within 1/2 to 1 1/2 year. In two cases, which were taken to be caseous tuberculous pneumonias — the patients died — were found saturated lobal opacities of the same atelectatic apperance as one of the cases of benign so-called epituberculosis. The demonstration of small round clearings looking like cavities does not give any data for prognosis, as they are not infrequently seen when benign opacities start clearing.

There seems little reason to maintain epituberculosis as a distinct picture of disease. Probably, the substratum for these lobal opacities is the same as for the less extensive benign opacities, viz. a perifocal reaction, at times complicated through atelectasis.

In some cases diffuse opacities with a mild course, often free from symptoms, appear at a later stage of the illness. These opacities are more transient, some-times with the appearance of pure collapses, at other times more satured without any atelectatic character. There are examples of such opacities appearing in conjunction with acute infectious diseases (measles — whooping cough). On the other hand, most of the children underwent such intercurring infections without any demonstrable exacerbation being revealed by X-ray examination.

The prognosis is relatively favourable, with a direct rate of lethality of 6 per cent in this material (120 children with an average age of 1 year and 7 months on admission) — 7 per cent, computing the rate of lethality of those cases only where X-ray examination revealed pathological conditions in the lung. 5 died of meningitis, 2 of them with a miliary spread in the lung, 2 of caseous tuberculous pneumonia. Even in the age group 0—6 months, only 2 died out of 18. There is, however, one instance showing that meningitis may shatter all expectations after the process apparently has come to rest.

Literature.

Armand-Delille & Lestocquoy: La Tuberculose pulmonaire et les maladies de l'appareil respiratoire de l'enfant et de l'adolescent. Paris 1933. — Beltle, J.: Zeitschrift f. Kinderheilkunde 1938, 60, 95. — Dale, T.: Der Wert der Röntgenuntersuchung in der Lungendiagnostik. Stockholm 1930. — Ebenius, B.: Nordisk Med. Tidsskrift 1936, 12, 2056. — Falkenfleth, G.: Nordisk Med. 1941, 9, 99. — Friderichsen, C.: Acta Pædiatrica 1939, 27, 1. — Frimann-Dahl & Waaler: Röntgenologische und pathologisch-anatomische Studien über den tuberkulösen Primärkomplex. Acta Rad. Suppl. 33, Oslo 1936. — Holm & Winge: Nordisk Med. 1940, 8, 2121. — Macpherson, A. M. C.: Primary tuberculosis of the lung in children. London 1939. — Rosenberg, P.: Acta Pædiatrica 1940, 27, 452. — Simon & Redeker: Praktisches Lehrbuch der Kindertuberkulose. Leipzig 1926. — Söderling, B.: Acta Pædiatrica 23, Suppl. II, 1939. — Ustvedt, Y.: Norsk Mag. f. Lægevidenskaben 1916, 1301. — Vannfält, K. A.: Nordisk Med. 1941, 9, 163. — Wallgren, A.: Tuberculosis in children. Nelson new loose-leaf Medicine, Vol. I, p. 337.

REPORT FROM THE LABORATORY OF THE COPENHAGEN BOARD OF HEALTH.

Comparative Studies on Feces of Healthy Breast-, Bottle- and Spoon-fed Infants.

By

CHR. ULDALL.

Since Escherich (1886) published his classical studies on intestinal bacteria in infants, numerous works have been published on the intestinal flora in adults as well as in children — even though most often with reference to various pathological conditions or to individual bacteria or bacterial groups. Still, attempts have been made also to estimate the total number of bacteria in the feces. From the Scandinavian countries a good many works have been published on this subject (*e.g.*, by Yllpö, Lunding, S. Orla-Jensen, O. Winther), and within the veterinary physiology and pathology this question has attracted considerable interest, especially among Danish investigators (*e.g.*, C. O. Jensen, M. Christiansen, E. Mejlbo). Measuring of the hydrogen ion concentration in the feces and the cause of its differing reaction in bottle- and breast-fed babies, besides experiments to modify or alter this reaction, has been the subject of many considerations and experiments — thus, for instance, in particular Baumann (in Germany) and Tisdall & Brown (in America) have been dealing with this question; and yet the full explanation of the difference in reaction of the feces has not been established conclusively; still, the latter authors carried out no less than 1300 determinations on infantile feces. More recently the interest in the entirely chemical analysis of the feces has been falling off. The studies on the chemical composition of the feces in infants was pursued most ardently at the beginning of the century (*e.g.*, BLAUBERG, HECHT, STRASSBURGER). Yet, later several American authors have reported some extensive studies on the determination of the fat content of the feces of infants (*e.g.*, HOLT, COURTNEY & FALE).

In the present paper I shall present the outcome of a combined chemical and bacteriological examination of the feces of normal infants. These studies comprise: Determination of the dry matter content of the feces, of the percental fat content of the feces, the reducing elements, and the nitrogen content. Further, the hydrogen ion concentration is estimated. In addition, I have estimated the number of living aërobic and anërobic bacteria, capable of multiplying, besides the so-called colon titer. Further, studies were carried out with a view to estimation of the occurrence of bacteria of the lactic acid group. Besides, studies were carried out with a view to the demonstration of pathogenic intestinal bacteria in the fecal specimens. Finally, in one experiment, the so-called fat and carbohydrate balance was determined in the case of a breast-fed of 3 months.

Technique.

The methods here employed for the chemical analyses are given partly by HEUPKE in his »Die Fæces des Mennchen», 1939. For practical reasons, the dry matter is determined on the total fecal output, which as a rule weighed from 10 to 30 g. After homogenization of the native feces, samples are taken for bacteriological examination and for determination of the hydrogen ion concentration. The remaining native feces are smeared out in a thin layer in a dish, and dried to constant weight, for about 40 hours in a drying oven at 98° C. At intervals, during this drying process, the feces are loosened from the side of the dish and powderized. Feces containing much fat require longer time for this process, but it proved practical in this way to obtain a constant weight. In spoon- and bottle-babies the portion of feces produced by a single bowel movement was often found to be sufficient. In breast-fed babies, on the other hand, it was necessary as a rule to collect the feces from several bowel movements. This naturally called for an inquiry into the question about the preservation of the feces.

Carbohydrate. For determination of the reducing elements, the STRASSBURGER method was employed. No other serviceable method appears to have been given in the literature available to me.

The weighed sample of feces is boiled with 2 % hydrochloric acid in a reflux cooler. After filtration, a part of the filtrate is boiled with FEHLING's solution. The precipitated cobber is dissolved in nitric acid, precipitated by evaporation after addition of concentrated sulphuric acid — in the form of cobber sulphate — and dissolved in distilled water. The amount of cobber is determined by titration — as retitration by means of ammonium thiosulphate and silver nitrate, with iron alum for indicator. The amount of sugar corresponding to the amount of cobber is read in PFLÜGER's table.

Fat. For determination of the fat content of the feces, it was decided as the quickest and least expensive method to try extraction with trichlor-ethylene ad modum GROSSFELD, modified by SEMERDIEW. Judging from the duplicate and comparative determinations, this method appears to be serviceable for determination of the total fat content of the feces, whereas the fractional analysis on later control experiments has proved it to be somewhat misleading.

The weighed, dried, sample of feces is heated to boiling with 10 cc. of concentrated hydrochloric acid, then cooled, and extracted by boiling for 10 minutes with technical trichlor-ethylene — which, as a rule, contains no evaporation rest — in an effective reflux cooler; and then it is cooled and poured into a separator-funnel. After standing for some length of time, the trichlor ethylene is poured off, and 25 cc. is pipetted off into a measured flask, and then it is »eveporated». The evaporation rest is weighed. The outcome is calculated after the following formula:

$$\frac{\text{Evaporation rest} \times 10{,}000}{\text{Sample} \times (25 - \text{evaporation rest/specific gravity of fat})} =$$

% of total fat. The specific gravity of the fat may be set approximately as 0.92, and it has to be included in the calculation, as the measured 25 cc. introduces a volumetric value.

For the fractional determination, the powderized feces were extracted with trichlor ethylene, as described above, but without any preceding acidification. The filtrate was evaporated, dried and weighed, then dissolved in neutralized alcoholic-ether, and titrated with n/10 alcoholic NaOH, with phenolphthalein for indicator. As the results obtained in this way did not agree with those reported by American authors, while the total determination showed good agreement, it was decided to look into the American method more thoroughly (as given by HOLT, COURTNEY & FALE). With the American method the dried and weighed fecal powder was acidified for 20 minutes with 10 cc. of 25 % HCl, on boiling water-bath, extracted in ROEHRIG tubes or in RÖSE-GOTTLIEB tubes with alcohol, ether and benzine. The extract was poured off, evaporated, dried and weighed, giving the total amount of fat. For fractionated determinations, the acidified fat was dissolved in benzene, and titrated with n/10 alcoholic NaOH, with phenolphthalein for indicator. In this way the amount of split fat is determined by multiplying the titer value by a constant, and the unsplit fat is determined as the rest. Further differentiation of the split fat in free fatty acid and soaps may be obtained by extraction of another sample from the same specimen of feces in SOXHLET's apparatus. But the authors did not think that this differentiation would be of any particular significance.

A priori it seems rather surprising that acid-treated fat — even after drying — might be suitable for the titration. But control tests with melted beef suet — free from soap — after the method given by HOLT, COURTNEY & FALE, and merely dissolved in ether-benzine, evaporated and dried, showed only a slight difference in the titer values for acid-treated and non-acid-treated fat (from 0.5 to 4.5 %). For additional surety, a specimen of dried and powderized feces was divided into 3 parts, one of which was treated after GROSSFELD's method, one portion after HOLT's method and one portion was extracted with ether in SOXHLET's apparatus. As will be seen from Table 1, the values showed good agreement in the determination of the total fat, whereas the figures for the fractionated determination with trichlor ethylene deviated considerably from the others.

Table 1.

	Trichlor ethylene		HOLT		HOLT + SOXHLET	
Total	40 %	(100 %)	39.5 %	(100 %)	38.5 %	(100 %)
Soaps	9.3 %	(38.7 %)		(82.6 %)	27.4 %	(82.3 %)
Acids	6.2 %				3.9 %	
Neutral fat	24.5 %	(61.3 %)		(17.4 %)	7.2 %	(17.7 %)

Table 1 shows the findings with the fat extract from the same specimen of feces examined after three different methods.

Determinations of the total fat with trichlor ethylene extract and after Holt, Courtney & Fale's method show good agreement, whereas the fractionated determinations show a great divergence. From the 3rd column it will be noticed that the amounts of soaps, acids and neutral fats determined after the Holt method combined with Soxhlet's apparatus and the titration on the Soxhlet extract correspond to the amount of split and unsplit fat obtained after the Holt method.

Thus is seems reasonable to assume that the treatment of the non-acidified specimen of feces with trichlor ethylene implies extraction of a good deal of soap, and the method does not seem suitable for fractionate fat determination, whereas it is very serviceable for determination of the total fat content of the feces.

In its technical form, trichlor ethylene is inexpensive, and it may be evaporated over open fire, as the vapours are non-inflammable and may be used several times if the vapours are condensed — what ought to be done invariably, as the vapours contain phosgen.

In the work presented in this paper, the fractional analysis was carried out on trichlor ethylene extracts. For the reasons given above, however, the findings in these studies are refuted on account of the circumstances mentioned. Later, in the Queen Louise Hospital for Children the writer has had an opportunity to carry out fractionated fat determination ad modum Holt, Courtney & Fale on non-breast-fed infants (up to the present, 7 cases). Here the fat was found chiefly to consist in split components (fatty acids and soaps), to a considerable less extent in neutral fat (4—27 % of the total fat). In one experiment the amounts of acids, soaps and neutral fat were determined. The total fat percentage was 52 (100 %), including soaps 44 (84.6 %), fatty acids 3.7 (7.2 %), and neutral fat 4.3 (8.2 %). The dried matter percentage was 21. The child was $2^1/_2$ months old and it was given 50 % milk + barley water, 130 g $\times$ 3, and 100 % buttermilk 130 g $\times$ 3.

Proteins. A complete determination of the proteins excreted with the feces is very time-consuming, requiring large amounts of material, and it appears not to be exactly practicable. For this reason the writer has carried out the nitrogen determinations after the Kjeldahl method. It is to be admitted, however, that the nitrogen determined in this way gives merely an approximate idea of the protein content of the feces, as the total nitrogen content will depend also on undigested remnants of food and on the intestinal secretions and bacterial flora. The greater part of the nitrogen content of the feces is claimed to originate from secretions, while about one-fourth originates from bacteria and the rest from undigestid food (HEUPKE).

Hydrogen Ion Concentration. The hydrogen ion concentration is determined electro-metrically. For this determination about 1 g of homogenized feces is stirred thoroughly with about 4 cc. of distilled water. This determination is carried out with a calomel-quinhydrone electrode, which measures accurately only at pH = 7.9; after this the measures become less accurate, the inaccuracy increasing with the rising pH. Still, it is practicable to use the reading for pH up to 8.5, or even 9.0. Before each measuring — and in several cases also afterwards — control determinations are made with the buffer solution of SØRENSEN. Generally, the difference has been 0.01, never exceeding 0.02.

In the male infants, as a rule, contact of the feces with the urine has been avoied by means of a KAPER's glass, if the pH of the urine is widely different from that of the feces. In the cases of female infants, however, the feces have sometimes been in contact with the urine, as, with a view to irritation of the skin, it did not seem quite safe to employ any KAPER's tubes or similar remedies.

Bacteriological Examination. The bacteriological examination of the feces has been carried out with the technique given by MEJLBO, NYGART & PLUM. In this way, the numbers of multiplying, anaërobic and aërobic bacteria are estimated — as well as the so-called colon-aërogenous titer. Further, examinations have been made for pathogenic intestinal bacteria of the paratyphoid group, besides particular examinations with a view to the occurrence of bacteria of the lactic acid group.

The technique adopted was as follows:

Weighing, on a piece of sterile paper, 0.5 g of faces, which is then shaken totally with 49.5 cc. of physiological salt solution. This suspension forms the basis for a number of dilutions. For cultivation from the dilutions I have used a pipette given by DEMETER with graduate marks for 0.5, 1.0 and 1.1 cc. For estimation of the total amount of aërobic bacteria, I have used a modified DRIGALSKI medium: ordinary beef extract agar with 0.5 % lactose and $^{2}/_{10}$ cc. per 100 g of agar of an alcoholic 1.6 % solution of bromochresol purple. Corresponding estimation of anaërobic and facultative anaërobic bacteria are carried out with milk agar medium. For the colon titration I have used gentian violet peptone lactose bile broth in double tubes (KESSLER & SWENARTON, J. Bact. *14:* 27, 1922). The colonies are counted and multiplied by the dilution figure. For this count of colonies, as far as possible, I have selected plates and tubes with a suitable number of colonies — preferably between 50 and 1000. In all these experiments the incubator temperature has been 37.5° C.

A colon titer is given as the weakest dilution with gas production. A number of apparently similar colonies on plates and in tubes were examined microscopically for diagnostic purpose, and when they turned out to be rods looking like acidophilus or bifidum, a few colonies were transplated in sterile milk; then the growth was noted, and the culture examined microscopically. For additional surety, subcultures were made on milk agar.

For examination for pathogenic intestinal bacteria a little feces is removed from the specimen with a platinum loop, left standing in tetrathionate broth (with a sediment of calcium carbonate); from this, subcultures were made on modified DRIGANSKI medium.

Accuracy of the Technique. In order to decide on the accuracy of the technique, a triple test was made, besides other control tests with additional known amounts of lactose and fat. The homogenized specimen of feces was divided into three parts, dried, and then examined for fat, reducing elements and nitrogen. As shown in Table 2, the variations were very small.

Table 2.

	a	b	c
Dry matter	26.7	26.9	27.0
Total fat	15.2	14.4	15.6
Reducing elements . .	8.5	8.2	9.0
Nitrogen	4.9	4.6	4.7

Other duplicate tests showed similar results. For additional control of the accuracy of the method, a dry and powderized specimen of feces was divided into two portions; in the control specimen the fat percentage was 14. The other portion of powderized feces was mixed as thoroughly as possible with 18 % fat. An analysis of this portion showed a total fat content of 29.8 %, that is, 2.2 % was missing. A similar test was made with lactose, giving 25.1 % reducing elements, that is, a deficiency of 1.1 %.

In comparison with other methods, the one adopted here shows good agreement with the shaking method (HOLT, COURTNEY & FALE), as the trichlor ethylene method gave 43 % total fat while a corresponding sample of feces treated after the HOLT method gave 41.5 %. In other similar tests the figures were respectively 42.6 and 39.9 %, and 32.5 and 32.6 %. In conclusion, in a single experiment I looked into the so-called balance for fat and approximate balance for carbohydrates, reckoning the reducing elements observed in the feces as carbohydrates — something that can be done only with reservation. »Balance» means here the proportion between the food elements ingested and the amounts excreted with the feces.

For a few days prior to these experiments the child was given exclusively mother's milk, without any addition of cod liver oil, fruit juice or iron. The amount of milk ingested in 24 hours was determined by weighing the child before and after each meal. At the morning meal, a noon meal and the evening meal, samples of 5—8 cc. of the mother's milk were taken at the beginning of the suckling, in the middle of the suckling period, and shortly before the meal was finished. These samples were used for estimation of the fat percentage. In addition, in each meal a sample was taken of 5 cc. for determination of the lactose percentage. It was not considered necessary to determine the lactose percentage on each specimen separately. The percentage was determined on the total amount. In the fat analysis, however, the per cent was determined for each sample, the average percentage for the individual meal and the fat per cent for the total amount of milk ingested. At the morning meal the fat per cents were 2.88—4.27—6.73, averaging: 4.63. At the noon meal the corresponding figures were: 3.98—6.42—7.09, averaging: 5.83. At the evening meal the figures were: 1.66—3.71—5.45, averaging: 3.61. Total average: 4.69 %.

The feces evacuated on the day of examination and the following 5 days were collected so completely as possible and examined for dry matter, fat, reducing elements, and pH (also the pH and specific gravity of the mother's milk was estimated). There was defecation on the day of examination, and on the 4' and 5' days. The fat per cent of the milk was estimated in the usual way (Röse-Gottlieb): a weighed amount of milk with addition of 1 cc. of ammonia, 25 cc. of alcohol and 25 cc. of ether in a Röse-Gottlieb tube. After shaking, the specimen is left standing for 24 hours; and the alcohol-ether is pipetted off and the fat evaporated, allowance being made for the column of the solution remaining on the pipetting. The lactose percentage was determined by polarization. On the day of examination, December 15, the child was given altogether 630 g of mother's milk, with an average fat content of 4.69 %, a lactose content of 5.75 %, pH = 6.5, and the specific gravity 1.031. Thus, the ingested

Table 3. Balance Test on a Breast-fed Infant.

	Date						Total output in 6 days	Average daily output	Intake	Output in per cent of intake
	15/12	16/12	17/12	18/12	19/12	20/12				
Total native feces . . .	15.26 g	0 g	0 g	0 g	6.9 g	5.48 g	27.64 g	4.61 g		
Dry matter	21.5 % = 3.28 g				20.5 % = 1.44 g	23.4 % = 1.28 g	6 g	1 g		
Total fat	35.3 % = 1.16 g				35.9 % = 0.52 g	36.7 % = 0.47 g	2.15 g	0.36 g	29.55	1.2
Reducing elements . . .	10 % = 0.33 g				12.6 % = 0.18 g	9.5 % = 0.12 g	0.63 g	0.11 g	36.23	0.3
pH	5.56				5.79	5.46				

The fecal output for 6 days and the amounts of fat and reducing elements excreted. There is seen to be a considerable variation in the daily amount of feces whereas the percentages of dry matter, total fat and reducing elements vary but little. The acidity is fairly constant.

amount of fat was 29.5 g, and the ingested amount of lactose 36.23 g. The daily fat excretion was on an average 0.36 g, and the excretion of reducing elements 0.11 g daily. Thus, the fecal fat output was found to make 1.2 % of the intake, and the excretion of reducing elements amounted to 0.3 % of ingested carbohydrate.

As will be noticed in Table 3, I have found it preferable to reckon with the average excretion for a suitable number of days (6), as the child did not have defecation every day. The intake of mother's milk is assumed to have been fairly constant from day to day.

Material. The present infant material originates from »Børnehjemmet af 1870»,[1] comprising 14 breast-fed infants, 12 infants getting milk mixtures, and 13 infants on a more mixed diet.

This material may be said to be so uniform as practicable, as the children have been getting a uniform diet, all the milk has been furnished from the same dairy, and the vitamin supplement to the diet has been the same preparation throughout.

Immediately after defecation, as far as possible, the entire portion of feces was scraped off from the diaper with a spatula and placed in a stoppered glass, put on ice, or, in some cases, stored in a DEWAR jar with carbon dioxide snow. As a rule the feces were examined a few hours later; in some cases, however, — especially breast-fed infants — where the fecal output was very slight, the feces have been stored for up to 72 hours. In order to investigate the effect of the storage at + 3° and — 60°, duplicate analyses were carried out as shown in Table 4. The homogenized specimen is divided into 3 portions, two of which are stored for 24 hours at respectively + 3° and — 60° while the third is analyzed at once. All the specimens of feces are dried for 35 hours at 98° in drying oven.

---

[1] I wish here to acknowledge my indebtedness to the personel of this children's home, especially Miss HOLM, nurse, for her assistance in the collecting of this material, and to the Superintendant for her kind permission to carry out these studies in the children's home.

Table 4. Influence of Storage Temperature on the Fecal Contents.

Sample No.	I.			II.			III.		
Temp. of storage	fresh	+ 3° C	− 60° C	fresh	+ 3° C	− 60° C	fresh	+ 3° C	− 60° C
Hours » »	0	24	24	0	24	24	0	24	24
pH	5.9	5.6	6.1	6.4	6.6	6.8	6.9	6.6	6.9
Dry matter	8.3	7.9	7.7	17.3	17.5	17.4	16.6	16.6	18.8
Total fat	7.8	8.4	7.7	10.3	11.3	10.6	16.5	15.2	16.0
Reduc. elements	10.0	11.4	9.0	8.7	8.3	8.2	9.3	7.6	9.7
Nitrogen	6.0	6.5	5.7	5.5	5.5	5.4	5.9	6.0	5.5
Bacterial counts (in millions).									
Colon bacilli	1/100	1/100	1/10	1/100	1/100	1/10	1/0.01	1/0.01	1/0.01
Anaërobic bact.		800	80	100	200	100	60	200	3
Aërobic »	1 130	1 900	750	360	290	77	2.8	2	1

The chemical analysis shows no particular variation, whereas the bacterial counts show a distinct fall on storage at − 60° C.

From Table 4 it appears as if the different experimental conditions mentioned have caused no particular difference in the outcome of the analytical results. For it has to be kept in mind, too, that several samples taken from the same homogenized portion of feces as a rule will not turn out exactly alike. On the other hand, it has been stated that the fat content of the feces decreases on cold storage; but this appears not to be the case here.

As to the bacteriological examination there is a distinct fall in the number of bacteria on storage at $-60°$, and a slight rise on storage at $+3°$. On account of this finding, I now went on to place the feces on ice and to fetch as soon as possible the portion employed for the bacteriological examination and pH determination while the rest was placed in the drying oven. The specimen of feces evacuated in the following 24 hours was then obtained, dried and mixed in mortar with the rest of the earlier specimen. The total portion was used for the chemical analysis. In this way, the percentage of dry matter was determined several times for each child; and it is the average of these determinations that is recorded in Table 4. The same applies to the pH determination.

Owing to the difficulty in obtaining a sufficient number of healthy breast-fed children with mothers living under the same conditions, on some of these children I have repeated the examination at intervals of one to two months. One child was examined both as bottle-fed and spoon-fed (No. 32= No. 34), and one spoon-fed infant was examined twice (No. 1 = No. 25).

Dry Matter. The components and amount of the feces are largely dependant on the quality and quantity of food taken in. Still, the elements in the feces originate in part also from secretions of the digestive tract and from the bacterial flora. The amount of feces is less in breast-fed infants than in bottle-fed, as mother's milk is utilized better than cow's milk. The amount is generally reckoned to be about 3 g of feces per 100 g of mother's milk (about 13—20 g of feces

Table 5. Spoon-fed Infants.

No.	Name	Reg. No.	Age in months	Weight in g	Cod liver oil concentrate (Decamin)	Cod liver oil	Fruit juice	Iron	Colour	Consistency	Smell	Urine	Remarks
1=25	M. L.	1957	11	9 940	—	+	+	+	green-black	formed	flat	(+)	1)
2	J. R.	1988	13	9 330	—	+	+	+	greyish	mushy	slightly stinking	—	
3	B. K.	1974	11	10 050	—	+	+	+	grey-yellow	formed	flat	—	
4	L. G.	1989	9	9 230	—	—	+	+	greenish	formed	flat	—	
5	J. A.	1953	16	10 800	—	—	+	—	grey	formed	flat	—	
6	G. L.	1942	15	10 800	—	+	+	—	grey-black	formed	slightly stinking	—	
7	J. H.	1990	10	10 800	—	+	+	—	grey-green	loose	slightly stinking	(+)	
8	K. P.	1977	9	9 380	—	+	+	—	grey-yellow	formed	flat	—	
9	K. P.	1997	11	8 100	+	—	+	—	greenish	formed	slight smell	—	1)
10	J. A.	1968	12	8 300	—	—	+	—	green-yellow	formed	slightly stinking	(+)	
20	D. H.	/	16	/	—	+	—	—	grey-brown	formed	flat	—	
25=1	M. L.	1957	13	10 600	—	+	—	—	grey-brown	formed	flat	—	
34	G. V.	2049	6	6 450	—	+	+	+	grey-black	formed	flat	—	2)

The diet has been the same for all these infants, consisting in bread-soup (whole rye bread), mashed potatoes, carrots, spinach, sago gruel and milk.

The vitamin A and D supplement is given as cod liver oil (5 g × 2) or cod liver oil concentrate (Decamin fortior) (gtt. 5 × 2).

Vitamin C is given in the form of juice, g 5 × 2 (orange juice, lemon, or tomato, depending on the season).

Iron is given as ferrous tartrate ctg 25 × 2.

1) In 2'mth., lact. acid for 3 weeks.

2) Examined also as bottle-fed (No. 32, Table 6).

daily) and about 5 g per 100 g of cow's milk (about 30—40 g of feces daily).

In the studies here reported, the total amount of fecal output in proportion to the intake of food was determined only in one experiment and here it was found to fall considerably below the cited figures. On the whole, it was my impression that the amount of fecal output of breast-fed children was distinctly less, as it was rather difficult to obtain sufficient amount of feces for these studies.

The average of the dry matter per cents shows no particular variation. As was to be expected from the consistency of the feces, it is lowest for spoon-fed children. The values here obtained correspond fairly well to those given by BAUMANN (20—34 % dry matter). All the chemical analyses are carried out on the dry matter. It may be that the dry matter percentage is somewhat too high. The feces have been scraped off from the diaper as soon as possible, but, in view of the fact that the subjects in these studies are healthy infants living in a children's home, it was considered unsafe to employ any oil-cloth inside the diaper as this may readily give rise to irritation of the skin on the buttocks.

Methods have been given, it is true, also for fat determination on native feces. But, by employing such methods, one would be deprived any real basis for comparison between the different groups, as the water content of the feces is subject to considerable variation. The percental content of the components assayed here may often be very high — as is evident from some of the experiments recorded — but from the balance experiments it will be seen that the loss of energy for the organism must be said to be minimal. In the last-mentioned experiment this loss amounted only to 1.2 % of the ingested amount for the fat, and 0.3 % for carbohydrates. Furthermore, the fats found in feces do not all originate from the food intake, a part of them comes from the gastro-intestinal secretion.

I his »Chemical Methods in Clinical Medicin», HARRISON (1937) states that the total fat content of the feces gives an

Table 6. Bottle-fed Infants.

The cow's milk is diluted with barley water. The vitamin and iron supplement is given as mentioned under Table 5.

No.	Name	Reg. No.	Age in months	Weight in g	Milk %	Milk mixture	Cod liver oil concentrate (Decamin)	Cod liver oil	Fruit juice	Iron	Colour	Consistency	Smell	Urine	Remarks
11	B. A.	2013	3 1/2	6 200	75	200×5	+	—	+	—	yellow-brown	crumpling	flat	(+)	[1]
14	G. P.	2019	4	6 000	75	200×5	+	—	+	+	green-yellow	formed	flat	—	
16	T. K.	2010	4 1/2	6 130	75	200×5	+	—	+	+	grey-brown	homogeneous	flat	—	[2]
21	L. A.	2003	4	6 250	75	200×4	—	+	+	—	yellow-green	formed	flat	(+)	[2]
22	P. D.	2008	4	6 580	75	200×5	—	+	+	—	green-yellow	formed	flat	—	[2]
23	B. S.	2035	3 1/2	5 390	75	125×5	+	—	+	+	green-yellow	formed	flat	(+)	[3]
24	N.	2030	1 1/2	4 190	60	150×6	+	—	+	—	yellow	formed	sour	—	[4]
29	B. P.	2041	4	6 070	75	200×5	—	+	+	—	yellow	firm	flat	—	
30	M. N.	2038	5	5 650	75	200×5	—	+	+	+	green-yellow	formed	flat	—	[5]
31	V. H.	2040	4	6 220	75	175×5	—	+	+	—	grey-yellow	formed	flat	—	
32	G. V.	2049	5	6 000	75	175×5	—	+	+	—	yellow	formed	flat	—	
33	H.	2059	1	3 660	50	120×6	+	—	—	—	yellow	formed	flat	—	

[1]) In 3'mth., lact. acid for 3 weeks. [2]) In 4'mth., lact. acid for 5 days. [3]) In 3'mth., lact. acid for 3 days. [4]) In 2'mth., lact. acid for 11 days. [5]) In 4'mth., lact. acid for 3 weeks.

expression for the absorption of the fats, while the amount of unsplit fat (neutral fat, sterols, pigments, etc.) indicates the effectiveness of the fat digestion. Previous fat analyses have shown considerably lower values than obtained with more recent methods, owing to defects in the earlier methods — something that was realized also by the earlier investigators. Thus, BIEDERT (1900) found 10—20 % fat in the feces of breast-fed infants, and UFFELMANN found it to be 14—25 %; still, HECHT (1910) thought that these figures were about 10 % too low. It seems reasonable to assume that the modern methods give a practically complete extraction of the fat (99 %, according to HOLT). The most recent comprehensive investigation of this kind has been carried out by HOLT, COURTNEY & FALE, and it is cited in the above-mentioned book by HARRISON. Fat analyses were carried out on 44, 94 and 62 specimens of feces from breast-fed, bottle-fed and spoon-fed infants respectively. The averages (34.5—34.1—18.7) correspond very well to my figures: 36.7—37.2—18.8 per cent total fat. In both investigations the maximum and minimum values deviate markedly from the average, so that it will be proper to insist upon the presence of 70 % fat in any random specimen of feces in order to be able with certainty to designate it as pathological.

Previous analyses with fractionated determinations stated that the fat consisted chiefly in neutral fat, but even SCHMIDT & STRASSBURGER (1915) suggested that the reverse may be the case, and in 1937, HARRISON asserted that the amount of unsplit fat (neutral fat) must not exceed one-third of the total fat content. As mentioned, the trichlor ethylene extraction does not correspond hereto, but a more thorough investigation appears to show that the American requirement is correct. So, the fractionated trichlor ethylene extraction method has to be given up as unsuitable. The analyses carried out subsequently by the present writer after the HOLT, COURTNEY & FALE method have given figures that agree very well with the American.

Table 7. Breast-fed Infants.

The diet consisted exclusively in mother's milk. Vitamin supplement and iron given as mentioned in Table 5.

No.	Name	Reg. No.	Age in months	Weight in g	Cod liver oil concentrate	Cod liver oil	Fruit juice	Iron	Colour	Con-sistency	Smell	Remarks
12	E. P.	2018	4	1 056	+	−	+	−	yellow	ointment	sour	
13	T. R.	2005	3	4 800	−	+	+	−	greenish	lose	sour	
17	J. R.	2037	3	4 600	+	−	+	−	yellow-green	ointment	sour	
18=12	E. P.	2018	$5^1/_2$	7 500	−	+	+	−	yellow	ointment	sour	
19	F. P.	2027	2	4 810	−	+	+	−	green-yellow	ointment	sour	
27=17	J. R.	2037	5	6 000	−	+	+	−	yellow	ointment	sour	
28	E. H.	2034	2	4 350	+	−	+	−	yellow-green	ointment	sour	
35	B. R.	2060	2	4 000	+	−	+	−	yellow-green	ointment	sour	
36	P. T.	2042	5	6 750	−	+	+	−	brown	pasty	flat	
37	L. N.	2071	$^1/_2$	2 900	+	−	+	−	green-yellow	ointment	sour	
38	M. J.	2055	3	6 900	−	+	+	−	green-yellow	granular	sour	
39	G. AA. L.	2062	2	4 200	−	+	+	+	green-black	pasty	slightly stinking	[1]
40=35	B. R.	2060	3	4 600	−	+	+	−	yellow	ointment	sour	

[1]) Prev. on mixed diet. Since $^{26}/_{11}$ on mother's milk excl.; examined in middle of December.

Carbohydrates. Sugars, that is, mono- or disaccharids, have never been demonstrated in the feces, although a single investigator (Blauberg) thinks he has found a trace. In the studies here reported, an attempt was made to demonstrate the presence of reducing elements in the extract after boiling with distilled water for $1^1/_2$ hours, it being fully realized that also substances other than sugars might give evidence of their presence (*e.g.*, protein split products). No demonstrable amounts of such elements were found, however.

After boiling with 2 % hydrochloric acid for $1^1/_2$ hours, for determination of the so-called starch reaction, a peculiar finding was noted. The amount of reducing elements calculated as glucose was found in the breast-fed infants to average 7.6 %, in the bottle-fed, 2 %, and in the spoon-fed, 15.6 %. That the percentage is greatest in spoon-fed children is obvious, as the more varying diet, including cereals, potatoes and vegetables, naturally will give reducing elements in the feces. But in children living entirely on mother's milk or on diluted cow's milk with an addition of glucose, one would not a priori expect to find starch or other higher sugars in the feces. Mucin is able to reduce Fehling's solution, but apparently it was not present in these feces from perfectly healthy children. Possibly bile pigments, which likewise are able to reduce Fehling's solution, were the cause of this finding, but the distinct and recurrent difference in breast-fed and bottle-fed infants is difficult to explain. Experiments to elucidate this question are being continued now, because, as far as I have been able to find out, no similar studies have yet been reported.

Nitrogen. The nitrogen determinations carried out here show no marked difference between the three groups. The figures are less variable than might be expected on account of the diverse origin of the nitrogen in the feces (food elements, bacteria, secretions). Perhaps some ammonia may be lost in the drying process (Van Slyke) so that the values recorded here are somewhat to low; but some investigators (*e. g.*, Harrison) claim that this loss is so small as to be insignificant.

Table 8. Examination of Feces from the Same Child on Milk Mixture and on Mixed Diet (No. 32 = 34), and from four Children receiving same diet but at different ages.

No.	Bottle 32 =	Breast 35	Breast 40 =	Spon 34	Breast 12 =	Breast 18	Breast 17 =	Breast 27	Spoon 1 =	Spoon 25
Age in months	5	2	3	6	4	$5^1/_2$	3	5	11	13
Stored at	+5°	+5°	+5°	+5°	−60°	−60°	--60°	+5°	+5°	+5°
For hours	10	2	2	2	72	72	72	3	1	2
pH	8.1	5.14	5.56	8.5	5.01	5.6	6.0	5.4	7.2	6.33
Dry matter	20.5	26.5	21.5	22.2	17.6	15.9	13.3	26.6	20.1	17.1
Total fat	18.1	43.1	35.3	9.5	37.0	25.0	31.0	53.0	9.3	8.8
Reducing elements	0.4	8.1	10.0	22.9	10.0	6.6	9.8	3.7	15.4	14.2
Nitrogen %		3.56	5.9	3.54	4.4	6.0	4.7	3.2	4.7	4.3
The following figures are given in millions.										
Colon-aërogen.	1/1000	1/1000	1/100	1/1000	1/100	1/10000	1/10	1/100	1/10	1/1000
Anaërobic	2000	1000	6000	3000	1800	800	120	2000	300	1200
Aërobic	5200	219	1230	7360	260	260	120	6000	740	1300
Lactic acid bacilli	−	+ Ac.	+ Ac.	−	−	−	+	−	−	−
Cooci	+		+	+	+	+	+	+	+	+
Proteus	−	+	−	−	−	−	−	−	+	−
Special bacteria	−	−	−	−	−	−	−	−	−	−

The examination of the first child shows the great variation in the amount of fat and reducing elements on the two diets. There is only a slight variation in the results of the bacteriological examination. The examination of the other four children shows only slight chemical variation, whereas the bacteriological findings are more variable.

Reaction. According to EITEL, SCHMIDT tried as the first to determine the hydrogen ion concentration of infantile feces. Like the classical test on urine, this test too was made by tasting the feces, thus it was ascertained that the feces of breast-fed infants tasted sour. Meconium, on the other hand, tasted rather sweet. Most later investigators have employed the electrometrical method (*e. g.*, YLLPÖ as the first in 1916, and EITEL in 1917). TISDALL & BROWN, however, emphasize the colorimetrical method as easier and just as reliable — something that is suggested indeed by their comparative studies on the two methods.

It is well-known that as a rule the feces of breast-fed infants give an acid reaction, while the feces of bottle-fed infants are alcaline. Exceptions to this rule are encountered now and then, however. In my experiments a specimen of feces from a bottle-fed baby gave an acid reaction (pH = 6.4). Other authors have reported similar occasional findings, *e. g.*, BAUMANN who states that the reaction of feces from bottle-fed infants varies between pH 5.67 and pH 8.35. Most investigators, however, have found exclusively alcaline reactions of such feces (YLLPÖ, EITEL, TISDALL). All the feces of breast-fed infants gave an acid reaction, agreeing in this respect with the findings of other investigators. Still, FREUDENBERG & HELLER found a single healthy breast-fed baby with alcaline feces (pH 7.4). These investigators also found the reaction to vary but little from day to day (cited after LEPPO) while most authors have found considerable variations — as seen in my experiments too. The feces of spoon-fed children showed as a rule a reaction at the neutral point, but varying in either direction.

Bacteriology. Various authors have tried in different ways to estimate the total number of bacteria in the feces. Originally, for instance, an attempt was made to estimate the number of bacteria by inocculating culture media with suspensions of varying dilutions, by weighing of the bacterial mass (STRASSBURGER) or by direct count on dilute suspensions (ETERLE, HELLSTRÖM, and others). The results obtained with these

Table 9. Examination of Feces of 13 Spoon-fed Infants.

No.	1	2	3	4	5	6	7	8	9	10	20	25	34=32	Max.	Min.	Aver.
Age in months	11	13	11	9	16	15	10	9	11	12	16	13	6	16	6	11.6
Stored at	+5°	−60°	−60°	fresh	−60°	−60°	−60°	fresh	+5°	+5°	+5°	+5°	+5°			
For hours	1	1	1 1/2		2	3	2		3	2	2	2	2			
pH	7.2	7.6	7.8	7.3	8.6		8.1	7.5	6.8	7.2	8.5		8.5	8.6	6.8	7.73
Dry matter %	20.1	20.8	23.3	20.8	20.3	20.4	19.0	24.2	23.6	25.0	23.5	17.1	22.2	25.0	19.0	21.8
Total fat %	9.3	40.7	11.2	25.8	32.7	16.9	30.1	14.5	21.3	18.3	12.8	8.8	10.28	40.7	8.8	18.8
Reduc. elements %	15.4	8.3	18.0		7.5	14.8	14.8	18.8	14.0	13.0	10.0	14.2	22.9—26.7	26.7	7.5	15.8
Nitrogen %	4.7	3.9		4.4	3.4	3.6	4.7	3.8	3.8	3.9	3.5	4.3	3.54	4.7	3.4	3.96
The following figures are given in millions.																
Colon-aërogen.	1/10	1/1	1/10	1/10	1/1	1/1	1/1	1/100	1/10	1/10	1/1	1/1000	1/1000	1/1	1/1000	1/100
Anërobic	300	3	11	3100	25	1000	130	750	200	600	210	1200	3000	3100	3	612
Aërobic	740	5	49	349	1.3	100	60	1000	417	900	73	1300	7360	8000	5	1634
	1040	8	60	3449	26.3	1100	190	1750	617	1500	283	2500	10360	11100	8	2246
Lact. acid bacilli	—	—	—	—	+	+	+	—	+	—	—	—	—	+ in 40 %		
Cocci	+	+	+	+	+	+	+	+	+	+	+	+	+	+ » 100 %		
Proteus	+	—	—	—	—	—	—	—	—	—	—	—	—	+ » 10 %		
Special bacteria	—	—	—	—	—	—	—	—	—	—	—	—	—	+ » 0 %		

methods could be only rough and approximate estimates, on account of the uneven distribution of the bacteria in the feces. In some studies by MEJLBO & PLUM, not yet published, the cultivation method has been further elaborated — but, of course, it can give an expression only for the number of viable bacteria present in the feces. This method was employed also in the studies here presented, and the culture media employed were picked out with a view to an equal growth of the various bacterial species present in the feces.

Opinions differ as to whether the bacterial flora in the feces of breast-fed children consists mostly of Bact. Bifidum or Lactobacillus acidophilus. In the present studies no differentiation is made between these two species; they are simply reckoned under the lactic acid group. Nor has any differential count been made on the different bacterial species, as this will be presented in the above-mentioned work by MEJLBO & PLUM; but I have looked into how often bacteria of the lactic acid group, Proteus bacilli, so-called »pathogenic intestinal bacteria» (typhoid, paratyphoid, dysentery) and micrococci could be demonstrated in the feces.

The large amount of bacteria of the colon-aërogenes group, which the colon titer is an expression for, is a striking finding in the breast-fed infants, being greater here than in the bottle-fed and spoon-fed infants. But the material is too small to allow of any definite conclusions. In the aforementioned work of MEJLBO, NYGART & PLUM the findings were different, however, as here the feces of the breast-fed infants showed a numerically preponderant flora of Gram-positive lactid acid bacteria (acidophilus, bifidum, streptococci). As the children in the present material are somewhat older, however, it may be that the apparently conflicting findings may still be compatible.

The greatest total number of bacteria was found in the feces of bottle-fed infants, while the difference between breast-fed and spoon-fed was only slight in this respect. In previous investigations, pathogenic intestinal bacteria have sometimes been found in healthy children (WOLLSTEIN, for instance,

Table 10. Examination of Feces from 12 Infants on Milk-mixture.

Nos. 22, 23 and 24 are not included in the calculation of the bacterial averages.

No.	11	14	16	21	22	23	24	29	30	31	32=34	33	Max.	Min.	Aver.
Age in months	$3^1/_2$	4	$4^1/_2$	4	4	$3^1/_2$	$1^1/_2$	4	5	4	5	1	5	1	3.7
Stored at	−60°	−60°	−60°	−60°	−60°	−60°	−60°	+5°	+5°	+5°	+5°	+5°			
For hours	2	$1^1/_2$	6	12	72	72	72	10	20	10	10	10			
pH	8.2	7.74	7.6	7.9	8.4	7.9	6.5	7.6	8.7	8.5	8.1	8.4	8.7	6.5	7.91
Dry matter %	36.4	22.5	22.6	21.0	20.7	28.7	25.5	23.6	25.0	25—27 26	22.5—18.5 20.5	21.6—23.9 22.8	36.4	18.5	24.6
Total fat %	30.4	51.0	52.0	37.0	9.3	43.8	57.0	14.2	53.7	57.3	18.1	16.4	57.3	16.4	37.2
Reduc. elements %	3.2	3.0	2.7	4.0	2.1	2.0	1.6	1.5	1.0	1.5	0.4	1.1	4.0	0.4	2.0
Nitrogen %	2.9	4.8	3.2	3.2	3.5	3.6	3.0	3.0	3.2	2.7		2.9	4.8	2.7	3.3
The following figures are given in millions.															
Colon-aërogen. titer	1/1	1/10	1/100	1/10	1/10	1/10	1/10	1/100	1/10	1/100	1/1000	1/1000	1/1	1/1000	1/259
Anaërobic	40	519	20	1000	1	500	3000	7900	300	3000	2000	6000	7900	20	2308
Aërobic	80	960	29	380	34	159	2570	8000	249	10000	5200	1250	10000	29	2002
	120	1470	49	1380	35	659	5570	15900	519	13000	7200	7250	17900	49	4310
Lactic acid bacilli	+	—	—	—	—	—	—	—	—	—	—	—	+ in ca. 9 %		
Cocci	+	+	+	+	+	+	+	+	+	+	+	+	+ » 100 %		
Proteus	+	+	—	—	+	+	—	—	—	—	—	—	+ » ca. 33 %		
Special bacteria	—	—	—	—	—	—	—	—	—	—	—	—	— » 100 %		

Table 11. Examination of Fece

Nos. 12, 18, 13, 17 and 19 are not included in the calculation

No.	12	18	13	17	27	15	19	28
Age in months .	4	$5^1/_2$	3	3	5	3	2	2
Stored at	−60°	−60°	−60°	−60°	+5°	fresh	−60°	+5°
For hours	72	72	72	72	3		72	1
pH	5.01	5.6	5.2	6.0	5.4	4.8	6.3	5.3
Dry matter % . .	17.6	15.9	33.7	13.3	26–26–28 26.3	17.2	31.1	21–22–2 22.3
Total fat % . . .	37.0	25.0	29.7	31.4	53.0	26.0		34.6
Reduc. elements %	10.0	6.6	7.2	9.8	3.7		4.3	10.0
Nitrogen % . . .	4.4	6.0	3.0	4.7	3.2	5.7	2.9	3.6

The following figur

Colon-aërogen. titer	1/100	1/10000	1/10	1/10	1/100	1/1		1/100
Anaërobic	1800	800	250	120	2000	16		2000
Aërobic	280	260	7	120	6000	73		149
	2080	1060	257	240	8000	89		2149
Lactic acid bacilli	−	−	+	+		+		
Cocci	+	+	+	+	+	+		+
Proteus	−	−	−	−	−	−		−
Special bacteria .	−	−	−	−	−	−		−
Colon								

found Shiga's dysentery bacillus in one case). The present studies reveal no pathogenic intestinal bacteria in the feces. Owing to the conditions mentioned above, the bacterial content of specimens of feces stored for a considerable length of time at − 60° is not reckoned within this account.

rom 14 Breast-fed Infants.

e bacterial averages because the storage temperature was too low.

35	36	37	38	39	40	Max.	Min.	Average
2	5	1/2	5	2	3	5.5	0.5	3.1
+5°	+5°	+5°	+5°	+5°	+5°			
2	2	2	2	2	2			
6/11—18/11 ?.14 4.89	6.48	18/11 22/11 4.9 5.96 2/12 6.39	4.94	5.79	5.56	6.39	4.89	5.5
26.8 26.2 26.5	30.1	21.7		24.9	21.5	33.7	15.9	23.2
43.1	46.1 45.4	35.5		47.8	35.3	53.0	26.0	36.7
8.7—8.1	5.5—4.96	11.4		6.6	10.0	11.4	3.7	7.6
3.56	5.5	3.6		—	5.9	6.0	2.9	4.3

e given in millions.

1/1000	1/1000	1/1	1/100	1/1	1/100	1/1	1/1000	1/270
1000	spr.	130	1300	11	6000	6000	11	1556
219	900	97	525	16	1230	6000	16	1023
1219		227	1825	27	7230	12000	27	2579
—	—	Bif: 30	Acid: +1000	—	Acid: +3000		+ in 50 %	
+	+	+100	+ 300	+11	+1000		+ » 100 %	
+	++	+	—	—	—		+ » 23 %	
—	—	—	—	—	—		— » 100 %	
					2000			

Summary.

In the present work, chemical and bacteriological studies were carried out on the feces of 39 healthy infants, 13 of whom were given a mixed diet, while 12 were given a milk mixture, and 14 received mother's milk; the average age of the infants in these three groups was respectively 11.6 months, 3.6 months, and 3.1 months.

Chemical Studies: The pH of the feces was found on an average to be 5.5 in the breast-fed infants, 7.91 in the bottle-fed, and 7.73 in the spoon-fed. The dry matter content was nearly the same for the three groups: 23.3, 24.6, and 21.8 %. The total fat content was not found to differ greatly in the breast-fed infants and the bottle-fed, but it was considerably lower in the spoon-fed. A distinct difference was found in the amount of reducing elements, this being smallest in bottle-fed infants (2 %), highest in the spoon-fed (15 %), and intermediate in the breast-fed (7 %).

The nitrogen content showed no particular variation.

The total fat content did not differ to any particular extent in breast-fed and bottle-fed children, being here respectively 36.7 % and 37.2 %, but it was found to be considerably lower in spoon-fed children (18.8 %).

In some cases (7) fractionated fat determination was performed after the method of HOLT, COURTNEY & FALE, which showed that by far the greater portion of the fat in the feces consists in split fats (acids and soaps) and only a small part of unsplit fat (neutral fat, etc.).

Bacteriological Studies: With the technique here employed the total number of bacteria per gram of feces was found to be highest in bottle-fed infants (5 214 millions), and not particularly different in spoon-fed infants (2 246 millions) and in breast-fed (2 579 millions). Lactic acid bacilli were found most often in breast-fed infants, more infrequently in bottle-fed. A colon titer was of about the same magnitude, although somewhat lower in spoon-fed infants than in breast-fed and bottle-fed.

Gram-positive micrococci were found on every examination in all three groups.

Pathogenic intestinal bacteria were not demonstrated in any instance.

Table 12. Summarizing Table of the Averages of the Examinations of Feces 14 Breast-fed, 12 Bottle-fed and 13 Spoon-fed Infants.

	Breast-fed Infants			Bottle-fed Infants			Spoon-fed Infants		
	Max.	Min.	Aver.	Max.	Min.	Aver.	Max.	Min.	Aver.
Age in months	5.5	0.5	3.1	5.0	1.0	3.7	15.0	6.0	11.6
pH	5.39	4.89	5 5	8.7	6.4	7.91	8.6	6.8	7.73
Dry matter %	33.7	15.9	23.0	36.4	18.5	24.6	25.0	19.0	21.8
Total fat %	53.0	26.0	36.7	57.3	16.4	37.2	49.7	8.8	18.8
Reducing elements %	11.4	3.7	7.6	4.0	0.4	2.0	26.7	7.5	15.8
Nitrogen %	6.0	2.9	4.3	4.8	2.7	3.3	4.7	3.4	3.96
The following figures are given in millions.									
Colon-aërogen. titer	1/1	1/1000	1/270	1/1	1/1000	1/259	1/1	1/1000	1/100
Anaërob. and facult. aërobic	6000	11	1556	7900	20	2308	3100	3	612
Aërobic	6000	16	1023	10000	29	2906	8000	5	1634
	12000	27	2579	17900	49	5214	11100	8	2246
Lactic acid bacilli	+ in 50 %			+ in 9 %			+ in 40 %		
Cocci	+ » 100 %			+ » 100 %			+ » 100 %		
Proteus	+ » 23 %			+ » 33 %			+ » 10 %		
Special pathogen. bacteria	— » 100 %			— » 100 %			— » 100 %		

In one experiment *the fat and carbohydrate (reducing elements) balance* was examined in a breast-fed infant, aged 3 months, weighing 4 800 g. The daily output with the feces was 1.2 % fat of the amount ingested within the same period (29.55 g) and 0.3 % reducing elements of the ingested amount of carbohydrate (36.23 g).

In conclusion I wish to acknowledge my indebtedness to Drs. MEJLBO and WINTHER, veterinary surgeons and to Dr. med. P. PLUM for their kind advices and suggestions in the planning and performance of these studies.

References.

1. BAUMANN: Monatschr. f. Kinderheilk. 1934. 60. 81. — 2. BLAUBERG: Experimentelle und kritische Studien über Säuglingsfaeces. Berlin 87. — 3. CHRISTIANSEN, M.: Bakt. af Tyfus-Coligruppen. D. Kgl. Danske Vidensk. Selskl. Skrift. Naturv. og matem. Afd. 8 Række, 1—3. — 4. DOLENCOURT et LAVUDON: Le Nourisson 19. 147 (1931). — 5. EITEL: Zeitschr. f. Kinderheilk. 1917—16—13. — 6. FRIEDBERGER u. PFEIFFER: Lehrbuche der Mikrobiologie. Jena 1919. — 7. FROST and HANKINSON: Lactobacillus acidophilus. Dawis Green Corp. Milton. U. S. A. — 8. HAWK and BERGEIN: Practical physiological Chemistry. New York 1937. — 9. HARRISON: Chemical Methods in clinical Medicin. London 1937. — 10. HECHT: Die Faeces des Säuglings u. Kindes. Berlin—Wien. 1910. — 11. HEUPKE: Die Faeces des Mennschen. 1939. Dresden—Leipzig. — 12. HOLT, COURTNEY and FALE: Am. J. Dis. Child. 1919. 17: 38—241—423 og 18:107—157. — 13. KORDATZKI: Taschenbuch der praktischen pH=Messung. München 1934. — 14. LEPPO: Act. pæd. Sc. Vol. XXVIII. Suppl. II. 1940. — 15. LUNDING: Act. med. Sc. 1928. 68. 97. — 16. MEJLBO, NYGART og PLUM: Ugeskr. f. Lg. 41. 6. 187. — 17. MEJLBO og NYGART: Nord. Med. 1939. 3. 2383. — 18. ORLA-JENSEN, S., ORLA-JENSEN, H. B. og WINTHER, O.: Zentralbl. f. Bakt. II 1936. 93, 321—343. — 19. ORLA-JENSEN, S.: The Lactic acid. bacteria. D. Kgl. Danske Vidensk. Selsk. Skrift. Naturv. og matem. Afd. 8 Række. V 2. — 20. SCHMIDT und STRASSBURGER: Die Faeces des Mennchen. Berlin. 1915. — SLYKE, V. and PETER: Quantitative clinical Chemistry. London 1937. — 22. SEMERDIEW: Zeitschr. f. Untersuch. d. Lebensmittel. Marts 1940. — 23. TISDALL and BROWN: Am. J. Dis. Child. 1924. 27, 312. — 24. TIDWELL and HOLT: J. Biol. Chemistry. 1936. 112, 605. — 25. YLLPÖ: Zeitschr. f. Kinderheilk. 1916—14—268.

AUS DEM KINDERKRANKENHAUS SAMARITEN, STOCKHOLM.

Erfahrungen bei der Rachitisprophylaxe frühgeborener Kinder.

II: Die Schutzdosis von Vitamin D_3 für Kinder mit einem Geburtsgewicht bis 2 000 g.

Von

NILS MALMBERG.

In meiner vorangehenden Arbeit mit obigem Titel (Acta Pædiatrica, Vol. XXIV, 1939) war darauf hingewiesen worden, dass die prophylaktische Behandlung gegen Rachitis möglichst bald nach der Geburt eingeleitet werden soll, am besten in der zweiten Hälfte der ersten Lebenswoche. Ferner hatte die Untersuchung ergeben, dass es nicht einmal bei so frühzeitig einsetzender Prophylaxe möglich war, durch Zufuhr von 2 700 I. E. D_3 pro die vorzeitig geborene Kinder mit einem Geburtsgewicht unter 2 000 g gänzlich vor röntgenologischen Rachitissymptomen zu schützen.

Diese Resultate standen mit den Erfahrungen anderer Untersucher, beispielsweise denjenigen von DAVIDSON[1] und Mitarbeitern in Amerika 1934 und 1936, im Einklang.

Damals war eine neue Untersuchungsserie in Aussicht gestellt worden, um zu prüfen, ob eine grössere D-Vitaminzufuhr bessere Resultate liefern könnte.

Zunächst wurde die Dosis auf das Doppelte der früheren, d. h. auf 5 400 I. E. pro die, gesteigert, welche in Perioden von 4—5 Wochen mit zweiwöchigen Intervallen gegeben wurden.

---

[1] Am. J. Dis. Childr., Bd. 48, 1934; ibid., Bd. 51, 1936.

Sehr bald fand ich indessen, dass auch bei dieser Dosierung röntgenologisch, freilich leichte, Rachitissymptome auftraten, weshalb ich zu dem Präparat D-Vimin der Astra-AG. in Södertälje überging, von dem 20 Tropfen, 10 000 I. E. D_3 entsprechend, pro die verabreicht wurden.

Die prophylaktische Behandlung wurde in dieser neuen Serie am 4.—7. Lebenstage eingeleitet. So erhielten gewisse der Kinder am ersten Dosierungstage 2 gtt., jeden Tag um 2 gtt. bis 20 gtt. steigend, womit fortgefahren wurde; bei anderen betrug die Anfangsdosis 5 gtt., mit täglicher Zulage von 5 gtt. bis zur Volldosis von 20 gtt. — Auf diese Weise ging ich zuwege, um die individuelle Toleranz der Kinder für das Präparat zu prüfen. Irgendwelche dyspeptischen oder sonstigen Symptome, welche eine Abweichung von dem Dosierungsschema veranlasst hätten, traten nicht auf. Die Kinder bekamen während der ersten Monate im allgemeinen Muttermilch oder Allaitement mixte mit Zulage von Citridomilch. — Röntgenuntersuchungen der Rippenknochenknorpelgrenzen, Hand- und Fussgelenke wurden mit 2—4, in späteren Lebensmonaten ca. 4—6 Wochen Abstand vorgenommen. In der oben zitierten Arbeit habe ich gemeinsam mit F. Knutsson die Bedeutung der Untersuchung der Rippenknochenknorpelgrenzen nachgewiesen; einmal waren Erscheinungen von Rachitis dort eher zu finden als an den Hand- und Fussgelenken, sodann können sich die röntgenologisch feststellbaren Rachitissymptome hinsichtlich ihrer Lokalisation auf die Rippenknorpelenden beschränken.

Die Serie enthält 22 Kinder, von welchen 4 ein Geburtsgewicht unter 1 500 g und 18 ein solches bis 2 000 g hatten. — Die untersuchten Fälle sind in der beigefügten Tabelle, nach dem Geburtsgewicht geordnet, zusammengestellt. Aus der Tabelle wird auch die Länge der Beobachtungszeit in Monaten ersichtlich, ferner die Wirkung der prophylaktischen Behandlung in bezug auf röntgenologische Rachitissymptome. Die Beobachtungsdauer beträgt bei 19 der Fälle 6—10 Monate; nur in 3 Fällen ist sie 3 ½ bzw. 5 und 5 Monate. Da bekannt ist, dass Rachitissymptome bei unbehandelten debilen Kindern schon während des ersten Lebensvierteljahrs auftreten, dürften auch die letzteren Beobachtungszeiten als hinreichend erachtet werden können.

Prophylaktisch behandelte frühgeborene Kinder.

20 gtt. D-Vimin = 10 000 I. E. D_3 pro die vom 4.—7. Lebenstage an.

Geburtsgewicht	Beobachtungszeit in Monaten	Röntgenologische Symptome (Rippen, Hand- und Fussgelenke)
1 150	8	0
1 200	9 1/2	0
1 250	8	0 (Spuren? an Rippen und Ulna, von kurzem Bestand)
1 450	10	0
1 580	3 1/2	0
1 600	10	0
1 640	5	0
1 650	8	0
1 660	7	0
1 700	8	0
1 710	8	0
1 770	5	0
1 780	6 1/2	0
1 790	8	minimale Rippensymptome von kurzem Bestand
1 860	8 1/2	0
1 880	6	0
1 930	7 1/2	0
1 930	9 1/2	0
1 950	6 1/2	0
1 960	8 1/2	0
1 970	8 1/2	0
2 000	6	0

4 Fälle 1 001—1 500 g
18 » 1 501—2 000 g

Wie aus der Tabelle hervorgeht, liessen sich nur in einem Fall ganz leichte, aber eindeutige röntgenologische Rachitiserscheinungen nachweisen; ein Kind mit einem Geburtsgewicht von 1 790 g bekam im Alter von 2 Monaten minimale Symptome kurzer Dauer am Thorax, dagegen keinerlei Erscheinungen an Hand- und Fussgelenken. — In einem anderen Fall, bei einem Kinde mit einem Geburtsgewicht von 1 250 g, war es im Alter von 3—3 1/2 Monaten zweifelhaft, ob die Bilder der Rippenknochenknorpelgrenzen und der Ulna als pathologisch zu bezeichnen wären.

Bei den übrigen 20 Fällen von 22 fehlt trotz dicht aufeinanderfolgender Untersuchungen jede Spur röntgenologisch wahrnehmbarer Erscheinungen seitens der Rippen, Hand- und Fussgelenke.

Auf die Frage des Wesens der periostalen Auflagerungen, meistens an der Tibia, bisweilen aber auch an anderen Röhrenknochen, hoffe ich bei späterer Gelegenheit zurückkommen zu können.

Von den 22 Kindern mit einem Geburtsgewicht bis 2 000 g in der vorigen Serie, welche 2 700 I. E. pro die erhalten hatten, wiesen nicht weniger als 13 Anzeichen von Rachitis auf. In der oben vorgelegten Reihe mit Zufuhr von 10 000 I. E. liess dagegen nur 1 Kind von 22 minimalste Symptome von kurzem Bestand erkennen, welche sich bei der üblichen Untersuchung von lediglich Hand- und Fussgelenken der Entdeckung entzogen hätten.

Eine Dosierung von 5 400 I. E. erwies sich als ungenügend.

Zusammenfassend dürfte man also auf Grund der vorliegenden Untersuchung sagen können, dass man mit einer Dosierung von 10 000 I. E. D_3 pro die, periodenweise von der zweiten Hälfte der ersten Lebenswoche an gegeben, bei Kindern mit einem Geburtsgewicht bis 2 000 g praktisch sämtliche derartigen Kinder vor gewöhnlichen, auch leichtesten Formen von röntgenologischen Rachitissymptomen an den Rippenknochenknorpelgrenzen, Hand- und Fussgelenken zu schützen imstande ist.

Diese Untersuchungen scheinen mir also dafür zu sprechen, dass bei kontinuierlicher, von kürzeren Perioden ohne D-Zufuhr unterbrochener Behandlung der Bedarf an D-Vitamin in Form von D_3 zur Prophylaxe bei frühgeborenen Kindern mit einem Geburtsgewicht bis 2 000 g bei ungefähr 10 000 I. E., womöglich etwas niedriger, aber jedenfalls über 6 000 I. E. liegt.

FROM THE MEDICAL DEPARTMENT OF THE HOSPITAL FOR CHILDRENS DISEASES, GOTHENBURG, SWEDEN.

The Neonatal Mortality in Sweden, from a Pediatric Point of View.

By

ARVID WALLGREN, M. D.

The infant mortality in Sweden has shown, broadly speaking, a continuous fall from 20—22 per cent in the middle of the eighteenth century and 15 per cent 100 years later to 3.9 per cent in the year 1940. This fall has not been equally pronounced in all periods of the first year of life. The earliest available statistical data capable of shedding light on this question are from the years 1860—1866, the rates of which for deaths during the first year of life were studied and worked up by the professor of pediatrics and statistician FREDRIC THEODOR BERG. A comparison between the rates then and now shows that the decline in mortality is least pronounced during the first period of infant life. (Table 1.)

Table 1.

Decline in mortality at different months of age in the first year of life from 1860/66 — 1932/38.

Months	1	2	3	4	5	6	7	8	9	10	11	12
1860—66	47.0	15.8	12.9	10.3	8.2	6.6	6.2	5.5	5.5	5.1	4.8	4.9
1932—38	25.2	3.9	3.2	2.6	2.0	1.8	1.7	1.5	1.4	1.3	1.3	1.0
Fall in %	*86*	*305*	*303*	*296*	*310*	*267*	*265*	*267*	*293*	*292*	*269*	*390*

This is so much the more significant as the mortality is quite especially high during the first period of life — the younger the infant the higher is the mortality, so it was earlier and so it still remains. It is this both relatively and absolutely high mortality during the first period of life that is designated »neonatal mortality» (the Frühsterblichkeit of

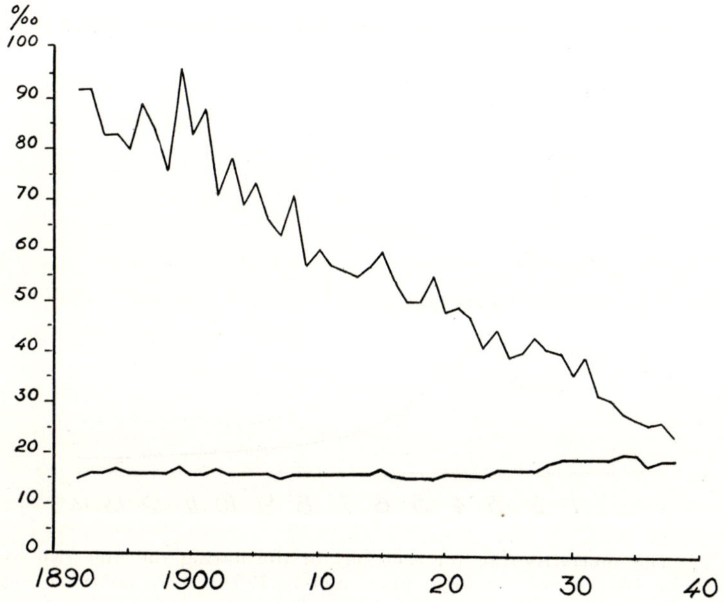

Fig. 1. Infant mortality in Sweden 1891—1935.

Lower curve = Neonatal mortality.
Upper curve = Post-Neonatal infant mortality.

the Germans, mortalité précoce of the French). This term has been given somewhat different interpretations, having been employed by different investigators to cover deaths during periods varying from the first three (von Pfaundler) to the first thirty (Cruickshank) days of life. As the majority interpret early mortality to mean deaths during the first week of life, the term »neonatal mortality» will be employed here in that sense.

Since 1891 Swedish official statistics have recorded the number of infant deaths for each day of life during the first month of life as well as for each month of life during the first year of life. These data have been studied by me in different ways and put into relation with the number of live children of the same period of age. In Fig. 1 the upper curve represents the post-neonatal mortality during the first year of life, the lower curve the neonatal mortality. The two

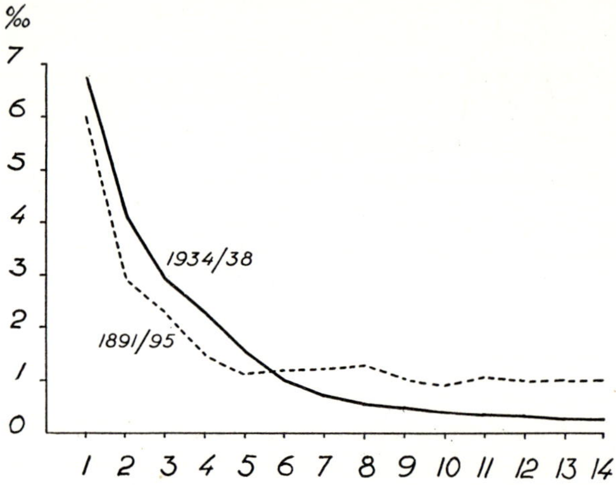

Fig. 2. The mortality-rate for each day of life during the first two weeks of life in 1891—1895 (broken curve) and in 1934—1938 (unbroken curve).

curves run quite a different course. Whereas the post-neonatal mortality curve, like the curve for infant mortality in general, drops continuously, the neonatal remains at about the same level; there are remarkably small variations from year to year.

Towards the end of the curve the neonatal mortality even shows a certain tendency to rise. This deterioration is very noticeable if a five-year period at the beginning of the curve is compared with a five-year period at its end. In Fig. 2 the unbroken curve represents the neonatal mortality for 1934—1938, the broken curve that for 1891—1895. It will be seen that the former has a higher course during the five first days of life, whereupon the curves cross and from and including the sixth day the curve for 1934—1938 is lower throughout. The difference between the neonatal mortalities shown by these five-year periods separated by fifty years is rather considerable. The percentage increase in mortality during the five first days of life is reflected in the figures 11.9—54.5 per cent, and the decrease in mortality after the fifth day of life in the figures 14.3—70.5 per cent. That this increased mortality during the first few days of life is not a chance phenomenon is indicated by the fact that the same observation has been made in other countries and is an experience that with few exceptions is no doubt fairly universal. Only the order of magnitude and the time of the transition from increaso to decrease of mortality varies.

This deterioration in the chances of survival for new-born children has quite naturally aroused serious apprehensions and has been the subject of keen debate, especially in pediatric and obstetric circles. The subject has been discussed at national and international conferences. The Health Section of the League of Nations has instituted an expert investigation into infant mortality, in which the neonatal mortality also received consideration, and articles on the subject appear at certain intervals in the medical periodicals. The question that presented itself was: what is the reason that early mortality has been so refractory to those economic, social-hygienic and psychological factors which have brought about the marked decline in mortality during the rest of the first year of life. No satisfactory explanation of this problem has been reached. This much seems certain, however, that the principal causes of death are not the same where neonatal infant mortality is concerned as where post-neonatal is concerned.

For the elucidation of the causes of neonatal mortality it is not without interest to study another group of deaths, viz. the stillborn. In Fig. 3 the upper curve represents the frequency of stillbirth during the last fifty years in Sweden, the lower curve represents the neonatal mortality. There is a remarkable agreement in the course of the two curves; stationary with a horizontal course at first, slow upward tendency towards the end. This similarity in the curves would appear to indicate that the causes of death are probably the same for the stillborn and the neonatal infants. Almost every statement referring to neonatal mortality in the following text will also apply to the mortinatality. The etiological agreement between mortinatality and neonatal mortality has induced some workers to combine these two groups of deaths under one head, perinatal mortality (v. PFAUNDLER). Some idea of the order of magnitude and the importance of this group, not least of all from the point of view of population, is obtained when one learns that the number of perinatal infant deaths

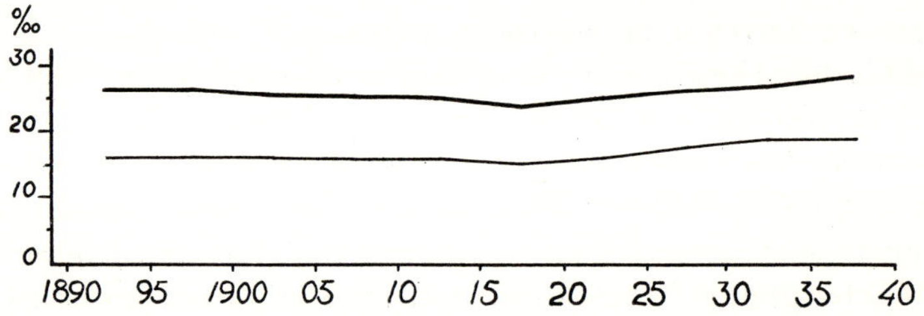

Fig. 3. Mortinatality (upper curve) and neonatal mortality (lower curve) in Sweden in 1891—1938.

is not unessentially higher than the number of infant deaths during the whole of the first years of life.

The causes of deaths occurring during the first week of life are not recorded separatedly in the Swedish official statistics. To get an idea of the causes of neonatal deaths it is therefore necessary to have recourse to the primary data sent in to the Statistical Central Bureau. Data collected in this way, however, would not be more than an approximate guide, as the causes of death recorded on the medical death certificates are, so far as the neonatal period is concerned, unreliable to quite a special degree, having as a rule been based, in the best cases, on clinical observation, in ordinary cases, on statements made by relatives or midwives. Often, the physician who issues the death certificate has not seen the child. When the nature of the disease causing death is not very obvious, the cause of death is doubtless classed as debilitas congenita, possibly as birth trauma. Especially debilitas congenita is undoubtedly often a diagnosis of convenience, and obviously need not mean that the children were premature at birth.

An example showing the need of caution when drawing conclusions from causes of death recorded on death certificates is a statement of BRODIN's that has reference to infant deaths in Gothenburg during the first two weeks of life. From the five-year period 1913—1917 to the five-year period 1933—1937 the infant deaths per thousand from debilitas congenita had diminished from 16.5 to 8.5, while the infant deaths per thousand from birth traumata and malformations during the same periods had increased from 0.67 and 0.88 respectively to 4.1 and 3.2 respectively. The other causes of death had kept at about the same level, 4.1 and 3.5 per thousand respectively. There can scarcely be any doubt that this change in the principal causes of death during the 25-year period concerned is more apparent than real and depends on increased knowledge of the significance of birth trauma and on more thorough examination and more frequent autopsies. It was during the period mentioned that YLPPÖS and SCHWARTZ's investigations caused attention to be focused upon birth trauma and its significance, and the great part this trauma plays as a cause of neonatal deaths has now received general recognition. This applies not only to the gross anatomical haemorrhages attending the trauma, but also and perhaps in a still higher degree to those necrotic changes and ganglion-cell degenerations which may be produced by even a transitory oxygen deprivation as a result of vasospasm, contusion, commotio, increase of intracranial pressure, or shock.

Obviously, the more thoroughly and expertly the examination of a deceased new-born child is carried out, the more accurately will the cause of death be established. Neither a subnormal weight nor a demonstrable congenital malformation should be accepted as cause of death unless a thorough post-mortem examination has ruled out other causes and it can be considered probable that the established disturbance was incompatible with life. A material of this character does not exist in Sweden. From some obstetric clinics records are available concerning causes of neonatal deaths at the clinic in question. Such death statistics, however, cannot be regarded as a norm for deaths in general during this period of age, since the indications for admission to an obstetric clinic obviously entail the collection there of complicated cases that must set their stamp on the causes of death during the neonatal period.

In order to arrive at a conception of the nature of those morbid states and disturbances which constitute causes of infant death during the first week of life a study may be made of the conditions in a rather large more or less self-contained community. As far as is possible an effort should then be made to ascertain from the doctors issuing the death certificates their reasons for classing the cause of death as they did. This has been done in Gothenburg since the year 1935. The resulting material comprises altogether 772 deaths, 436, or 55 per cent, of which occurred during the first week of life. The majority of the cases were submitted to post-mortem examination and most of the others were followed clinically and the disease causing death diagnosed during life.

The 436 neonatal deaths during the years 1935—1941 are distributed as follows (Fig. 4): Prematurity 47.2 per cent, birth traumata 24.7 per cent, malformations 13.8 per cent, infections 8.3 per cent, diseases typical of the neonatal period 5.5 per cent, and other diseases 0.5 per cent. Broadly viewed, therefore, it can be said that the neonatal mortality was mainly caused by disturbances that arose prior to birth (prematurity and malformations), less often during birth (birth traumata), and rarely after birth (infections and other diseases). The post-neonatal deaths in infancy are distributed as follows: infections 64.9 per cent, malformations 18.5 per cent, birth traumata 1.8 per cent, prematurity 4.8 per cent, diseases typical of newly born children 0.8 per cent, and other diseases 9.2 per cent. The post-neonatal infant mortality can thus be broadly considered to be mainly due to diseases arising after birth (infections and other diseases), less often prior to birth (prematurity and malformations), and rarely during birth (birth traumata).

It is evidently prematurity that determines the level of the neonatal mortality. The share premature children had in the number of infant deaths is greater than is indicated under the head prematurity as cause of death, as some fifty other of the infants that died were underdeveloped at birth although

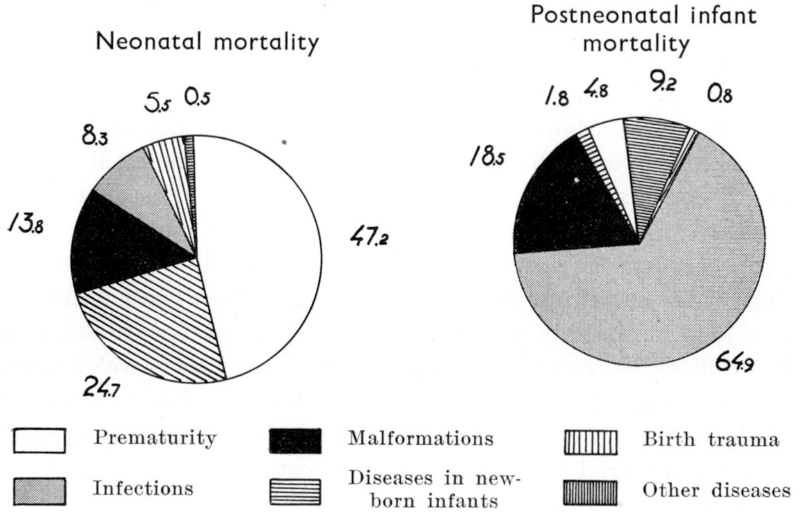

Fig. 4.

the immediate cause of death had been other than prematurity. A new-born infant that has attained a very unsatisfactory degree of maturity may die within a few minutes or hours without any other cause than prematurity. The less under-developed the infant is, the greater are its chances of survival, and other causes than prematurity are frequently responsible for its death. Then, however, it is necessary that such a cause of death should be verified anatomically and that it really can be assumed to be incompatible with life. These other causes are chiefly birth traumata and malformations, in a less degree also infections.

The three last-mentioned states of disease will not infrequently compete with prematurity as causes of death, and sometimes it may be impossible to decide whether the death has been caused by prematurity or by some other anomaly. Strictly speaking, it can be fairly immaterial whether the cause is prematurity as such or some other disease in a premature child, for prematurity in itself may be a predisposing factor to the origin of the diseases mentioned as well as of other morbid states. Disturbances associated with birth trauma take effect more especially in underdeveloped infants — premature infants have lowered capillary resistance (Ylppö) and consequently haemorrhages are more apt to arise, and their capillary system is undeveloped (Räihä) with the result that vascular injuries are more likely to be attended by a deficient supply of oxygen with degeneration of the ganglion cells as a consequence. Malformations, too, seem to occur more frequently in premature than in other infants, probably owing to the fact that certain malformations (e. g. hydrocephalus) are apt to cause premature delivery. The fact that premature children, in addition, possess less resistance to infections is well known. On account of all this it is often an expression of a purely subjective judgment which cause of death, prematurity or some other, is entered on the death certificate.

What has been said shows that it is scarcely possible to conceive of an essential improvement in the neonatal mortality without a marked reduction of premature births. In order to proceed rationally to that end the causes of premature birth must be elucidated. Unfortunately, our actual knowledge of the causes of prematurity is highly deficient. A lot of exogenous and endogenous factors are known, or believed to be known, which are considered capable of giving rise to subnormal weight, immaturity, and lowered viability. In most cases, however, the cause is unknown. There undoubtedly remains very much arduous research-work before we advance so far as we can reach with our present resources in the direction of elucidating the causes of prematurity. It would be an extremely valuable step towards combatting neonatal mortality and stillbirth if in each individual case of premature birth an effort was made to determine as far as possible the reason why pregnancy was terminated too early in that case. Competent, tactful and judicious investigation of the mother's state of health, home conditions and conduct during the whole course of pregnancy ought in many cases to give at least probable information as to the presence of any existing deleterious influences that may have induced the premature birth.

To prevent, discover and treat such conditions as may lead to premature birth, to ensure for the prospective mother such good conditions of life that she will not, through overexertion, privations of various kinds, or careless conduct, endanger her own health or the life of the fetus, or bring about a premature termination of her pregnancy, these are the things it is hoped the prenatal care centres in Sweden will accomplish. As yet, however, the influence this institution has had in these respects is scarcely discernible. It is still quite a new organization, it has as yet reached so few pregnant women, and, at any rate in many places, it is not managed with such enthusiasm for its object and in so rational a manner as would be desired. An awakening is here required in order that the prenatal care centres may achieve what we expect of them. Cursory routine must yield place to individual assistance given with zeal and really imbued with solicitude for those seeking help.

It may be of interest to give some attention to the requirements which, following the Children's Bureau standards, are adopted in the U. S. A. for the antenatal care of pregnant women, viz. supervision over the condition of the mother beginning not later than the fifth month of gestation, periodic blood preassure readings, regular chemical and microscopic examinations of the urine, WASSERMANN or KAHN tests, the taking of internal pelvic measurements, determination of the position of the fetus and the existence of heart tones, a complete physical examination, attention to diet and elimination, and advice as to exercise, work, recreation and rest. Antepartum care must meet these requirements to be considered as adequate, otherwise the expectant mother is not regarded to have received proper care. If the same demands were prescribed for prenatal care in our Swedish antenatal centres, the number of properly pre-cared for women would be very small.

It is my definite opinion that a demand must be raised for regular visits to be paid to the homes of expectant mothers by experienced nurses or midwives in order to learn the resources of the home and what means the prospective mother has of taking care of herself in the manner prescribed, as well as to discover and adjust any faults in the mother's antenatal conduct and to assist and sustain her in every way. There are many details and worries that can be discussed betten in the privacy of the mother's home with a person in whom she has or will acquire confidence than during a short visit to the physician.

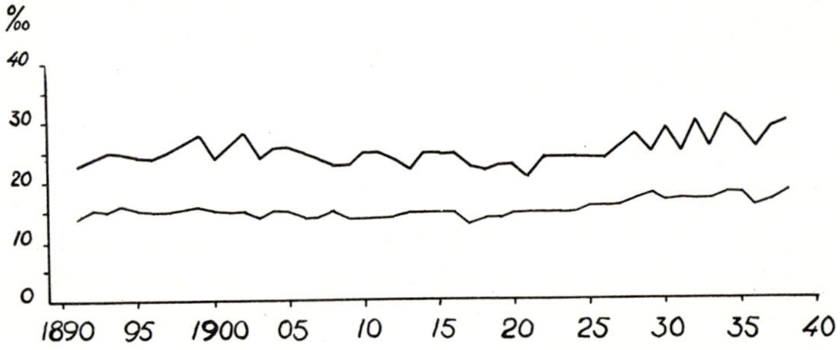

Fig. 5. Neonatal mortality in Sweden in 1891—1938 in legitimate (lower curve) and illigitimate (upper curve) infants.

That a rational social-medical care of pregnant women can essentially improve the chances of survival for new-born infants is shown by reports from various countries, among them the U. S. A. (The Maternity Center Assoc.) and Germany (Theisen). That it would also contribute in Sweden to reducing neonatal mortality and mortinatality seems to be borne out by a comparison between illegitimate and legitimate children. It will be seen from the curves in Fig. 5 that the immediate prospects of survival for illegitimate children are much inferior to those for the legitimate. Of a similar nature is the relation between stillborn legitimate and stillborn illegitimate infants. It is universally considered that the reason for the poorer chances of the illegitimate infants is to be sought, among other things, in the poorer possibilities the unmarried mothers have of looking after themselves, their greater tendency to negligent conduct, their lack of interest in motherhood, the increased tendency to abortion, and the more frequent first pregnancies.

In some measure the illegitimate children and their mothers will presumably always be handicapped, but their position can undoubtedly be substantially improved in many ways. If it could be so arranged that unmarried prospective mothers were able to enjoy the same benefits as the married, if their standard of living could be improved, the risks to life run by their new-born infants would be lessened and the neonatal mortality reduced. To a large extent the inferior position in life of the illegitimate children is bound up with economic factors. The very large part these play in infant mortality is apparent from observations made at different places; the mortality is lower for children in families belonging to the higher income classes than in those with lower incomes (Edin).

It is no doubt generally known that the first pregnancy as compared with those following nearest after it more often terminates in stillbirth, or premature birth, or with delivery complicated in some other way. When natality is low the number of first births is greater than when natality is high. As is known, the birth-rate has now been on a steady decline in our country for the last few decades; that is to say, the primigravidas have proportionately been increasing in number. Possibly it is in this fact that we have to seek an explanation of at least the rising tendency of the stillbirth rates and neonatal death rates. A lower neonatal mortality rate would undoubtedly result if an increased nativity set in. It is possible, and it is to be hoped, that a better enlightenment of the people to the risk of depopulation that threatens, a change in our people's view of life, and State aid, will bring about an increase of births and with it a decline in the frequency of first births, of stillbirth, and of neonatal mortality.

A measure that would assuredly lead to an improvement in the chances of survival for new-born children would be improved neonatal care, especially of the premature children. In communities where there are pediatrists, the supervision of the care of the children at the lying-in establishments should be entrusted to them. A further development of that collaboration between obstetricians and pediatricians which already exists in several places, a better understanding and increased interest among our medical officers for the rational care of debile children, greater skill and training in the management of them on the part of our midwives and nurses, these are the objects to be desired in this connexion. It should be borne in mind that more valuable than a first-class equipment and the best environmental conditions are good knowledge and experience in infant care, love of these tiny human beings, and enthusiasm for the task of preserving them in life and health.

I shall not go into the more obstetric aspect of the matter, but I cannot omit mentioning the possibility that there is an element of risk in the use of anaesthetics and analgetics in the shape of their effects on the health of the fetus and the postpartum conditions. From certain reports it is to be presumed that these agents have a noxious effect on the fetus through depression of the respiratory centre, as a result of which neonatal asphyxia is more likely to occur. (Courville, Schreiber, Cole, Kimball and Daniels). Others, however, have made observations that argue against the existence of such a risk. (Kotz and Kaufmann.) Before proceeding to adopt an increased use of anaesthetics in deliveries it would be a wise plan to investigate this question fully.

The violent resuscitation efforts that were formerly in general recourse against neonatal asphyxia undoubtedly caused, according to present-day views, more harm than good, and it ought therefore to be a very desirable step to abandon these methods altogether and to replace them with more rational and less deleterious measures. With reference to neonatal care in other respects mention may be made of just one method that has received so much attention of late, viz. the prophylactic administration of vitamin K to mother and child. It has been considered probable that the administration of this vitamin has, among other things, the effect of diminishing at least the late haemorrhages due to birth trauma by lessening the hypoprothrombinaemia during the neonatal period. It can scarcely be asserted that any such effect has so far been verified to be produced by the prophylactic administration of vitamin K, but our experience is as yet too small. I do not believe, however, that we should expect too much from this measure, not least of all for the reason that the dangers menacing fetus and child from birth trauma do not consist merely of gross anatomical haemorrhage but also of other intracranial lesions (ganglion-cell degeneration through oxygen deficiency). That the administration of vitamin K cannot with certainty prevent another serious form of bleeding during the neonatal period, melena neonatorum, is well known. The influence that a generally adopted administration of vitamin K is likely to have will probably never be so great as to be registrable in the form of an established decline of the neonatal mortality in our country.

Bibliographique.

ANDERSSON, N. A. and LYON, R. A. Am. Journ. Dis. Childr. Vol. 58. 586. 1939. — ANDERSSON, N. A., BROWN, E. W. and LYON, R. A. Am. Journ. Dis. Childr. Vol. 61. 72. 1941. — BERG, F. TH. Statistisk Tidskrift. Vol. 3. 1869. — BRANDER, T. Finska Läkaresällskapets Handl. Vol. 81. 1010. 1938. — Monatschr. f. Kinderheilk. Vol. 77. 11. 1939. — Centralbl. f. Gynäkologie. Vol. 61. 1645. 1937. — BREESE, B. B. Journ. of Pediatrics· Vol. 12. 648. 1938. — BRODIN, Å. Nord. Medicin. Vol. 4. 3659. 1939. — BUNDESEN, DAHMS, FISHBEIN and HARMON. Journ. Americ. Med. Ass. Vol. 107. 270. 1936. — BUNDESEN, FISHBEIN, DAHMS and POTTER. Journ. Americ. Med. Ass. Vol. 109. 337. 1937. — BUNDESEN, FISHBEIN, DAHMS, POTTER and VOLKE. Jorn. Americ. Med. Ass. Vol. 111. 134. 1938. — CLIFFORD, S. H. Journ. Americ. Med. Ass. Vol. 103. 1117. 1934. — DEBRÉ, JOANNON and CRÉMIE-ALCAN. Rev. d'Hygiène. Vol. 54. 1. 1934. — EDIN, K. Quoted by RIETZ. — *Enquète* Internationale de la Section d'Hygiène de la Soc. des Nations. 1930. — EPSTEIN and GERSTL. Med. Klinik. 1932. — HESS, J. H. Premature and Congenitally Diseased Infants. Philadelphia. 1922. — Journ. Americ. Med. Ass. Vol. 107. 400. 1936. — Journ. Pediatrics. Vol. 8. 104. 1936. — Journ. Americ. Med. Ass. Vol. 115. 1542. 1940. — HJÄRNE, U. Hygiea. Vol. 99. 609. 1937. — KALL, G. Gesundheitsfürsorge f. d. Kindesalt. Vol. 4. 145. 1929. — KOHN, J. Gesundheitsfürsorge f. d. Kindesalt. Vol. 7. 42. 1932. — KOTZ and KAUFMANN. Journ. Americ. Med. Ass. Vol. 113. 2035. 1939. — LICHTENSTEIN, A. Erste Konferenz des Internat. Verbandes für Vorbeugende Pädiatrie. Haag. 1931. — LUNDQVIST, B. Acta Obstetrica et Gynecologica. Vol. 9. 331. 1930. — MEYER-HOUSELLE, O. Gesundheitsfürsorge f. d. Kindesalt. Vol. 4. 130. 1929. — MOLL. L. Gesundheitsfürsorge f. d. Kindesalt. Vol. 3. 1928. — PECKHAM, C. H. Journ. Pediatrics. Vol. 13. 474. 1938. — PFAUNDLER, M. VON. Zeitschr. f. Kinderheilk. Vol. 57, 60 and 62. — POTTER, E. Journ. Americ. Med. Ass. Vol. 115. 996. 1940. — POTTER, E. and ADAIR, F. L. Journ. Americ. Med. Ass. Vol. 112. 1549. 1939. — REPLOH, H. Gesundheitsfürsorge f. d. Kindesalt. Vol. 5. 292. 1930. — RIETZ, E. Acta Pædiatrica. Vol. 9. 1930. Supplement. III. — ROTT, F. Gesundheitsfürsorge f. d. Kindesalt. Vol. 4. 138. 1929. — RYDBERG, E. Acta pathologica et microbiologica. Supplement. X. 1932. — RÄIHÄ and SALMI. Acta Pædiatrica. Vol. 15. 1934. — SAXL, O. Monatschr. f. Kinderheilk. Vol. 64. 136. 1935. — SCARZELLA, M. Stato attuale della assistenza agli immaturi nelle collettività ospedaliere. Torino. 1939. — Atti del XVII Congresso Italiano di Pediatria. Roma. 1939. — SCHWARTZ, P. Monatschr. f. Kinderheilk. Vol. 34. 1926. — SCHWARZ, E. Medicina Italiana. Vol. 9, 1940. — SCHMINKE, R. Gesundheitsfürsorge f. d. Kindesalt. Vol. 6. 41. 1931. — SISSON, W. R. Journ. Americ. Med. Ass. Vol. 115. 2040. 1940. — Statistiska Meddelanden. — SZÉNÁSY, J. Gesundheitsfürsorge f. d. Kindesalt. Vol. 8. 198. 1933. — SÖDERLING, B. Nord. Medicin. Vol. 8. 2000. 1940. — THEISEN, E. Gesundheitsfürsorge f. d. Kindesalt. Vol. 6. 422. 1931. — Ibid. Vol. 4. 544. 1929. — TOVERUD, K. Norsk Magaz. f. Lægevidenskab. 1933. — WILCOX, D. A. Americ. Journ. Dis. Childr. Vol. 52. 848. 1936. — YLPPÖ, A. Monatschr. f. Kinderheilk. Vol. 34. 502. 1926. — ZELTNER, E. Gesundheitsfürsorge f. d. Kindesalt. Vol. 6. 29. 1931.

FROM THE STATE SERUM INSTITUTE (DIRECTOR: J. ØRSKOV, M. D.), DEP. V, THE KOMMUNEHOSPITAL, COPENHAGEN (CHIEF PHYSICIAN: T. KNUDTZON, M. D.) AND THE PEDIATRIC DEP. OF THE SUNDBY HOSPITAL (CHIEF PHYSICIAN: C. FRIDERICHSEN, M. D.).

Pneumococcal peritonitis typed by precipitation of the urine.

By

CHR. R. ROESGAARD.

The effective treatment of pneumococcal peritonitis, aiming to institute an adequate chemo- and serotherapy as early as possible, has always been hampered by the difficulty in obtaining the material for typing of the infecting pneumococci. Hitherto, only one method was known for this purpose: *opening of the peritoneum*, either by puncture or by laparotomy. But as both of these procedures are considered rather risky, it will be an advance if the typing can be accomplished in some other way.

Cultures from the throat and vulva or from the feces give but slight information or none at all.

Blood cultures give valuable information in those cases where they yield a growth of pneumococci. But this method of examination takes a good deal of time, and hence it is of no value as a guidance for the early institution of serum treatment.

The method that will be mentioned in the following, and which permits of type diagnosis on the urine is based on the serological demonstration of the pneumococcus carbohydrate excreted with the urine.

In 1917 Dochez & Avery described the occurrence of soluble pneumococcal substances in the blood and urine of patients suffering from lobar pneumonia and showed that these substances could be recognized by precipitation with homologous immune sera — in other words, that they were type-specific.

These type-specific substances, which on subsequent thorough chemical investigation proved to be polysaccharides, make up the main part of the pneumococcus capsule; on multiplying of the cells they diffuse into the surrounding medium, and they are liberated on disintegration of the cells.

The observations reported by DOCHEZ & AVERY have been confirmed by several authors, *e. g.*, by BLAKE, QUIGLEY, CRUICKSHANK, and also through an investigation that is being carried out in the State Serum Institute.

The observations made under this work with regard to the excretion of these carbohydrates with the urine in pneumonic patients invited to further studies on the urine from patients with other pneumococcal infections, above all the urine from patients with pneumococcal peritonitis, as a priori it seemed reasonable to expect a rather considerable excretion of the carbohydrates in such an extensive infection.

The method which has been tried out and elaborated in its details here in the Institute may be outlined briefly as follows:

Two modifications are employed: ring precipitation and mixture precipitation.

After the first method, the ring precipitation, the centrifuged clear urine is cautiously placed on top of the undiluted type-specific pneumococcus sera in small tubes. The positive reaction appears as a whitish ring or disk at the border between the two fluids in the tube, where the corresponding antibody and carbohydrate get in contact. If the urine contains a fairly large amount of the carbohydrate, the reaction will appear within 10 minutes.

The other method, the mixture precipitation, is more sensitive but also more slow. Here the diluted type-specific sera are mixed with the urine. The tubes are placed in ice-box, and the result is read after 30 minutes, 2 hours, and 18—20 hours. The positive reaction appears as a diffuse opacity or as a sediment.

Simultaneously with these tests, 40 cc. of centrifuged urine is evaporated to about 3 cc. The type-specific carbohydrate is precipitated in the concentrate by addition of 10 volumes absolute alcohol. The precipitate is separated by centrifuging, dried and suspended in 4 cc. of distilled water, whereafter the fluid is clarified by rapid centrifuging. With regard to the concentration of the type-specific carbohydrate, then, this fluid represents the urine concentrated 10 times. This solution is then used for a mixed precipitation test, which is carried out as outlined above for voided urine.

By making a series of urine dilutions — 1 : 1, 1 : 2, 1 : 4, 1 : 8 and so on, with 0.5 cc. in each tube — and by adding 0.5 cc. of homologous diluted serum to each tube, one may obtain an impression of the carbohydrate concentration of the urine from the number of dilutions with a positive reaction after standing for 18—20 hours. This concentration is expressed by the *carbohydrate titer*, which here signifies the reciprocal value of the highest urine dilution giving a positive reaction.

The patient material comprises two cases:

Case 1.

Girl, 9 years old. Admitted to Dep. V, the Kommunehospital, $^{19}/_{3}$—$^{20}/_{3}$ 42, †. (Rec. No. KH., V 487/42.)

The past history of the patient was of no interest in this connection. The present illness commenced 4 days before admission, with frequent vomiting of mucous fluid and slight abdominal discomfort. On the day before admission her condition was aggravated: The vomiting, which had subsided somewhat, was again becoming more frequent and severe, and the pain in the abdomen was accentuated. No bowel movement or flatulence for 4 days. Considerable emaciation. Maximum temperature: 38°.2; on the day of admission: 37°.4.

On admission the patient was very exhausted, pale, with a dark ring round the eyes. *Skin*: Dry and cool. *Tongue*: Parched. *Abdomen*: Not distended, not moving with the respiration; no conspicuous veins in the flanks; percussion note somewhat tympanitic throughout. Some tightening of the abdominal musculature on palpation in the right iliac region. Slight tenderness all over, most marked in the right iliac region. *Rectal* exploration gave an impression of a fairly large, soft intumescence pressing against the wall of the rectum. Marked tenderness corresponding to the anterior wall. *No other abnormality* revealed by the examination. Temperature, on admission: 37°.3. Pulse: 116.

The general condition of the patient was so poor that it did not seem safe to submit her to an operation. She was given 1 liter glucose-saline at once, and stimulants every other hour (ephedrin and nicordamin) plus chemosept.

The diagnosis was uncertain. A perforated appendicitis with diffuse peritonitis seemed most likely. But, as a possibility of a pneumococcal peritonitis was ventilated, too, a specimen of venule blood, swabs from the throat and vagina and urine were sent to the Pneumococcal Department of the State Serum Institute.

As the condition of the patient showed no improvement in the evening, and as the process appeared to to progressive, an *explorative laparotomy* was performed under ether anesthesia, notwithstanding the exhausted state of the patient. Opening of the peritoneum revealed a considerable amount of thick, creamy pus, especially in the small pelvis, and patches of fibrinous exudate on the intestines. The appendix looked normal and was not removed. — A specimen of the peritoneal pus was sent to the Serum Institute at once.

As later it was reported from the Serum Institute that *Type 1 carbohydrate* had been demonstrated *in the urine,* and pneumococci of Type 1 in the peritoneal pus, the patient was given 200,000 units of rabbit antipneumococcal serum Type 1, intravenously. In the course of the day she had received 3 g. of chemosept.

The patient died two hours after the operation.

Autopsy Diagnosis: Bilateral empyema of the lungs; Atelectasis of the lower lobe of the left lung (slight) from compression; Fibrinopurulent peritonitis (marked degree); Subacute enlargement of the spleen (slight).

Laboratory Tests: Cultures from the blood, throat and vagina gave growth of Type 1 pneumococci. Cultures from the urine gave no growth of pneumococci (all specimens taken before the death of the patient). The ring precipitation test on the urine turned out positive after 3 minutes. The mixture precipitation test showed a Type 1 carbohydrate titer of 8.

Case 2 (Described in detail by Emilie Faber).

Girl, 6 years old. Admitted to Pediatric Dep., the Sundby Hospital, $^{15}/_{8}$—$^{21}/_{9}$ 40, †. (Rec. No. Sundby Pediatric Dep. 533/40.)

Two months prior to her admission the patient had been suffering from diarrhea and fever for 4—5 days. Two weeks before admission she again commenced to have frequent bowel movements, with thin, slimy and fetid stools. She had only vomited once. 6 days before admission she had high fever, pain round the umbilicus and delirium. No cough.

The patient was admitted to the Surgical Dep. of the Sundby Hospital, under the diagnosis: empyema, but was transferred at once to the Pediatric Dep. under the diagnosis: pleurisy (right) and intestinal infection(?).

On admission to this clinic the patient was exhausted, intoxicated, somewhat emaciated, and her respiration was groaning. *Face:* Congested with cyanotic hue. *Tongue:* Rather dry and coated, with the tip free. *Heart:* No abnormality. *Lungs:* Changes suggestive of pneumonia of the right inferior lobe with pleurisy. *Abdomen:* Pinhead-sized petechiae here and there; slight distention and slight diffuse tenderness and defensive rigidity. No localized tenderness, intumescence or enlargement of organs. *No other abnormality* revealed by the examination. Temperature on admission: $40^{\circ}.0$. Pulse: 120. Respiration: 64.

According to the above findings, this was a case of sepsis manifest by pulmonary, pleural and peritoneal symptoms. A specimen of venule blood and a swab from the throat were sent to the State Serum Institute at once, and treatment was commenced with sulfapyridin.

X-ray examination on the day after admission showed pneumonia of the right lower lobe, pleurisy and encapsulated empyema.

From the Serum Institute it was reported that the swab from the throat had yielded pneumococci of Types 15 and 34. Five days later the blood specimen was reported to have given growth of Type 1 pneumococci.

During these days the pneumonic symptoms had been subsiding gradually, but on the 14th day of illness the patient again got worse. Auscultation revealed pericardial friction sounds. Clinically as well as roentgenographically a pneumonic process could be demonstrated in the lower part of the left lung. For this reason, the patient was given rabbit antipneumococcal serum Type 1, but only 40,000 units were injected as she suddenly presented violent symptoms of serum shock. The sulfapyridin therapy, which had been discontinued on the preceding day, was now continued again.

About the 24th day of illness the abdominal symptoms became more pronounced: the abdomen was more distended and there was an intense, diffuse tenderness, with defensive rigidity, besides dullnes on percussion over the declive parts.

It was then decided to resume the serum therapy, this time with horse immune serum, in order to avoid shock.

From the 29th to the 33rd day of illness the patient was given altogether 40,000 units intraperitoneally and 440,000 units intravenously, under the guidance of repeated antibody determinations on the blood (for details, see EMILIE FABER). Notwithstanding the large dosage, no lasting antibody excess was obtained in the blood.

On the 32nd day of illness, Type 1 carbohydrate was demonstrated in the voided urine by the ring precipitation test. The reaction was positive at once, immediately after the contact of the two agents.

In the mixture precipitation test the carbohydrate titer was found to be 16.

On the 33rd day of illness Type 1 pneumococci were demonstrated in the peritoneal pus (obtained by incision puncture). On the 36th day of illness a swab was made from the vagina; it yielded no pneumococci. During the following week the peritoneal symptoms were the predominant clinical features. The patient died on the 43rd day of illness.

Autopsy Diagnosis: Diffuse fibrinopurulent peritonitis (pneumococcal); Seropurulent pericarditis; Bilateral fibrinous pleurisy with adhesions; Congestion of the lungs; Parenchymatous degeneration of the liver; Subacute enlargement of the spleen; Congestion of the kidneys.

Epicrisis.

The material comprises two patients: two girls, 9 and 6 years old. Both patients entered the hospital with peritonitis and Type 1 pneumococcus sepsis; in addition, No. 2 had pleuropneumonia on the right side.

In the first case the lesion took an atypical course, as both diarrhea, which is considered a characteristic symptom, and elevation of the temperature were absent.

On laparotomy it was evident that the lesion was a pneumococcal peritonitis, and hence the abdomen was closed at once. After typing of the infecting organism on the urine and peritoneal pus, serum therapy was instituted, but the patient died a couple of hours after the operation.

In the second case the condition of the patient appeared

to improve under treatment with sulfapyridin. About the 14th day of illness, however, pneumonia developed on the left side, and now serum therapy was instituted. About the 24th day of illness the peritonitis flared up again. In spite of large doses of serum, the patient died on the 43rd day of illness.

Both patients excreted Type 1 carbohydrate with the urine. In No. 1 it was demonstrated on the day of admission. The ring precipitation test gave the *type diagnosis after a reaction period of 3 minutes.* In No. 2 the test was not made till the 32nd day of illness. *The reaction was positive instantaneously.*

Discussion.

The above observations confirm the results of previous investigations: in extensive pneumococcal infections the type-specific carbohydrates are excreted with the urine in serologically demonstrable amounts.

On the basis of the findings here presented, correlated with the experiences from examination of the urine of pneumonic patients, I think it is safe to state that in such an extensive infection as pneumococcal peritonitis *it will be practicable in almost every instance to make the type diagnosis on the urine at a very early juncture.*

So, when one is faced by a case in which the possibility of pneumococcal peritonitis cannot be excluded, a type determination on the urine should be carried out as soon as possible.

This examination requires preferably 50 cc. of voided urine (minimum 10 cc.), which is sent to a special laboratory equipped for such work. If only the carbohydrate concentration of the urine has reached a fair degree (titer $\geqq 8$), the type diagnosis can be made in about 10 minutes, whereas it will take at least 3 hours if the urine has to be concentrated. Concentration of the urine should always be carried out in cases where the reaction on the voided urine is weak or negative.

Employment of the urine precipitation test in suspect cases of peritonitis will make it possible *1)* to spare the patients with pneumococcal peritonitis an operation, and *2)* to institute type-specific serum treatment early in the disease — two points of decisive importance to a favorable course of this lesion.

Summary.

After mention of the methods employed so far for the typing of pneumococcal peritonitis — each of which is encumbered with drawbacks — a method is outlined for *type-determination on the urine* of these patients.

A report is given of the examination of the urine from two patients with Type 1 pneumococcal peritonitis: *in both cases it was possible within 10 minutes to make the type diagnosis on the urine.*

In conclusion, the significance of the reaction to the prognosis is pointed out.

The test makes it possible to institute a specific serum treatment without any debilitating operation.

References.

Blake, F. G.: Arch. Int. Med. *21*: 779, 1918. — Cruickshank, R.: J. Path. & Bact. *46*: 67, 1938. — Dochez, A. R. & Avery, O. T.: Proc. Soc. Exper. Biol. & Med. *14*: 126, 1917. — Faber, Emilie: Nord. Med. *13*: 870, 1942. — Quigley, W. J.: J. Infect. Dis. *23*: 217, 1918.

FROM THE PEDIATRIC SERVICE OF CENTRALLASARETTET, LINKÖPING, SWEDEN.

Physiological Enlargement of the Spleen in the Newborn Child.[1]

By

Y. ÅKERRÉN.

The current opinion that a palpable, i. e. enlarged, spleen in a newborn child is pathological is certainly incorrect. Both my own investigations and the works of MENSI, LEMEŽ and POLLITZER have shown that a palpable spleen is a common finding in clinically healthy newborn children. A palpable spleen is thus neither pathognomoic for syphilis nor a very suspicious sign of this disease, as often claimed. It is clear that syphilitic enlargement of the spleen is generally more marked both as to size and consistency than the physiologic form and, therefore, more easily observed than the latter, which is usually not discovered unless a particularly careful examination is made. Systematic palpations of the spleens in healthy infants reveal a surprising number of positive findings. Practice is undoubtedly of great importance in this respect.

The Writer's Results.

Of 144 clinically healthy infants examined daily throughout the newborn period, 111, or 77 per cent, showed enlarged

[1] A preliminary report on the subject was made at the Seventh Nordic Pediatric Congress at Oslo in 1938 and appeared in the Transactions of the meeting. The present work is intended to give both a brief recapitulation of the direct results of my studies on the occurrence of palpable spleen in healthy newborn children and a more detailed discussion of the significance of the observations made.

spleen on at least one of the examinations. The results appear in more detail in the following table.

Table.

Distribution of positive and negative palpation findings on the first 7 days after birth.

Day	Negative findings	Positive findings	Positive findings in per cent	No. of children examined
1	104	40	27.8 ± 3.74	144
2	86	58	40.3 ± 4.09	144
3	67	77	53.5 ± 4.16	144
4	76	68	47.2 ± 4.16	144
5	90	54	37.5 ± 4.03	144
6	104	40	27.8 ± 3.74	144
7	108	34	24.0 ± 3.58	142

Note: Two of the 144 were discharged on the seventh day and were not, therefore, examined on that day.

The table suggests that the positive palpation findings reach their maximum on the third day of life. Can this maximum be established statistically, or is it a matter of coincidence? If the values secured are assumed to have varied due to chance only, all the figures should lie within a range of variation which could be calculated theoretically. An average of 36.9 per cent of the individuals examined daily showed a palpable spleen. The material consisted of 144 subjects, except on the seventh day, when there were 142. The standard deviation for the average figure is, therefore, ± 4 per cent. The range of variation will thus extend from 49 per cent down to 24 per cent. But one of the figures (the value on the third day) represented 53 per cent, which is clearly beyond the range of variation which could be governed by coincidence. Here, therefore, we have an established maximum, which does not depend on chance. In addition, if the variability were governed by chance only (the fact that the figures vary must inevitably depend partly on chance), no special trend would be obtained in the figures. But the figures do show a trend, first rising to a maximum and then decreasing. Seven values might happen to be arranged in this way by accident, but this is hardly likely. Thus there are two reasons to justify the conclusion that *the spleen is more often palpable on the third day of life than on the first and seventh days.*

Before turning to a discussion of the significance and interpretation of my observations, I shall treat the objections which may be made to the primary observations from various viewpoints.

Mistaking the spleen for some other organ is scarcely possible. The technique of palpation is based on the displacement of the spleen by the respiration and on its characteristic form, with a marked lower pole, as well on its position under the left costal margin. Neither the left lobe of the liver nor the left kidney can be mistaken for the spleen.

I have refrained from establishing the outlines of the spleen by percussion, since this method, like percussion of the spleen in general, is notably unreliable, particularly in infants. LEMEŽ, to whose work on the spleen in the newborn I shall return, did carry out percussion of this kind, but did not, as far as can be judged from his presentation of the facts, attribute any importance to this phase of examination in the diagnosis of enlargement of the spleen.

Naturally it may be asked whether the finding of a palpable lower splenic pole, for that is all one feels in the examination in question, really signifies enlargement of the spleen and not merely a dislocation of the spleen. Dislocations of the spleen are undoubtedly exceedingly rare in clinically healthy individuals; in his treatise on differential diagnosis, FEER speaks of a low-lying spleen in cases of extensive pleural exudation. He says the normally sized spleen can be felt even in cases of very relaxed abdominal walls. I have not observed such lack of muscular tone in any of the healthy infants in the present series.

One may also ask what influence the state of fulness of the abdominal organs has on the observations. In reply I may say that all the examinations were made at the same time of the day and after the same interval since the last meal (2 to 3 hours), if any (the infants ate nothing for the first twenty-four-hours of life). Nevertheless the contents of the stomach and intestines must have varied considerably with regard to both food and gas as well as to fecal matter. Neither pronounced meteorism nor abdominal distention were present in any case, however, and it was never difficult to introduce the fingers to a suitable depth under the left costal margin in order to find the spleen. It therefore appears very unlikely that such factors had any effect on the findings. The same must also apply to the possibility of the physiologic loss of weight, with any effect it may have on the consistency of the tissues, being of importance in this connection. The temperature of the environments might also be imagined to affect the size of the spleen. All the children, except a few just delivered, were examined in the same well-heated room, lying in bed, and immediately after their garments had been removed. Thus uniform conditions prevailed on the whole from the point of view of temperature also.

All the children in the series were born at term and were of normal weight (not less than 2 900 Gm.). They were free from signs of disease during the whole newborn period. The health of the mothers and the course of the deliveries were also normal (nothing is known as to possible anemic conditions in the mothers). The Wassermann test was not made, but many years of experience as head of the Pediatric Service at this hospital have taught me that congenital syphylis is practically unknown in these parts.

I am not unaware that the method for determining the size of the spleen, upon which the primary data are based, is far from perfect. Attempts were made to do this roentgenologically, but did not yield satisfactory results. In general, it seems to be difficult to measure the spleen, and this applies to animals too. Barcroft fixed metal clips to the margins of the spleen in animals, but was unable to secure reliable measurements even by this means. In infants, therefore, we must probably be content for the time being with the subjective palpation method.

Earlier Investigations on Physiologic Enlargement of the Spleen in the Newborn.

In my preliminary report I only mentioned earlier investigations by MENSI and, mainly, POLLITZER, who, like I, observed splenic enlargement in healthy newborn children. I refer to the comparison between these authors' results and mine, which I made in the above-mentioned report. At that time I had not read the important work by LEMEŽ on erythema neonatorum toxicum, in which the author, in agreement with his teacher MAYERHOFER's theory, tried to prove that this form of erythema is allergic in origin. In this connection, LEMEŽ studied both the leukocyte picture and the condition of the spleen during the period immediately after birth. He examined »systematically» the spleen in 75 healthy children up until, if possible, the fourteenth day of life. A palpable spleen was observed in 51 of the 75, or about 70 per cent, a figure which corresponds well with the one I found in my material. The size of the spleen was stationary in 27 of these 51 cases, or in 52 per cent of the cases showing splenic enlargement. In the remaining 24 enlarged cases, LEMEŽ considered he could observe an enlargement of the spleen which at the most brought the organ to within 1 1/2 fingers (according to LEMEŽ one finger is the equivalent of 1.5 cm.) of the costal margin. This swelling was seen twice on the second day of life, five times on the third, ten times on the fourth, three times on the fifth and once each on the sixth, seventh, ninth and eleventh days. Another swelling (*Nachschubanschwellung*) in the second week of life was found by LEMEŽ twice on the eighth, three times on the ninth, twice on the tenth and once on the eleventh day of life. In the great majority of cases, LEMEŽ found the spleen to be palpable first on the second or third day, less frequently not until the fourth day of life. The last mentioned points agree more or less well with my observations, in which the frequency of positive palpation findings rose steadily until the third day and showed a comparatively small, statistically unestablished difference between the third and the fourth day. With regard to the second week of life, no comparison can be made, because my investigations ended with the seventh day of life. LEMEŽ wrote, however, that the splenic swelling usually lasted through the second week of life and that in a great many cases it remained stationary during the whole period of examination These claims might appear to contrast somewhat with my findings, which show a continuous decrease in the frequency of positive palpation findings after the third to fourth day. However, LEMEŽ's examinations during the second week of life do not appear to have been particularly extensive, since at one place he wrote: »Da sich meine Untersuchungen zum grösseren Teil nur auf 7—8 Tage beschränken mussten.» LEMEŽ stated, it is true, that his examinations were »systematic», but it does not appear clearly whether he did daily palpations. The leukocyte picture is illustrated by curves on which the size of the spleen is also marked, but in no place is the latter given for each day, but only for several, at the most five times during the first fourteen days of life. On the whole, LEMEŽ's description of the results of his splenic palpations is rather unclear, so that it is difficult to form an exact conception of his observations.

LEMEŽ considered that he could differentiate between a splenic tumor reaching to within one-third of a finger of the costal margin and one reaching to within one-fourth of a finger, which seems a somewhat bold claim. One should undoubtedly excercise great restraint in reporting small variations in the size of the palpable spleen. It is true that I attempted to distinguish the very marked positive palpation findings from those in which the spleen was only faintly palpable, but I have purposely placed only slight emphasis on this probably very subjective differentiation. The only difference I stressed in my presentation is the one between positive and negative findings.

To summarize, I think I may say that there is no great difference between LEMEŽ's and my observations regarding the occurrence of splenic enlargement during the first week of life. LEMEŽ seems to have found a decrease in the frequency of positive findings during the second week of life.

The Nature of the Physiologic Enlargement of the Spleen.

A few details regarding the anatomy of the spleen will first be given. According to HELLMAN, whose material although small is the only series of cases published which is reliable from the point of view of absence of infection and other complicating factors, the average weight of the spleen in the dead newborn child is 9 Gm. with rather small variations. If one inspects a spleen of this size *in situ* in a newborn child or one just past the newborn stage at autopsy, one finds it hard to believe that it could ever have been palpable. However, as BARCROFT pointed out, there is a considerable difference between the size of the spleen *in vivo* and *post mortem*, because most of the blood in the living spleen leaves it upon death. And, according to HUECK's experiments on cadavera the human spleen can absorb approximately three times its weight of fluid. This circumstance in itself indicates that a palpable spleen in a healthy newborn child is a spleen well-filled with blood.

In his investigation on the quantitative anatomy of the spleen, HELLMAN found that in newborn children the white pulp, i. e. the lymphoid apparatus, constitutes 15 per cent of the dead organ, while the red pulp, i. e. the portion containing the greater part of the spleen's blood vessels and blood stores constitutes about 85 per cent. An increase in the quantity of the white pulp to a degree sufficient to produce a palpable enlargement of the organ probably never occurs under physiologic conditions. The only reasonable solution, therefore, is an enlargement of the red pulp and the only probable cause of the latter becoming enlarged under physiologic conditions is a collection of blood, i. e. an accumulation of red corpuscles in it.

LEMEŽ claims that swelling of the spleen during the newborn period is due to an accumulation of leukocytes in the spleen. Like other workers, LEMEŽ found a rapid decrease in the leukocyte count in the same period from the high values characterizing the time just after birth to the low values reached on the third to fourth day of life. LEMEŽ advanced no anatomical or other proof that this drop in the leukocyte count is due to an accumulation of leukocytes in the spleen.

Changes in the distribution of the white corpuscles among the different vascular areas in the body are undoubtedly of great importance in the appearance of leukopenic conditions and in this respect the spleen plays a not unimportant part (cf. VEJLENS). However, it seems highly improbable that an accumulation of leukocytes under non-infectious circumstances would lead to swelling of the spleen. Even in cases of infectious tumor of the spleen, an accumulation of blood, mainly erythrocytes, appears to be regarded as the most important factor. I refer to LAUDA's work on the subject.

In the course of my investigations, I occasionally observed that a previously palpable spleen became smaller or impossible to palpate in connection with vigorous crying, and the same was true to an even greater degree in several experiments with adrenalin injections. As is known, adrenalin produces a contraction of the spleen and evacuation of its blood stores.

The Spleen's Function as a Blood Reservoir.

My explanation of the origin of the physiologic enlargement of the spleen in the newborn is closely linked up with BARCROFT's theory, now generally accepted, of the reservoir function of the spleen. According to BARCROFT, the spleen is a store for red corpuscles. This depot functions as follows: Under certain conditions it fills with blood, mainly erythrocytes, while under others it empties its whole supply of blood into the circulating blood stream. The latter activity of the reservoir function occurs mainly in connection with an increased need for oxygen transport, e. g. on increased motor activity, in anoxemia of different kinds, etc. On transition from conditions of increased oxygen transport to conditions with smaller oxygen requirements, e. g. from motor activity to rest, from anoxemia or hypoxemia to a better oxygen supply, a number of the erythrocytes return to the reservoir. In this way there is a continuous alternation between filling and evacuation of the blood reservoir of the spleen, an alternation which is also influenced by other factors than the ones mentioned here.

The Erythrocyte Picture and the Cause of the High Hemoglobin Values in the Newborn.

The extensive literature on this matter was quite recently reviewed by Wetzel (1938) and Wollstein (1938) and with regard to hemoglobin by Gräfinghoff (1938). The old view that both polyglobulism and high hemoglobin values are present in the newborn is only partly correct. There is probably no true polyglobulism in infants immediately after birth, but, on the other hand, the content of hemoglobin per volume unit of blood is high and considerably higher than in healthy adults. These values appear even higher when compared with those found in healthy infants from the age of three months onward. Macrocythemia, i. e. a condition with large red corpuscles and larger absolute quantities of hemoglobin per erythrocyte than usual, is thus present at this time (Magnusson, Faxén, Vahlquist).

A hemoglobin content as high as that in newborn children is only found in other ages under pathologic conditions, e. g. in heart disease of the congenital cyanosis type. In diseases of this kind the high hemoglobin content is reached through polyglobulism, while in the newborn child the same result is attained through macrocythemia.

An unusual form of polyglobulism appears under special living conditions, to wit, at high altitudes. It is generally believed that the cause of this form of polyglobulism is the low oxygen tension in the mountain atmosphere. Through the increased erythrocyte content in the blood the quantity of hemoglobin per volume unit of blood rises and more favorable conditions for the transport of oxygen are attained. Corresponding to the polyglobulism, there is increased activity of the bone marrow, which finds expression in a rise in the reticulocyte content of the blood, among other things. The polyglobulism and the bone marrow changes associated with it constitute a part of the compensation mechanism. On transition from a normal height above sea level to the mountains, a more or less rapid change in the direction of polyglobulism occurs in the blood. If the transition takes place too rapidly, the characteristic mountain sickness, which is a sign of imperfect adaptation, appears.

Ziegelroth was the first to apply views borrowed from the theory of the polyglobulism found at high altitudes to the hematologic picture of the newborn and to the hematologic process occurring during the newborn period. Since then, E. Volhard, Anselmino and Hoffmann, and Goldbloom and Gottlieb have presented similar views. It is mainly through Haselhorst's and Stromberger's pioneer investigations on the oxygen tension and oxygen content of the fetal and maternal blood in man that we have learned that there is considerable hypoxemia in the blood of the umbilical vein, which comes directly from the placenta, the respiratory organ of the fetus. The oxygen tension and oxygen content correspond to what would be found in a person living 10,000 metres above sea level. The hypoxemia in the blood that corresponds functionally to the pulmonary venous blood under extra-uterine conditions, is further accentuated by the special circulatory conditions during fetal life, when the blood most heavily charged with oxygen is mixed before, during and immediately after its passage through the heart with blood with a lower oxygen content. Barcroft (1938) calculated that the blood which reaches the brain of the sheep fetus during the last third of its intra-uterine life has an oxygen tension corresponding to stratospheric conditions. The high hemoglobin values in the newborn child thus in all probability have the same origin as mountain polyglobulism. From a functional viewpoint it is of no importance whether the increased hemoglobin content per volume unit of blood is the result of polyglobulism or macrocythemia.

The Effect of the Transition from Intra-uterine Life on the Reservoir Function of the Spleen.

When the organism requires an increased oxygen transport or when hypoxemia is present for various reasons, a mobilization of the blood in the spleen and other reservoirs takes place. In the opposite case, e. g. in connection with a transition from hypoxemia to optimal oxygen supply, the reverse must occur and the stores, including that of the spleen, be filled with blood. For the whole reservoir function is reversible, with an alternation between filling and evacuation. The accumulation of blood is probably particularly marked when, as is the case during fetal life, pronounced chronic hypoxemia is present with an accompanying increase in the hemoglobin content of the volume unit of blood. Thus in all probability *the transition from intra-uterine to extra-uterine life is associated with an intensive filling of the blood store of the spleen. The simplest interpretation of the splenic enlargement which so often occurs during the newborn period is that it is the result of an accumulation of blood in the blood store of the spleen.*

In this connection I shall discuss my primary observations against the background of this hypothesis. It may seem odd from this point of view that the positive palpation findings increased in frequency up to the third day after birth. A certain period must be expected to elapse after birth, however, before the whole adjustment from intra-uterine to extra-uterine conditions has been completed. The functional closure of the foramen ovale and of the ductus arteriosus may often not occur immediately on birth, but may require a little time; the same applies to the full dilation of the pulmonary parenchyma. The extensive accumulation of blood in the skin, which certainly exists in connection with the physiologic erythema in the newborn and which often reaches its maximum at the end of the first day of life or the beginning of the second, may also be imagined to affect the amount of blood collected in the spleen. With regard to all these factors, it must be taken into account that the speed at which one change or another occurs is subject to individual variations. Hence it appears reasonable that some time elapses after birth before the frequency of positive palpations reaches its peak.

The accumulation of blood in the spleen during the newborn period is a dynamic, not a static phenomenon. The whole nature of the reservoir mechanism is dynamic. And this has made itself felt in my investigations. It happened not infrequently that in one and the same child positive palpation findings were made one day, not the next and again the next day. It is reasonable to suppose that, during the newborn period as at other times, there is a constant alternation between filling and emptying of the blood store of the spleen. But the high frequency of splenic enlargement which is found during the newborn period and which reaches its maximum on about the third day of life seems to me to show that the blood store is more often filled at this time than later in life. Other investigations on which I am now engaged but which are not yet sufficiently comprehensive, suggest that in clinically healthy children the spleen is palpable considerably less frequently after the newborn period than during it. LEMEŽ too clearly considered that in the majority of his cases the splenic enlargement disappeared later.

I cannot find any special circumstance that would particularly favor demonstration of the spleen in the newborn by palpation. The tone of the abdominal muscles is certainly not less pronounced at this time than later, and rachitic or other conditions affecting the shape of the thorax or the functions of the musculature or the suspensory apparatus have not yet had time to make themselves felt.

It may also be asked why in some children the spleen is never palpable at all. In my series, 23 per cent of the children did not have a palpable spleen at any of the examinations during the first week of life. There are several ways of explaining this. One possibility is that due to the alternation between emptying and filling of the store, it is natural that with a relatively limited number of examinations one will happen to palpate invariably at times when the spleen is comparatively empty of blood, which may account for the apparent deviation in these children. If the examinations are made frequently enough one may expect to find a palpable spleen on some occasion in these children too. Other factors also may play a part. One of these is the amount of blood in the newborn child, which probably varies according to the individual. The time when the cord is severed has a not insignificant effect on the quantity of blood. The size of the spleen, or rather the size of its storage space, must obviously be assumed to vary somewhat.

A further possible explanation of these observations is provided by POLLITZER's assumption that some children have a constitutional microsplenia while others have a constitutional splenomegalia. Enough investigations have not yet been conducted, however, for it to be decided whether this explanation is the correct one, and if so to what extent.

Icterus Neonatorum and the Increased Blood Destruction during the Newborn Period.

I shall not here enter into a detailed discussion of the problem of icterus neonatorum, but shall confine myself to a short summary of questions of interest at the present time. The most popular theory on icterus neonatorum proceeds from the assumption that hyperbilirubinemia, which occurs in all newborn children, is entirely or substantially a result of an increased destruction of erythrocytes. This conception is based on the belief that the high hemoglobin values per volume unit of blood in the newborn child is a consequence of intrauterine hypoxemia. Through the transition to the optimal oxygen supply of extra-uterine life, the compensatory macrocythemia becomes unnecessary functionally. As a part of the organism's adaptation to the changed conditions of life, there is an increase in the rate of blood destruction, which in turn gives rise to hyperbilirubinemia, i. e. to blood jaundice and, in most cases, skin and mucous jaundice also, although of varying intensity. The theory was first presented by ZIEGELROTH, worked out in greater detail and motivated by E. VOLHARD, and made known mainly by ANSELMINO and HOFFMANN'S publications in Germany and GOLDBLOOM and GOTTLIEB'S publications in the United States.

The proofs of this postulated increase in the rate of blood destruction have been assembled most completely by VOLHARD, who lists three signs of blood destruction: (1) the fact that the absolute elimination of bile pigment is greater during the newborn period than between the ages of two and three months (YLPPÖ); (2) the fact that the intensity of the bilirubinemia increases the richer the child is in blood, e. g. following late severance of the umbilical cord, late expression of the placenta, etc.; (3) the fact that immediately after birth polyglobulism is present, which disappears during the newborn period; (4) in addition we have LUCAS and DEARING'S investigations, which, although not mentioned by VOLHARD, seem to show that there is a relatively large amount of circulating blood in the newborn child and that this is considerably smaller in the two-week old child, at the same time as the hemoglobin content per volume unit of blood has also decreased. All these points suggest considerable destruction of blood.

VAHLQUIST has written a penetrating and in many ways a justified criticism of this theory of icterus neonatorum. I shall not discuss VAHLQUIST'S argumentation in any detail and instead shall only touch on it briefly. His discussion can be summed up in the claim that there are no changes in the composition of the blood during the newborn period which cannot be explained by a substantial decrease in the formation of new erythrocytes. Thus, according to VAHLQUIST, there is no need to assume that there is an increased destruction of blood in order to explain icterus neonatorum. If the hemolytic theory were found to be without sufficient foundation, this would, VAHLQUIST believes, constitute indirect support for the hepatic theory. It should be mentioned in this connection that many of the workers who have considered an increased destruction of blood during the newborn period to have been proved have, nevertheless, believed in the existence of a hepatic factor, a relative excretory insufficiency for bilirubin, in the newborn child (LEPEHNE, VOLHARD and others).

VAHLQUIST was undoubtedly right when he claimed with regard to Point 2 that the connection between late cutting of the cord or late expression of the placenta and the intensity of icterus neonatorum has not been adequately proved (cf. KRAMANN and HOFFMANN).

With regard to Point 3, we must agree with VAHLQUIST, since many recent investigations have not confirmed the polyglobulism in the newborn which heretofore has been regarded as axiomatic (WINTROBE and SCHUMACHER, HÓRVATH and HOLLÓSI, MURGRAGE and ANDERSEN, SACHS et al., VAHLQUIST). On the other hand, many recent investigations indicate that a progressive reduction in the hemoglobin content of the capillary blood takes place from birth until the age of about two weeks (LUCAS, DEARING, HOOBLER and others). WINTROBE and SCHUMACHER, HÓRVATH and HOLLÓSI, MURGRAGE and ANDERSEN, SACHS et al., and VAHLQUIST found that in the venous blood there is no important reduction in the hemoglobin values during the first two weeks of life, while the reverse applies to the capillary blood. Most of the older studies have concerned the capillary blood only.

This difference between the venous and the capillary blood during the newborn period is remarkable from many points of view. During all other ages under physiologic conditions the erythrocyte and hemoglobin contents are the same in the capillary and the venous blood. I shall not go into this matter, however.

Lucas and Dearing's frequently cited investigations on the quantity of circulating blood during the newborn period have been checked by Robinow and Hamilton using a new technique. These workers found fairly constant values for the volume of blood during the newborn period. Their figures were only very slightly higher in proportion to the body weight than those in adults and considerably lower than the ones found by Lucas and Dearing.

In his discussion of various arguments presented as support for the claim that the destruction of blood increases during the newborn period, Volhard pointed out that the investigations which demonstrated an increased iron content in the internal organs after birth or after the end of the newborn period do not constitute proof of an increased destruction of blood. Nor do more recent investigations in this field, conducted by Adler and Adler, prove this, as was also pointed out by Vahlquist.

Vahlquist made a study of the serum iron during the newborn period to see whether this would reveal anything conclusive regarding the hematologic phenomenon. Vahlquist found relatively high serum iron values in the newborn, which decreased greatly during the first day and then rose again rather sharply, although not to the height reached just after birth (average values in the blood of the umbilical vein, 159.8 γ; at one day, 51.5 γ; at six days, 114.4 γ; and at fourteen days old, 124.9 γ). The high value just after birth is not only present following ordinary deliveries, but following caesarean deliveries also. It cannot, therefore, as Vahlquist believed, be due to trauma during the child's passage through the birth canal. The rapid drop which occurs just after birth Vahlquist considered to be connected with the cessation of the placental circulation and of the supply of iron from the maternal organism. The rise which then follows can be interpreted in different ways. For example, it may be said to depend not only on an increased destruction of blood (experimental acute hemolysis with the help of intravenous injections of distilled water or the administration of phenylhydrazine entails pronounced although temporary increases in the serum iron), but also on a change in the relationship between the formation and destruction of erythrocytes (VAHLQUIST). Hepatic factors may also play a part.

GOLDBLOOM and GOTTLIEB considered they were able to produce experimentally a condition analogous to icterus neonatorum. Upon their return to ordinary atmospheric conditions following a stay in a low pressure chamber, GOLDBLOOM and GOTTLIEB's experimental animals showed a hyperbilirubinemia which these workers considered to be closely related to icterus neonatorum genetically. These experiments are not convincing, however. A closer study of the reports of the experiments reveals, namely, that in about one-half of them the bilirubin content of the blood had already begun to rise toward the end of the stay in the low-pressure chamber. Hence this argument in support of the increase in the rate of blood destruction in the newborn as the cause of icterus neonatorum also does not hold water (VAHLQUIST).

A review of the above points reveals that the apparently well-founded theory of a greatly increased destruction of blood during the newborn period has not been definitely proved. But this naturally does not signify that it has been disproved. Further thorough investigations are certainly necessary to clear up this matter. I would point out here, however, that there are two arguments which can be presented as rather strong evidence of the validity of the accepted theory. One of them is VOLHARD's Point 1 above. Admittedly it may be objected that the total amount of hemoglobin in the organism is probably somewhat greater in the newborn child than in the infant of two to three months old and that the fact of greater export of bile pigment in the newborn child than in the two or three-month old child is not indicative of a particularly pronounced destruction of blood. But the circumstance that this export of bile pigment occurs despite hepatic insufficiency (for if icterus neonatorum is not mainly due to increased blood destruction, there remains no other reasonable explanation than an insufficiency in the excretion of bile pigment) puts the matter in another light. A state of hepatic insufficiency with increased export of bile pigment is, however, something of a paradox. Further, in view of LEPEHNE's observations, according to which the bile of most newborn children shows pleiochromia, it seems difficult to explain icterus neonatorum as essentially due to hepatic insufficiency alone.

I think one is safe in assuming that the hemolytic-hepatic theory, which presupposes both hepatic insufficiency and increased destruction of blood as the cause of icterus neonatorum, still provides the most satisfactory explanation.

The Cause of the Increased Destruction of Blood in the Newborn.

If, as pointed out above, despite VAHLQUIST's criticism of the prevailing theory, one must continue to consider it probable that the destruction of blood increases during the newborn period, the question arises as to the cause of this increase. Oddly enough, this question has not received any attention. The increased destruction of blood has simply been regarded as a phenomenon of adaptation. It is the transition from hypoxemia to optimal oxygen supply which causes the destruction of the functionally superfluous hemoglobin. This purely teleologic explanation does not solve the problem of *how* this blood destruction takes place. The presence of an enlarged spleen due to an accumulation of blood in the stores is of not insignificant interest in this connection.

The Connection Between the Reservoir Function of the Spleen and its Hemolytic Function.

It has long been assumed, mainly on the basis of observations made under pathologic conditions, that the spleen is an organ with a hemolytic function — probably the organ most important in the destruction of erythrocytes. It is principally the therapeutically successful spleen extirpations in congenital family icterus which have prepared the way for this theory. Great pains have been taken to solve the problem of how the erythrocytes are destroyed and of the part played in the process by the spleen. LAUDA's monograph on the function of the spleen reveals how little we know or, rather, knew about this subject.

BERGENHEM and FÅHRÆUS in a publication followed later by others by them and by other associates of FÅHRÆUS (BERGENHEM, 1938; MELLGREN, 1938; FÅHRÆUS, 1939) opened up entirely new perspectives on these questions.

The point of departure for these workers was FÅHRÆUS' observation that native blood, particularly blood with a high rate of sedimentation, becomes changed when stored motionless at or near body temperature, in that the sedimentation rate and rouleaux formation decrease substantially. At the same time the erythrocytes become more spherical. BERGENHEM and FÅHRÆUS showed that this process, which they called the stabilization process, is caused by changes both in the plasma (or serum) and in the erythrocytes. The change in the plasma depends on the formation of lysolecithin, which takes place through the action of a lecithinase on the plasma or serum lecithin. Lysolecithin, a substance with strongly hemolytic properties, is known as the substance through which the hemolytic action of cobra venom is transmitted. Independent of the formation of lysolecithin in the serum and plasma, the red corpuscles, which are separated from the blood fluid and heated to body temperature, are so changed that when they are again suspended in their native plasma at ordinary room temperature, their rate of sedimentation has become substantially reduced. The stabilization process makes itself particularly strongly felt when plasma or serum and corpuscles are again mixed after having been kept separated at body temperature. Due to the change in form in the direction of spherocytosis undergone by the erythrocytes and the formation of lysolecithin which takes place at the same time, the stabilization process can be regarded as a prelude to hemolysis.

If these experimental plasma and corpuscle changes at body temperature are to take place, the corpuscles and plasma must be kept separated from one another. What is the significance to physiology of these conditions demonstrated *in vitro*? Are circumstances in the organism such as to allow this separation process with the accompanying hemolysis or pre-hemolysis?

BARCROFT's theory of the reservoir function of the spleen drew FÅHRÆUS' attention to the spleen as an organ in which the conditions for intravital separation of corpuscles from plasma appear to prevail. The conditions for this separation process in the spleen were thrown into even higher relief by KNISELY's important investigations on the blood circulation in the living spleen. Through his observations *in vivo*, KNISELY showed that the venous sinuses run between the finest branches of the arteries and the veins and that the passage of the blood through them is regulated by the sphincters situated both at the arterial and venous ends of the sinuses. Through the alternate opening and closing of these sphincters, the sinuses are either filled with corpuscles or empty of them. The filling of the sinuses takes place as follows: first the venous sphincter is contracted while the blood is still flowing in from the arterial end, whereupon closely packed corpuscles are collected in the sinus, which is thereby filled as a sausage skin is stuffed. At the same time the plasma filters through the wall of the sinus. When the sinus is completely filled with erythrocytes the arterial sphincter also closes and the corpuscles are entirely separated from the plasma. KNISELY observed that this process sometimes lasted as long as nine hours, a period of time more than adequate for the completion of the stabilization. After having been out of the blood circulation for a longer or shorter period, the sausage-like mass of corpuscles is released by the sudden opening of the sphincters and emptied into the efferent vein and the blood again passes as usual through the patent sinus as through an ordinary vessel. KNISELY's investigations thus reveal that the spleen acts as a separator for the blood. The conditions for intravital blood separation, with the hemolytic effects on the blood demonstrated by BERGENHEM and FÅHRÆUS *in vitro*, are thus present in the spleen.

That blood changes of hemolytic or pre-hemolytic nature really do occur in the spleen under physiologic conditions has been shown in several ways. Thus the venous blood of the spleen presents both spherocytosis and reduced rouleaux formation, as compared with the arterial blood (BERGENHEM and FÅHRÆUS, BERGLUND, MELLGREN). MELLGREN was also able to demonstrate directly in venous blood from the spleen, which he secured during the emptying of reserve blood from cat spleens, distinct hemoglobinemia, which further increased if the blood was stored at body temperature. Thus, when the blood is collected in the stores of the spleen and thanks to the separation of corpuscles from plasma which this accumulation implies, it undergoes a change of hemolytic tendency. Through his important investigations, FÅHRÆUS and his school evolved an original and fruitful theory for the function of the spleen as a hemolytic organ.

As pointed out above, the physiologic enlargement of the spleen in the newborn is in all probability caused by a large accumulation of blood in the blood depots of the spleen. The conditions for a relatively extensive destruction of red corcorpuscles are therefore present, according to FÅHRÆUS' theory. In further agreement with this theory, it is generally believed that extensive destruction of erythrocytes takes place during the newborn period. The facts thus seem to bear out the theory perfectly.

Although, as I have already stated, many of the arguments to the effect that an increased destruction of blood occurs in the newborn do not stand up against searching criticism, there remain many reasons which indicate that this conception is justified. The tendency toward a large accumulation of blood in the spleen, which appears to characterize the newborn period, together with FÅHRÆUS' theory of hemolysis, provides a simple explanation of the mechanism of the physiologically unique blood destruction which is assumed to occur during the newborn period.

Summary.

1. An enlarged spleen, in other words, one that is distinctly palpable, is remarkably common in healthy newborn children. Of 144 healthy newborn children examined daily for the first seven days of life, 117 (77 per cent) showed a palpable spleen on at least one occasion.

2. The positive palpation findings reached a pronounced and statistically established maximum on the third day of life. The frequency of enlarged spleen rose evenly until the third day, after which it declined steadily.

3. The physiologic enlargement of the spleen is in all probability caused by an accumulation of blood in the spleen. This is borne out both by anatomic data and by the variations in the palpability of the spleen, which can be observed in one and the same individual from day to day, as well as by the fact that the spleen can be made impalpable by the injection of adrenalin.

4. The extensive accumulation of blood in the spleen can in all likelihood be explained by the circumstance that the blood stores of the spleen become filled to capacity in the newborn child in connection with the transition from the persistent and pronounced hypoxemia of intra-uterine life to the optimal oxygen supply of extra-uterine life.

5. Together with FÅHRÆUS' theory of the hemolytic function of the spleen, these observations and the interpretation given them provide an explanation of the increased destruction of erythrocytes which is believed to take place in the newborn child and which is regarded as one of the main prerequisites for the appearance of icterus neonatorum.

Bibliography.

ADLER, K. & ADLER, M.: Zeitschr. f. Geburtsch. u. Gynäk. 101, p. 128 (1931). — ÅKERRÉN, Y.: Act. Pæd. 24, p. 23 (1939) Proceedings of the 7th North. Ped. Congr. (1938). — ANDRESEN, M. I. & MURGRAGE, E. R.: Am. J. Clin. Path. 8, p. 46 (1938). — ANSELMINO, K. J. & HOFFMANN, F.: Arch. f. Gynäk. 143, p. 477 (1931). — ——: Arch. f. Gynäk. 147, p. 69 (1931). — BARCROFT, J.: Ergebn. d. Physiol. 25, p. 818 (1926). — ——: The Architecture of Physiological Function. Cambridge 1934. — ——: The Brain and its Environment. New Haven 1938. — BERGENHEM, B.: Act. Path. et. Microbiol. scand. Suppl. XXXIX (1939). — —— & FÅHRÆUS, R.: Zeitschr. f. d. ges. exp. Med. 97, p. 555 (1936). — BERGLUND Å.: Hygiea 92, p. 677 (1930). — FÅHRÆUS, R.: Lancet, Sept. 16, p. 630, 1939. — FAXÉN, N.: Act. Pæd. 19, Suppl. I. (1937). — FEER, E.: Diagnostik der Kinderkrankheiten. 4 Aufl. Berlin 1931. — GOLDBLOOM, A. & GOTTLIEB, R.: Am. J. Dis. Child. 38, p. 57 (1929). — ——: J. Clin. Invest. 8, p. 375 (1929—30). — GRÄVINGHOFF, W.: Handb. d. Anat. d. Kindes. I, p. 123. München 1938. — HADEN, R. L. & NEFF, F. C.: Am. J. Dis. Child, 28, p. 458 (1924). — HASELHORST, G. & STROMBERGER, K.: Zeitschr. f. Geburtsh. u. Gynäk. 98, p. 49 (1930). — HELLMAN, T.: Zeitschr. f. Konstitutionslehre. 12, p. 270 (1926). — HORWÁTH, Z. & HOLLÓSI, C.: Am. J. Dis. Child. 49, p. 689 (1935). — HUECK, W.: Centralbl. f. allg. Path. u. Path. Anat. Ergänz.-heft.: verhandl. d. Deutsch. Path. Ges. 23. Tag. 19—21. apr. 1928, p. 6. — KNISELY, M. H.: Anat. Rec. 65, p. 23 (1931). — KRAMANN, H. & HOFFMANN, W.: Arch. f. Gynäk. 169, p. 659 (1939). — LAUDA, L.: Zeitschr. f. Kinderheilk. 45, p. 689 (1927—28). — LEMEŽ, L.: Zeitschr. f. Kinderheilk. 45, p. 689 (1927—28). — LEPEHNE, G.: Monatschr. f. Geburtsh. u. Gynäk. 60/61, p. 277 (1922—23). — LUCAS, W. P. & DEARING, B. F.: Am. J. Dis. Child. 21 p. 96 (1921). — ——, HOOBLER, H. F., COX, A., JONES, M. R. & SMYTH, F. S.: Am. J. Dis. Child. 22, p. 525 (1921). — MAGNUSSON, J. H.: Act. Pæd. 18, Suppl. I (1935). — MELLGREN, J.: J. Physiol. 94, p. 483 (1939). — MENSI: cited by POLLITZER. — POLLITZER, R.: Il Lattante, 1, p. 601 (1930). — SACHS, A., LEVINE, V. E., GRIFFITH, W. O. & HANSEN, C. H.: Am. J. Dis. Child. 56, p. 787 (1938). — VAHLQUIST, B.: Nord. Med. 7, p. 1516 (1940). — ——: Act. Pæd. 28, Suppl. V. (1941). — VEJLENS, G.: Act. Path. et Microbiol. scand. Suppl. XXXIII (1938). — VOLHARD, E.: Ergebn. d. inn. Med. u. Kinderheilk. 37, p. 465 (1930). — WETZEL, G.: Hand. d. Anatomie d. Kindes, I, p. 58. München 1938. — WOLLSTEIN, M.: Handbook of Hematology, ed. by DOWNEY. II, p. 923. London 1938. — YLPPÖ, A.: Zeitschr. f. Kinderheilk. 9, p. 208 (1913). — ZIEGELROTH, P.: Münch. Med. Wochenschr. 73: II, p. 1440 (1926).

AUS DER PÄDIATRISCHEN KLINIK DES KAROLINISCHEN INSTITUTS AM NORRTULLS KRANKENHAUS, STOCKHOLM. VORSTAND: DOCENT J. HENNING MAGNUSSON.

Missbildungen der Harnwege mit familiärem Auftreten von Doppelureter bei Kindern.

Von

ERIK FRISELL.

Angeborene Missbildungen im Bereich der oberen Harnwege kommen in erheblich grösserem Umfang vor und spielen beim Zustandekommen krankhafter Zustände des Urogenitalapparats eine viel wichtigere Rolle, als man früher wusste. Erst nach Einführung unserer neuzeitlichen urologischen Hilfsmittel ist dieser Sachverhalt klar erkannt worden. Hierdurch wurde auch freie Bahn für die wesentlich wirksamere Therapie geschaffen, welche chirurgische Eingriffe bei gewissen dieser Fälle darstellen.

Unter den verschiedenen Formen derartiger Missbildungen bilden Nierenbecken- und Harnleiterverdoppelungen die grösste Gruppe. Diese kommen in zwei — anatomisch betrachtet — voneinander abgrenzbaren Formen vor:

1. Vollständige Verdoppelung des Ureters, Ureter duplex, mit 2 Nierenbecken, 2 Harnleitern und 2 Ostien in der Blase, wenn beide Ureteren in diese münden. So verhält es sich gewöhnlich, aber in seltenen Fällen kann der eine, oder sogar beide, Harnleiter extravesikal münden.

2. Unvollständige Verdoppelung des Ureters, Ureter bifidus oder Uretur fissus, mit 2 Nierenbecken und 2 Harnleitern, die sich an irgendeiner Stelle auf dem Wege zur Blase hinab, nach Braasch aber am häufigsten im oberen Drittel, vereinen und mit einem gemeinsamen Ostium in die Blase münden.

In der Regel wird ein doppelter Harnleiter von einem doppelten Nierenbecken begleitet. Bei einer geringen Anzahl von Fällen sind abweichende Verhältnisse beschrieben worden, diese sind aber sehr selten (Mertz).

Der definitive Ausscheidungsapparat bildet sich bei den Vertebraten in einem frühen Stadium der Embryonalentwicklung aus zwei getrennten Anlagen, der sog. Ureterknospe und dem metanephrogenen Gewebe. Aus der ersteren entsteht der endgültige Harnleiter sowie die ableitenden Nierenkanälchen, aus der letzteren, dem metanephrogenen Gewebe, die sezernierenden Teile der Niere. Die Ureterknospe entwickelt sich aus der Rückseite des Wolffschen Ganges unmittelbar kranialwärts von der Einmündungsstelle in die Kloake als ein kleiner Zapfen und wächst stielartig in Richtung auf das obenerwähnte metanephrogene Gewebe hin aus. Sie verschmilzt mit diesem, und gleichzeitig teilt sie sich an ihrem freien Ende unter Bildung eines Nierenbeckens. Im weiteren Verlauf der Entwicklung werden die Einzelheiten in der eigentlichen Niere ausgebildet.

In gewissen Fällen kann auf einer oder beiden Seiten eine doppelte Ureterknospe angelegt werden. Von diesen beiden Anlagen kann entweder die eine im »Knospenstadium» verbleiben und die andere sich entwickeln (Weigert), oder beide können zu Harnleitern auswachsen. Diese finden den Weg zum metanephrogenen Gewebe hin, wo sich jede derselben wie beim Vorliegen des normalen, einfachen Ureters weiterentwickelt. Die dabei entstehende Doppelniere bildet gewöhnlich eine Einheit mit 2 getrennten Nierenbecken und Harnleitern, aber es existieren sämtliche Übergänge bis zu 2 ganz getrennten Nieren. Einen prinzipiellen Unterschied zwischen den anatomischen Endstadien gibt es also nicht. Eine zusammenfassende Bezeichnung für diese Formen von Anomalie ist Ureter duplex.

Die unvollständige Harnleiterverdoppelung, Ureter bifidus oder Ureter fissus, kommt nach Broman, Chwalla u. a. dadurch zustande, dass sich eine einfache Ureterknospe spaltet und die beiden Ureteräste jeder für sich in der oben beschriebenen Weise auswachsen. Über die näheren Einzelheiten bei diesem Vorgang sowie über eine Verwandlung der Duplexanlage in Ureter fissus oder vice versa gehen die Ansichten auseinander.

Die Angaben, welchen man im Schrifttum über das Vorkommen reno-ureteraler Missbildungen begegnet, stammen teils von Obduktionsmaterial, teils aus der Klinik. Eine Zusammenstellung einer Reihe von zugänglichen Obduktionsstatistiken ergibt, dass reno-ureterale Missbildungen in ca. 2 % der Obduktionsfälle vorliegen. Ureterverdoppelungen sind in ca. $^{1}/_{2}$ % der Fälle gefunden worden (siehe Tab. 1). Geht man zum klinischen Material über, so wird man finden, dass die entsprechenden Zahlen hier etwas höher liegen. Das ist ganz natürlich, da ja Individuen mit reno-ureteralen Missbildungen leichter Erkrankungen der Harnwege ausgesetzt werden als andere und daher öfter Gegenstand der Untersuchung werden als Personen im Durchschnitt.

In diesem Zusammenhang sei auf eine Zahlenangabe aus einer Arbeit von GUIZETTI u. PARISET in Virch. Arch. 204 (1911) hingewiesen, die man im einschlägigen Schrifttum immer wieder falsch zitiert sieht. Diese Autoren haben in einem Material von 20 000 Obduktionen renale Missbildungen in 0,44 % gefunden. Diese Zahl wird nun überall, wo sie vorkommt, als ein Ausdruck für das prozentuale Vorkommen reno-ureteraler Missbildungen zitiert. Dies ist irreführend; die betreffenden Autoren haben nämlich betont, dass keine Fälle von Doppelureter in die Statistik aufgenommen worden sind.

In Tab. 2 sind einige Literaturangaben über das Vorkommen der verschiedenen Formen von Doppelureter zusammengestellt. Dass die Art des Materials etwas wechselt, spielt ja in diesem Zusammenhang keine grosse Rolle. Aus der Tabelle geht hervor, dass Doppelureter viel öfter einseitig (80 %) als doppelseitig (40 %) vorliegt. Ferner erweist sich Ureter duplex als etwas häufiger (106 + 349 = 455, d. h. 56 %) als Ureter fissus (44 %). — Nur ein Autor hat Fälle gefunden, bei welchen ein Ureter duplex und ein Ureter fissus gleichzeitig vorlagen. Wären diese Fälle wirklich die einzigen in

Tab. 1.

Vorkommen von reno-ureteralen Missbildungen bzw. vom Doppelureter.

Autor	Material von	Anzahl Fälle	davon reno-ureterale Missbildungen in Fällen	Anzahl Fälle mit Doppelureter		
				insgesamt	in Prozent der Anzahl: untersuchter Fälle	in Prozent der Anzahl: reno-ureteraler Missbildungen
v. Gelderen	Obduktion	8 500	—	55	0,65 %	—
Roscher	desgl.	5 527	144 = 2,6 %	23	0,41 %	16 %
Motzfeld	desgl.	4 500	[1] 79 = 1,8 %	23	0,50 %	28 %
Rugbee u. Wollstein	desgl. (Kind)	4 903	104 = 2,1 %	—	—	—
Clarke, Lowsley u. Kingery	desgl. (Kind)	4 215	52 = 1,5 %	—	—	—
Schippers	desgl. (Kind)	390	22 = 5,6 %	—	—	—
Kohl	desgl.	833	—	27	3,2 %	—
Schmutte	Klinik (urolog. Abt.)	2 000	128 = 5,1 %	31	1,55 %	24 %
Burghele	Klinik	795	24 = 3,0 %	13	1,63 %	54 %
Mathis	Klinik (urolog. Abt.)	500	9 = 1,8 %	4	0,80 %	44 %
Barclay u. Baird	Röntgen	500	18 = 3,6 %	13	2,60 %	72 %
Bazzocchi u. Bernabeo	Klinik	—	35	17	—	49 %
Boeminghaus	desgl.	—	25	12	—	48 %
Herman	Operation	1 141	—	10	1,7 %	—
Lowsley	desgl.	600	—	15	1,3 %	—

diesem Material, so würde das bedeuten, dass die Kombination in 2 % sämtlicher Fälle vorkommt. Wahrscheinlich hat jedoch eine solche Kombination öfter bestanden, ohne dass die be-

[1] Hierbei sind keine kongenitalen Zystennieren mitberücksichtigt, weshalb die Zahl 1,8 % etwas zu klein und die Zahl 28 % etwas zu gross ist.

Tab. 2.

Vorkommen verschiedener Formen von Doppelureter.

Autor	Material von	Anzahl Fälle	doppelseitig			einseitig		
			duplex	fissus	zusammen	duplex	fissus	zusammen
MERTZ	Literaturzusammenstellung	276	51=18,5 %	9= 3,5 %	[1]74=27 %	140=50 %	62=23 %	202=73 %
PAPIN	desgl.	213	36=17,5 %	12= 5,6 %	48=23 %	107=50 %	58=27 %	165=77 %
BRAASCH u. SCHOLL	Klinik	144	8= 5,5 %	1= 0,7 %	9=6,2 %	36=25 %	99=68,7 %	135=94 %
HAWTHORNE	desgl.	63	3= 5 %	2= 3 %	5= 8 %	20=32 %	38=60 %	58=92 %
DOSZA	desgl.	33	3= 9 %	3= 9 %	6=18 %	17=51 %	10=31 %	27=82 %
SCHMUTTE	desgl.	31	2= 6 %	0 %	2= 6 %	15=48 %	14=46 %	29=94 %
ROSCHER	Obduktion	23			5=22 %			18=78 %
CAPORALE	Klinik	19	1= 5 %	1= 5 %	2=10 %	12=64 %	5=26 %	17=90 %
BARCLAY u. BAIRD	Röntgen	13	2=15 %	4=31 %	6=46 %	2=15 %	5=39 %	7=54 %
Gesamtmaterial		(792) 815	106=13 %	32= 4 %	157=20 %	349=44 %	291=37 %	658=80 %

[1] Diese Zahl enthält 14 Fälle, bei welchen Ureter duplex auf der einen und Ureter fissus auf der anderen Seite vorlag.

treffenden Autoren es für nötig hielten, dies besonders zu verzeichnen.

Was die Geschlechtsverteilung betrifft, so haben Autoren mit grossen Statistiken gezeigt, dass reno-ureterale Missbildungen bei Frauen häufiger angetroffen werden als bei Männern. Ferner hat es den Anschein, als ob bei den einseitigen Fällen Missbildungen auf der linken Seite öfter vorlägen als auf der rechten.

Über familiäres Auftreten der reno-ureteralen Missbildungen und über die Vererbung der Anlage ist sehr wenig bekannt. Eine Ausnahme stellen indessen Missbildungen vom Typ der kongenitalen Zystenniere dar, bei welchen eine deutliche Erblichkeit vorzuliegen scheint. GRUBER hat in neuerer Zeit aus dem Schrifttum rund fünfzehn Familien gesammelt, bei den sich derartige Anlagen als erblich erwiesen hatten, und zwar als sowohl rezessive wie dominante Eigenschaft.

Die familiär auftretenden Fälle von Nierenbecken- und Ureterverdoppelung sind sehr selten. Soweit Verf. finden konnte, sind in der Literatur nur 4 derartige Familien beschrieben (unter Vorbehalt für eine Arbeit des Russen MKRTYTEHIANTZ in Med.-biol. j. 5, 1929, über dieses Gebiet, die z. Z. hierzulande nicht zur Verfügung steht).

Zwei von diesen Familien sind von dem Schweizer RITTER erwähnt und später nebst einer dritten Familie von seinem Schüler STEINLEIN ausführlicher behandelt worden. Die vierte Familie, hier X. genannt, wurde von KAREŠ aus Prag beschrieben. Hier folgt ein kurzer Bericht über die aktuellen Daten aus diesen Familien sowie ein Diagramm über jede einzelne derselben (Fig. 1, Familie W., M., L. und X.).

1. Familie W.

Tochter S.: Ureter fissus dext., Ureter duplex sin.

Knabe K., Sohn der S.: Ureter duplex dext., linke Niere und Harnleiter o. B.

Sohn D.: rechte Niere und Ureter o. B., Ureter duplex sive fissus sin.

Sohn O.: rechte Niere und Ureter o. B., Ureter duplex sive fissus sin.

Ausserdem kamen bei dem Vater A. and zweien der Söhne andere pathologische Zustände vor, Hydronephrose bzw. Wanderniere bzw. Enuresis.

2. Familie M.

Sohn A.: doppelseitige deutliche Zweiteilung des Nierenbeckens.

Tochter H.: doppelseitige deutliche Zweiteilung des Nierenbeckens.

Tochter A.: angedeutete Zweiteilung des rechten Nierenbeckens, Ureter fissus sin.

Ausserdem kamen in der Anamnese der Mutter chronische Pyelitis und Nierenschmerzen vor.

3. Familie L.

Tochter M.: Zweiteilung des rechten Nierenbeckens, linke Niere und Harnleiter o. B.

Sohn E.: rechte Niere und Ureter o. B., Ureter fissus sin.

Sohn H.: angedeutete Zweiteilung des rechten Nierenbeckens, linke Niere und Ureter o. B.

Beiläufig sei hier noch erwähnt, dass STEINLIN in einer weiteren Familie H. bei einer Geschwisterschar von 9 Kindern 1 mit Ureter fissus unilateral., 5 mit erweiterten Nierenbecken auf einer oder beiden Seiten sowie 2 mit Bauchschmerzen unklarer Genese fand.

4. Familie X.

Sohn Y.: Ureter fissus bilateral.

Sohn Z.: Ureter fissus dext., linke Niere und Harnleiter o. B.

Zu diesen früher veröffentlichten vier Familien mit Auftreten von Doppelureter bei mehreren Mitgliedern kommt nun eine fünfte, die Familie Ö. (siehe Fig. 1), von der zwei Schwestern während der letzten Jahre in der hiesigen Kinderklinik Behandlung erhalten haben. Beide Schwestern wurden unter der Diagnose rezidivierende Pyelozystitis behandelt, bis die Urographie zutage brachte, dass bei beiden doppelte Nierenbecken und Harnleiter vorlagen.

Die Ältere der Schwestern wurde später mit gutem Erfolg operiert. Die Untersuchung der übrigen Familienmitglieder liess sich nicht durchführen.

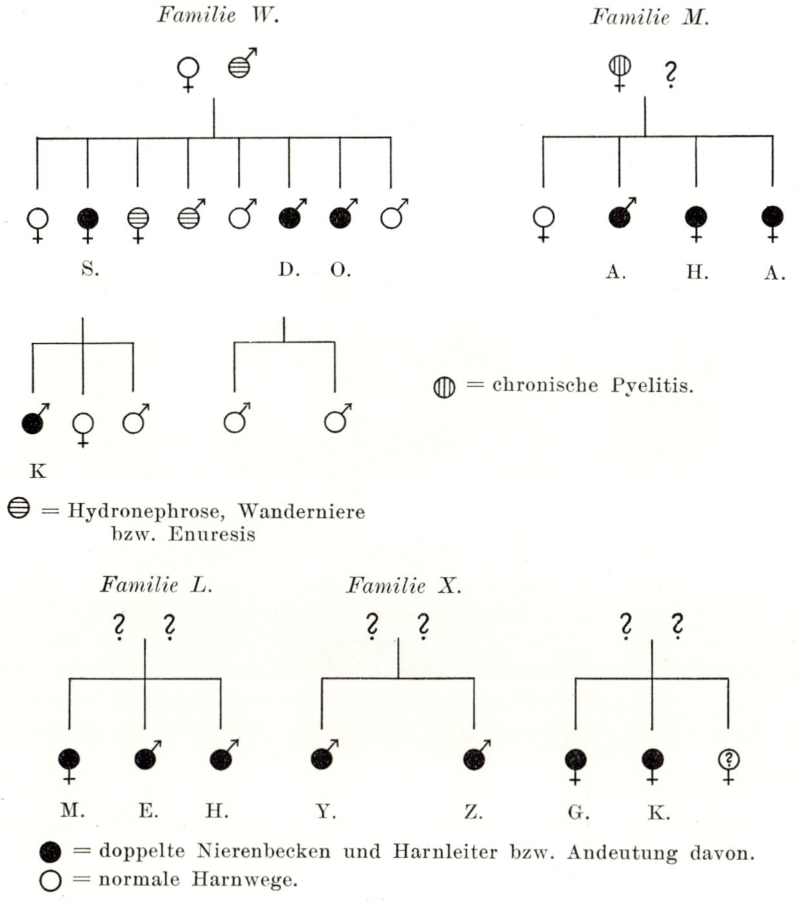

Fig. 1.

Fall 1. (Abb. 2 a u. 2 b).

G. Ö., Mädchen, 5 Jahre 5 Mon. Zweites Kind von dreien (sämtlich Mädchen). Geburtsgewicht 3 840 g. Partus o. B. Mischnahrung. Entwicklung o. B.

Seit dem Alter von 4 Mon. verschiedene Male Harnwegsinfektionen mit Fieber bis 40°. Klinisch und poliklinisch in der hiesigen Kinderklinik unter der Diagnose Pyelocystitis recidivans behandelt. Der Urin war im allgemeinen eiweissfrei, im Sediment wurden weisse Blutkörperchen und Bact. coli gefunden. Im Alter von knapp 3 Jahren hatte das Kind binnen 4 Mon. drei

Attacken der Erkrankung und wurde daher zur Beobachtung in Kronprinsessan Lovisas Vårdanstalt aufgenommen.

Zystoskopie und Ureterenkatheterismus (HINDMARSH): Blase von normalem Aussehen, fasst 200 ccm. Auf der linken Seite zwei dicht aneinander gelegene Harnleitermündungen, welche wie die auf der rechten Seite normal aussehen. In alle drei Ureteren lassen sich Kathether unbehindert einführen.

Röntgenuntersuchung. Bauchübersicht: Nieren machen den Ein-

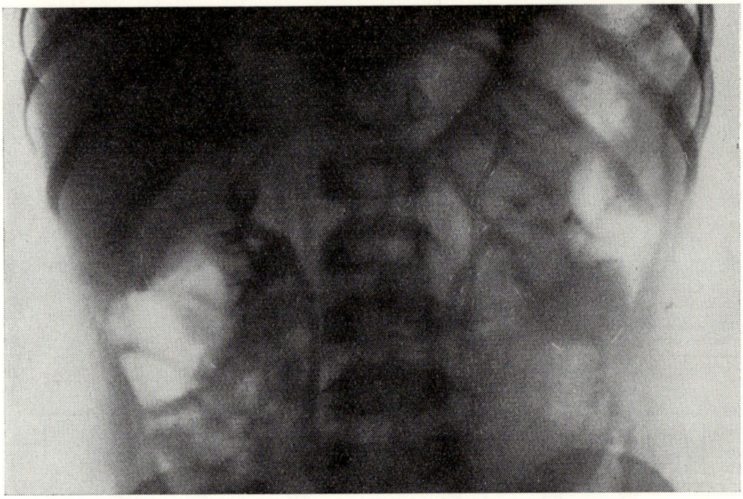

Abb. 2 a (Fall 1). Auf der linken Seite sieht man innerhalb des Nierenschattens 2 ganz getrennte Nierenbecken mit je 1 Ureter.

druck normaler Form und Grösse. Von den beiden Kathetern erreicht der eine die Mitte der Lendenwirbelsäule, der andere den unteren Teil des Sacro-iliacalgelenks.

Bei *Kontrastinjektion* füllt sich auf der rechten Seite ein normalgrosses Nierenbecken ohne Deformierung oder Füllungslücke. Calices grazil. Bei Injektion durch den einen, als »oberen» bezeichneten Katheter auf der linken Seite wird ein kleines, kranial in der Niere gelegenes Nierenbecken gefüllt. Bei Injektion durch den anderen Katheter wird ein etwas missgestaltetes, kaudal innerhalb der Niere liegendes Nierenbecken mit ziemlich plumpen Kelchen dünn ausgefüllt. In keinem der Becken sind Füllungslücken nachweisbar (SAHLSTEDT).

Diagnose: Ureter duplex sin.

Das Mädchen wurde dann von Prof. SÖDERLUND operiert (Serafimerlazarett, J.-Nr. 1041/39): Heminephrectomia mit Resektion des unteren Nierenpols mit zugehörigem unterem Nierenbecken auf der linken Seite. — Die oberen zwei Drittel der Niere bildeten eine Erweiterung mit der Grösse, Form und Farbe einer normalen

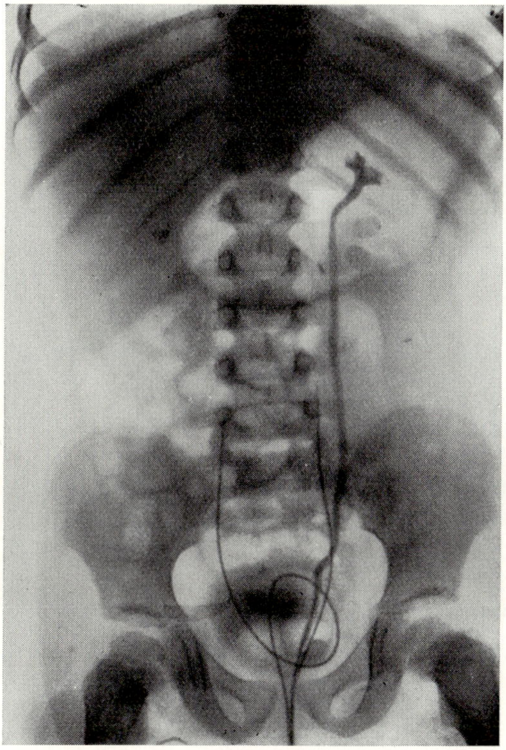

Abb. 2 b (Fall 1). Die Katheter sind durch die 3 Ureterostien in der Blase, 2 auf der linken und 1 auf der rechten Seite, eingeführt. Das obere Nierenbecken mit zugehörigem Ureter auf der linken Seite ist mit Kontrastmittel gefüllt.

Niere, während der durch eine schwache, aber deutliche sanduhrähnliche Einschnürung von dem oberen Teil getrennte Nierenpol mehr bläulich und härter war; derselbe machte den Eindruck, schlechter durchblutet zu sein als die obere, gesunde Partie.

Das untere Nierenbecken und der zu diesem gehörende Harnleiter waren mässig erweitert; jenes erstreckte sich bis gerade an die sanduhrförmige Einschnürung heran. Die zur oberen und unteren »Niere» ziehenden Gefässe waren voneinander getrennt (zur oberen verlief eine grobe Art. renalis, die untere wurde von zwei sehr dünnen Arterien versorgt). Der kranke Teil der Niere wurde an der obenerwähnten Einschnürung mittels Diathermie entfernt. *Pathalogisch-anatomische Diagnose:* pyelonephritische Narbenniere (Prof. HENSCHEN).

Postoperativer Verlauf völlig komplikationsfrei. Während der beiden seit der Operation vergangenen Jahre hat das Mädchen keinerlei Beschwerden gehabt.

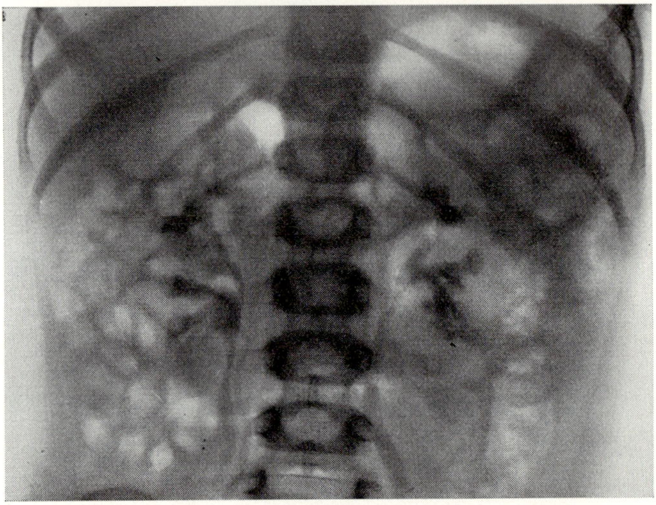

Abb. 3 a (Fall 2). Auf der rechten Seite sieht man innerhalb des Nierenschattens 2 ganz getrennte Nierenbecken mit je 1 Ureter. Zweiteilung des linken Nierenbeckens.

Fall 2. (Abb. 3 a u. 3 b).

K. Ö., Schwester von G. Ö., 3 Jahre 6 Mon. Drittes Kind von dreien. Geburtsgewicht 3 620 g. Partus o. B. Mischnahrung. Entwicklung o. B.

Ganz gesund bis zum Alter von 3 Jahren, wo das Kind einmal an einer heftigen Allgemeininfektion mit Fieber bis 40° und Nackenstarre erkrankte. Nach einer Woche Genesung.

Zwei Monate später kurze Attacke von hohem Fieber (etwa 40°) und Eiter im Urin. Mit Harnantiseptika behandelt, binnen einer Woche gesund. Nach 3 Wochen wieder kleine Temperaturzacken. Wurde zunächst daheim in derselben Weise behandelt, später aber zur Beobachtung in die hiesige Kinderklinik aufgenommen.

Laut Krankengeschichte war das Kind in den letzten Monaten etwas unruhiger geworden, hatte aber normal zugenommen. Im Status nichts Besonderes. M. S. R. 35 mm. Tuberku-

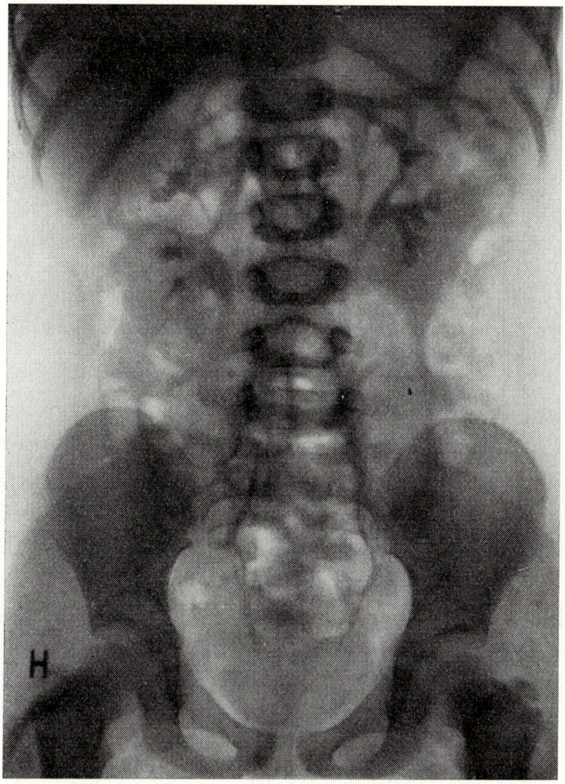

Abb. 3 b (Fall 2). Unmittelbar vor der Einmündung in die Blase vereinen sich die beiden Harnleiter auf der rechten Seite zu einem Ureter, welcher in die Blase mündet.

linprobe nach Moro neg. Im Urinsediment 3—4 weisse Blutkörperchen.

Röntgenuntersuchung (Ausscheidungspyelographie): Nieren von gewöhnlicher Form, Grösse und Lage. Konkremente nicht nachweisbar. Bei der Urographie gleichzeitige Ausscheidung auf beiden Seiten. Links füllt sich ein zweigeteiltes Nierenbecken mit einem kleinen gemeinsamen Sammelteil. Linker Harnleiter normal. Rechts ist das Nierenbecken in ein kleineres oberes und ein etwas grösseres unteres mit getrennten Ureteren geteilt, welche sich unmittelbar vor der Mündung in die Blase vereinen. Harnleiter normal weit. Calices auf beiden Seiten normal. Keine Hydronephrose. Normale Blasenkonfiguration (JONSELL).

Diagnose: Ureter fissus dext., Zweiteilung des linken Nierenbeckens.

Zur eventuellen Operation in das Serafimerlazarett (Prof. SÖDERLUND) verlegt.

Zystoskopie: Die rechte Uretermündung weist eine leicht gerötete Schleimhaut auf. Links o. B. Keine Anzeichen von Zystitis. Rechter Harnleiter lässt sich wie gewöhnlich katheterisieren. *Retrograde rechtsseitige Pyelographie* (Katheterspitze liegt in der Höhe des Querfortsatzes von L V): bei Injektion des Kontrastmittels füllt sich nur ein kleineres Nierenbecken.

Eine Operationsindikation wurde da nicht als vorliegend erachtet, weshalb das Kind entlassen und die Entscheidung über einen eventuellen Eingriff vertagt wurde.

Es handelt sich hier also um zwei Schwestern im Alter von 3—5 Jahren, aus einer Familie von 5 Personen (Eltern und 3 Töchter), welche wiederholter Pyelozystitisattacken wegen infolge von Verdacht auf Harnwegsanomalie geröntgt wurden und beide doppelte Nierenbecken und Harnleiter aufwiesen. Eine der Schwestern wurde mit gutem Erfolg operiert. Die übrigen Familienmitglieder sind nicht untersucht.

Zusammen mit früher veröffentlichten gleichartigen Fällen sind mithin 5 Fälle bekannt, in welchen Doppelureter als Anomalie bei mehreren zu derselben Familie gehörigen Individuen aufgetreten ist. Das Material ist jedoch zu klein, um demselben irgendwelche Aufschlüsse über eine etwaige erbliche Übertragung der Anlage zur Missbildung entnehmen zu können. Es ergeben sich auch keine Hinweise darauf, dass die Missbildung bei den familiären Fällen bei dem einen Geschlecht öfter als bei dem anderen erscheinen würde (♀ 6, ♂ 8 Fälle).

Aller Wahrscheinlichkeit nach ist jedoch das familiäre Auftreten doppelter Harnleiter erheblich häufiger, als es aus diesen fünf Fällen hervorgeht. Nur ein Teil dieser Missbildungen machen Erscheinungen, und zwar namentlich bei den Fällen, wo sie mit anderen Missbildungen im Bereich der

Harnwege, z. B. mit Ureterstrikturen, kombiniert sind. Vielfach werden sie auch rein zufällig entdeckt. Liesse man die Harnwege bei sämtlichen Geschwistern und den Eltern von Patienten mit Doppelureter konsequent untersuchen, eine Methode, der STEINLIN die Entdeckung des von ihm veröffentlichten Materials zu verdanken hat, so würde man wahrscheinlich multiples Vorkommen von Anomalien mit Harnleiterverdoppelung bei mehreren Mitgliedern einer Familie in einer viel grösseren Anzahl von Fällen finden, als jetzt bekannt sind.

In der Praxis wird diese Harnwegsanomalie sich oft hinter Fällen von chronischen Pyurien verbergen, welche falsch gedeutet und niemals gänzlich geklärt worden sind. Dies gilt auch für viele von denjenigen rezidivierenden Pyurien, bei welchen die Krankheitsattacken nur mit jahrelangen Zwischenräumen auftreten. Es sind in erster Linie diese sekundären Symptome, welche zur Entdeckung von derartigen Anomalien führen.

Zusammenfassung.

Nach Definition der beiden Anomalien Ureter duplex und Ureter fissus wird eine kurze Übersicht über die wahrscheinliche Entwicklung dieser beiden Missbildungen gegeben. In der folgenden Erörterung wird an Hand von Literaturmaterial gezeigt, dass doppelte Ureteren in ca. 0,5 % der Sektionsfälle, in klinischem Material aber erheblich häufiger vorkommen. Eine familiäre Häufung von Doppelureter ist im Schrifttum viermal beschrieben worden. Hierzu fügt Verf. eine fünfte Familie. Es handelte sich um zwei Schwestern, die Symptome in Form von rezidivierenden Pyelozystitiden hatten, und von welchen die eine nach Operation beschwerdefrei wurde. Abschliessend äussert Verf. die Vermutung, dass familiäres Auftreten von Doppelureter nicht so ungewöhnlich sei, wie es den wenigen veröffentlichten Fällen nach den Anschein hat. In vielen Fällen macht die Ureterverdoppelung sicherlich keine Symptome und entzieht sich daher der Entdeckung.

Schrifttum.

Barclay u. Baird: Lancet 2: 1169: 1935. — Bazzochi u. Bernabeo: Ann. ital. di chir. 18: 671: 1939. — Boeminghaus: Arch Klin. Chir. 170: 754: 1932. — Braasch u. Scholl: Surg. Gynec. a. Obstretr. 35: Nr. 4: 1922. — Broman: Normale und abnorme Entwicklung des Menschen, Wiesbaden 1911. — Burghele: Lyon Chirurgical 30: 385: 1933. — Caporale: Archiv. d. mal. d. reins 10: 357: 1936. — Clarke, Lowsley u. Kingery: Zit. n. Schippers. — Char, Shih u. Wen: J. Urol. 36: 305: 1936. — Chwalla: Zit. n. Johanning u. Hawthorne. — Dosza: Ztsch. f. Urol. Chir. 26: 1929. — Eisendraht: Ann. of Surg. 77: 450: 1923. — Gelderen: Virchows Arch. 263: 1889. — Gruber: Z. Urol. 31: 9: 1937. — ——: Med. Klin. 31: 833: 1935. — Guizzetti u. Pariset: Virch. Arch. 204: 1911. — Hawthorne: Canad. M. A. J. 34: 21: 1934. — Herman: Ztsch. f. Urol. Chir. 26: 505: 1929. Hryntschak: Ztsch. f. Urol. Chir. 9: 87: 1922. — Ionel: J. d'Urol. 39: 408: 1935. — Johanning: Medicinsk Revue 11: 1938 (Beilage). — Kareš: Casopis lékaru Ceských 77: 1247: 1938. — Kohl: Z. Urol. 24: 561: 1930. — Kreutzmann: J. Urol. 38: 67: 1937. — Lowsley: Zit. n. Herman. — Mathis: U. S. Navy Med. Bull. 32: 183: 1934. — Mertz: Urol. a. Cutan. Rev. 22: 551: 1918. — Motzfeld: Beitr. z. path. Anat. u. z. allgem. Pathol. 59: 1914. — Papin: J. d'Urol. 23—24: 127: 1927. — ——: Zit. n. Eisendrath. — Ritter: Helvetica Medica Acta 2: 169: 1935—36. — Ritchie: Canad. M. A. J. 38: 170: 1938. — Roscher: Acta Chir. Scandinav. 70: 493. — Rugbee u. Wollstein: Zit. n. Schippers. — Schippers: Bull. de la soc. de pediatr. de Paris 7: 480: 1925. — Schmutte: Ztsch. f. Urol. Chir. 27—28: 1929. — Steinlin: Dissertation, Zürich 1936. — Weigert: Zit. n. Johanning.